Advanced Practice in Nursing

Under the Auspices of the *International Council of Nurses (ICN)*

Series Editor
Christophe Debout
GIP-IFITS
Health Chair Sciences- Po Paris/IDS UMR Inserm 1145
Paris, France

This series of concise monographs, endorsed by the International Council of Nurses, explores various aspects of advanced practice nursing at the international level.

The ICN International Nurse Practitioner/Advanced Practice Nursing Network definition has been adopted for this series to define advanced practice nursing: "A Nurse Practitioner/Advanced Practice Nurse is a registered nurse who has acquired the expert knowledge base, complex decision-making skills and clinical competencies for expanded practice, the characteristics of which are shaped by the context and/or country in which s/he is credentialed to practice. A master's degree is recommended for entry level."

At the international level, advanced practice nursing encompasses two professional profiles:

Nurse practitioners (NPs) who have mastered advanced practice nursing, and are capable of diagnosing, making prescriptions for and referring patients. Though they mainly work in the community, some also work in hospitals. Clinical nurse specialists (CNSs) are expert nurses who deliver high-quality nursing care to patients and promote quality care and performance in nursing teams.

The duties performed by these two categories of advanced practice nurses on an everyday basis can be divided into five interrelated roles:

Clinical practice
Consultation
Education
Leadership
Research

The series addresses four topics directly related to advanced practice nursing:

APN in practice (NPs and CNSs)
Education and continuous professional development for advanced practice nurses
Managerial issues related to advanced practice nursing
Policy and regulation of advanced practice nursing

The contributing authors are mainly APNs (NPs and CNSs) recruited from the ICN International Nurse Practitioner/Advanced Practice Nursing Network. They include clinicians, educators, researchers, regulators and managers, and are recognized as experts in their respective fields.

Each book within the series reflects the fundamentals of nursing / advanced practice nursing and will promote evidence-based nursing.

More information about this series at http://www.springer.com/series/13871

Janet S. Fulton • Vincent W. Holly
Editors

Clinical Nurse Specialist Role and Practice

An International Perspective

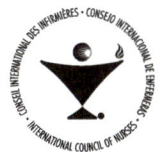

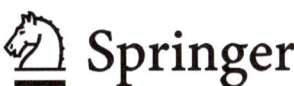

Editors
Janet S. Fulton
School of Nursing
Indiana University
Indianapolis
IN
USA

Vincent W. Holly
Indiana University Health, IU Hospital
Bloomington
IN
USA

ISSN 2511-3917   ISSN 2511-3925   (electronic)
Advanced Practice in Nursing
ISBN 978-3-319-97102-5   ISBN 978-3-319-97103-2   (eBook)
https://doi.org/10.1007/978-3-319-97103-2

This Springer imprint is published by the registered company Springer Nature Switzerland AG
The registered company address is: Gewerbestrasse 11, 6330 Cham, Switzerland

Preface

Across the world, nursing developed as a profession influenced by local, regional, and national policies, politics, norms, and traditions. Regardless of the path taken by the profession in any one country, nurses are universally committed to the health and well-being of the public we serve. As nurses, we strive to assure care and comfort for our fellow humans by preventing or reducing risk of disease and harm, relieving distressing symptoms, promoting physical and cognitive functioning, and maximizing quality of life. Nursing interventions are universal in scientific grounding yet unique in application. All nurses, regardless of educational preparation, regulatory title, or professional credentials, are dedicated to that one same mission.

Responding to the public's need for expanded, advanced, and complex care interventions, the nursing profession is creating clinicians to practice at advanced levels and in expanded scopes. Advanced practice nurse roles are established in some countries and evolving or still emerging in other countries. These advanced nurses have expert knowledge, complex decision-making abilities, and enhanced skills. First prepared as a generalist registered nurse, advanced practice nurses hold graduate degrees and other credentials necessary for authority to practice. In places where graduate nursing degrees are not available, transition programs are filling the gap between generalist education and advanced practice education.

The clinical nurse specialist is one of several advanced practice nursing roles. Other advanced practice nursing roles include the nurse practitioner, nurse anesthetist, and, in some countries, the nurse midwife (depending on educational preparation and scope of practice). A few countries, including Australia, the United Kingdom, and Hong Kong, use the title Clinical Nurse Consultant (CNC) to designate a practice role consistent with CNS practice. We recognize that a "nurse specialist," defined by the International Council of Nurses as a nurse prepared beyond the level of a generalist and authorized to practice in a specialty area with advanced expertise, has extensive experience, completed specialized courses, and/or on-the-job training. "Specialist nurses" are an important step in developing the advanced role of clinical nurse specialist.

In 2000, the International Council of Nurses created a special interest group for advanced practice nurses, the International Nurse Practitioner/Advanced Practiced Nursing Network, giving advanced practice nurses in differing roles an opportunity to network, collaborate, and move forward together. Clinical nurse specialists are engaged in the network. Advanced nursing roles have a common core that is molded by the country in which practice occurs. This book explores practice competencies, educational qualifications, credentialing, and regulation for clinical nurse specialists in 15 different countries across North America, Europe, Asia, Africa and Middle East, and Oceania. Chapter 1 provides an overview and a brief look at the role. Chapter 2 explores conceptual models and frameworks and their usefulness in explaining the clinical nurse specialist role and practice. Chapter 3 examines global differences and commonalities among clinical nurse specialist core practice competencies. Chapter 4 explores clinical nurse specialist at the graduate-level education including mechanisms for accrediting academic programs. Chapters 5 through 19 examine clinical nurse specialist by country, including the United States, Canada, United Kingdom, Ireland, Finland, France, Germany, Japan, China, Taiwan, Turkey, Saudi Arabia, Nigeria, Australia, and New Zealand. Each chapter includes a brief history of the clinical nurse specialist role, a definition, conceptualization of practice/practice competencies, educational requirements, and credentialing. Challenges and opportunities are discussed, and each chapter concludes with an exemplar of clinical nurse specialist practice in that country.

The editors are extremely grateful to the contributing authors for sharing their expertise. Each author made a best effort to distill a broad amount of information into a concise, up-to-date chapter. We recognize that each author offered a summary of their understanding of the CNS role in their country, which may lead to debate and discussion among nurses in their home country. Thus, we view this work as an opportunity for increased dialogue not only among countries but also within countries. An in-depth understanding of the educational systems and laws regulating nursing in each country and within intra-country jurisdictions is beyond the scope of this book. It is apparent that educational systems and credentialing mechanisms are unique to each country. Often the language differs but the meanings are similar. To help see the similarities across clinical nurse specialist role and practice, we created a few tables to summarize information. We close the book with a chapter that outlines the challenges and opportunities we see for clinical nurse specialist practice going forward.

We call to your attention the fact that the content of this book was prepared prior to the release of the 2020 ICN *Guidelines on Advanced Practice Nursing*. These guidelines provide general principles for defining advanced practice nursing and for shaping practice of clinical nurse specialists and nurse practitioners. As nursing moves forward with further defining and refining advanced practice roles, the ICN guidelines offer a path forward. Consider these guidelines as you review the chapter content.

The emergence of advanced practice nursing roles is an important and essential initiative for the nursing profession in fulfilling the social mandate to meet the public's need for nursing services. In moving forward with developing advanced roles, we should acknowledge the important contributions all nurses make to the health of the populations we serve, support our colleagues at all levels and in different roles, and to seek pathways for more nurses to advance their education.

Indianapolis, IN, USA   Janet S. Fulton
Bloomington, IN, USA   Vincent W. Holly

Contents

Part II   North America

Part I

General Considerations

Global View of the Clinical Nurse Specialist Role

Garrett K. Chan and Vincent W. Holly

Abstract

A clinical nurse specialist (CNS) is an advanced practice nurse who has acquired knowledge, skills, and aptitude at greater depth and breadth than generalist preparation registered nursing. Globally there are varying descriptions of the CNS role and practice. In the United States and Canada, the term CNS is used, whereas in other countries the role may be titled, for example, Clinical Nurse Consultant. As titling continues to evolve, the core criterion for a CNS is advanced formal nursing preparation at the postbaccalaureate level. CNS practice focuses on managing complex and vulnerable patients and populations, providing education and support for nurses and interprofessional staff, and creating change and innovation in healthcare systems for improved patient/population outcomes. A global need exists for the role of the CNS, and educational and regulatory support is required to fully implement the role in many countries and settings. Common concerns varying in importance by country include securing title protection, defining scope of practice, determining core practice competencies, establishing educational requirements and curriculum, securing professional certification, and obtaining authority to practice regulation. Continuing efforts to assure public access to CNS services are essential for the successful integration of the CNS role into the professional healthcare expertise contributing to the health and well-being of persons globally.

G. K. Chan
School of Nursing, University of California, San Francisco, CA, USA
e-mail: garrett.chan@ucsf.edu, garrett@healthimpact.org

V. W. Holly (✉)
Critical Care Services, Indiana University Health Bloomington Hospital, Bloomington, IN, USA
e-mail: vholly@iuhealth.org

© Springer Nature Switzerland AG 2021
J. S. Fulton, V. W. Holly (eds.), *Clinical Nurse Specialist Role and Practice*,
Advanced Practice in Nursing, https://doi.org/10.1007/978-3-319-97103-2_1

Keywords

Clinical nurse specialist · CNS · Advanced practice nurse · Nurse specialist
Specialist nurse · Clinical specialist

1.1   Introduction

Clinical nurse specialist is one of four advanced practice nursing roles developed to
provide advanced nursing care to specialty populations. Other advanced nursing
roles include nurse practitioner, nurse-midwife, and nurse anesthetist. Globally,
advanced practice nursing is recognized as nursing practiced beyond generalist registered nurse practice with advanced knowledge and skill derived from postbaccalaureate education. Advanced practice nursing is a natural evolution and extension
of nursing practice with unique roles representing greater depth and breadth than
generalist registered nurse preparation. Advanced practice nursing roles have varying levels of recognition depending on country and regulatory authority to practice
within a defined scope.

Clinical nurse specialists hold a graduate degree in nursing that prepared graduates for the advanced role of clinical nurse specialist. In countries where graduate
nursing degrees are not available, transition programs are filling the gap between
generalist education and advanced practice education. The 2020 ICN Guidelines on
advanced practice nursing provide a recommended path forward for nursing education to progress from generalist nurse to specialist nurse to clinical nurse specialist.

The foundation of CNS practice is direct patient care focusing on complex and
vulnerable population. CNS practice includes both advanced clinical practice and
practice that advances nursing care for improved clinical outcomes by providing
interprofessional education, individual mentoring, and leadership for evidence-
based practice for a specialty area. In addition, CNS practice includes addressing
system-level organizational structures and operating procedures to remove barriers
and facilitate nursing care for specialty populations. Examples of specialty populations for CNS practice are seen in Table 1.1.

Advanced practice roles are established in some countries while evolving and
emerging in other countries. While many countries use the term Clinical Nurse
Specialist, some countries use other titles for practice roles that match to the
CNS. Titles in other countries include Certified Nurse Specialist (Japan), Senior
Specialist (Saudi Arabia), Nurse Consultant (Australia, Saudi Arabia), Nurse

Table 1.1 Types of specialty care (National Association of Clinical Nurse Specialists 2019)

Specialty area	Population examples
Developmental age group	Neonatal, pediatrics, older adults
Disease/pathology	Diabetes, cancer, tuberculosis
Clinical problem	Pain, wounds, stress
Care delivery setting	Critical care unit, emergency care, surgery
Type of care	Rehabilitation, palliative care

Specialist, or Specialty Nurse (China). These various titles reflect a role that require advanced education beyond the generalist nurse and specify an advanced nurse with expert knowledge, complex decision-making abilities, and enhanced skills. Countries developing the role of the CNS are looking to standardize titling, education, competencies, and regulation. Regardless of title all roles should have advanced educational preparation, beyond the RN level, and focus on a specialty area of nursing practice. The level of development of the CNS role is different globally where the role may be just emerging or may be more established with educational standards, title protection, and accepted regulatory authority to practice.

1.2   History of the CNS Role and Practice

Often the CNS role was developed long before a formal definition or title was applied. Chapters in this book discussing CNS practice in different countries illustrate the evolution of the role on different timelines and following different paths. In the United States, the idea of an expert clinical nurse emerged in the 1940s and further developed through 1965, when Hildegard Peplau first used the term clinical nurse specialist. She described the CNS, an advanced practice nurse as having expertise in nursing practice in the care of complex patients. Peplau proposed graduate education in nursing at a minimum of the master's level to prepare CNSs (Peplau 2003). The impetus for creating the CNS role was the findings of several national studies about nursing, the most significant being the 1948 Brown report (Brown 1948). This report noted the lack of scientific principles in nursing education and the limited opportunity for development of in-depth clinical expertise in nursing practice. Nursing leaders suggested that nursing needed expert nurses at the bedside to lead the advancement of nursing practice. In-depth expertise was becoming specialized, and the CNS was the nursing profession's response to providing leadership in clinical practice. The need for expert nurses leading clinical practice continues to exist today. We see this as countries continue to develop the CNS role and as other countries are in the beginning stages of CNS role implementation.

The CNS role has emerged as a response to societal needs for improved nursing care. Each chapter includes a brief history of the development of the CNS role in each respective country. Many of the described efforts began without formal frameworks in place. Over the years these initiatives in various countries recognized the need to establish a framework for practice or are currently developing the role definitions and model for practice.

Several countries identified the late 1990s and early 2000s as a time of focused activity to establish the CNS role. Ireland's National Council for the Professional Development of Nursing and Midwifery, in 2001, published CNS definitions, core functions, and a framework establishing pathways for nurses to become CNSs. Japan first referenced the CNS role in 1987. In 1996, Japan began certifying CNSs and in 1998 began accrediting master's level CNS education programs. In 2007, the Japanese Association of Certified Nurse Specialists was formed. New Zealand introduced the role in the 1970s; by the late 1990s, the role started to proliferate. In

1998 the Ministerial Taskforce report highlighted the CNS role and its impact on patient outcomes. The report recommended recognition and endorsement of the CNS role as well as specific competencies consistent with the title. The CNS role continues to proliferate today.

Other countries started developing the role in the 2000s and are in the process of establishing the role. Finland first implemented the CNS role in 2001 and has seen rapid growth over the past 5 years. Although the CNS role is not title protected or regulated, work is well underway developing CNS competencies providing guidance for frameworks in role and practice implementation. The Ministry of Health of the People's Republic of China outlined China's nursing development plan in 2005. This plan initiated the development of the CNS. By 2007, the Ministry of Health clarified the criteria for CNS training programs, including length of training, content, and evaluation standards. Further opportunities include establishing competencies, regulation standards, and titling.

1.3 Definitions of Advanced Practice Nurse and Clinical Nurse Specialist

No one global definition for the CNS exists; however, similarities are evident when looking at the different organizational (e.g., International Council of Nurses, National Council of State Boards of Nursing) and country-specific definitions (e.g., Canada, Finland, United Kingdom, United States). Some of the definitions address all advanced practice nursing roles and are not specific to the CNS.

The International Council of Nurses describes the CNS as "a nurse with advanced nursing knowledge and skills, educated beyond the level of a generalist or specialized nurse, in making complex decisions in a clinical specialty and utilising a systems approach to influence optimal care in healthcare organizations" (International Council of Nurses 2020).

Further, the ICN Nurse Practitioner/Advanced Practice Nurse Network (NP/APNN) defines an APN as:

> …a registered nurse who has acquired the expert knowledge base, complex decision-making skills and clinical competencies for expanded practice, the characteristics of which are shaped by the context and/or country in which s/he is credentialed to practice. A master's degree is recommended for entry level (International Council of Nurses (ICN) 2008).

The United States has been moving toward the universal use of the term Advanced Practice Registered Nurse (APRN) to designate that the advanced practice nurse is first a registered nurse. The National Council of State Boards of Nursing (NCSBN), an independent organization of nursing regulatory bodies, defines the APRN as a nurse who meets the following criteria:

1. Completed an accredited graduate-level APRN role-based education program
2. Holds national certification in the role and population
3. Acquired advanced clinical knowledge and skills in providing direct care to patients
4. Practices with a greater depth and breadth of knowledge, increased complexity of skills and interventions, and greater role autonomy than a registered nurse
5. Assumes responsibility and accountability for health promotion and/or maintenance as well as the assessment, diagnosis, and management of patient problems, including use and prescription of pharmacologic and non-pharmacologic interventions
6. Completes clinical experience of sufficient depth and breadth to reflect the intended license
7. Holds a license to practice as an APRN in one of the four APRN roles: certified registered nurse anesthetist (CRNA), certified nurse-midwife (CNM), clinical nurse specialist (CNS), or certified nurse practitioner (CNP) (National Council of State Boards of Nursing (NCSBN) 2008)

These definitions are important as they both describe APN practice as being nursing practice that extends beyond the preparation and practice of a registered nurse and gives expanded authority in which to practice through legal recognition of regional or national credentialing. In the United States, the definition of a CNS should meet the criteria established for all APRNs, as do all advanced nursing roles.

Country-specific definitions of a CNS generally are consistent with these definitions. For example, the Canadian Nurses Association defines the CNS as a "registered nurse who holds a graduate degree in nursing and has a high level of expertise in a clinical specialty" (Canadian Nurses Association 2014). CNS practice in Canada is described as impacting three levels: the patient or client, nurses and interprofessional teams within practice settings, and organization/systems.

Finland has a functional definition for the CNS, as described in Chap. 9:

Clinical nurse specialist is an experienced master's or doctoral prepared registered nurse whose central focus of practice is advanced clinical nursing. The aim of the role is to support healthcare organizations to achieve their strategic goals, to assure and increase the quality and effectiveness of patient care, and to improve the merging of evidence-based practice and scholarship activities. Clinical nurse specialist role domains are advanced clinical practice and practice development, consultation and staff education, transformational leadership and scholarship activities. The role actualize through direct and indirect evidence-based patient care influencing positively to the patient care, nursing profession, organization, scholarship, and the community at large.

In Chap. 7, Leary defines the CNS in Scotland as:

A clinical nurse specialist is a registered nursing professional who has acquired additional knowledge, skills and experience, together with a professionally and/or academically accredited post-registration qualification (if available) in a clinical specialty. They practice at an advanced level and may have sole responsibility for care episode or defined client/group.

In the United States, the National Association of Clinical Nurse Specialists (NACNS) defines the CNS as (National Association of Clinical Nurse Specialists 2019):

> CNSs are licensed registered nurses who have graduate preparation (master's or doctorate) in nursing as a clinical nurse specialist. They have unique and advanced level competencies that meet the increased needs of improving quality and reducing costs in our health care system. They provide direct patient care, including assessment, diagnosis and management of patient health care issues.
>
> The essence of CNS practice is advanced clinical expertise in diagnosis and intervention to prevent, remediate or alleviate illness and promote health with a defined specialty population.
>
> CNS practice is the translation of advanced clinical expertise, expert knowledge, complex decision-making skills and clinical competencies necessary for expanded practice to directly provide and influence care and outcomes of individuals, categories of patients and/ or communities.
>
> CNS practice also transforms systems (such as health care institutions and systems, political systems and public and professional organizations) to mobilize and change these systems through expertly designed and implemented nursing interventions.

All the definitions require two criteria for the CNS role. First the definitions included advanced formal education, recommended at the graduate level, and second, the definitions specified expertise in a specialty area of nursing. These criteria are basic to the CNS role preparation.

Characteristics delineating CNS practice were summarized by Fulton and Holly (International Council of Nurses 2020) to reflect the following:

- Clinical nurse specialists (CNSs) are professional nurses with a graduate level preparation (master's or doctoral degree).
- CNSs are expert clinicians who provide direct clinical care in a specialized area of nursing practice defined by developmental age, clinical setting, a disease/ medical subspecialty, type of care, or type of problem.
- Clinical practice for a specialty population includes health promotion, risk reduction, and management of symptoms and functional problems related to disease and illness.
- CNSs provide direct care to patients and families, which may include diagnosis and treatment of disease.
- CNSs practice patient-/family-centered care that emphasizes strengths and wellness over disease or deficit.
- CNSs influence nursing practice outcomes by leading and supporting nurses to provide scientifically grounded, evidence-based care.
- CNSs implement improvements in the healthcare delivery system (indirect care) and translate high-quality research evidence into clinical practice to improve clinical and fiscal outcomes.
- CNSs participate in the conduct of research to generate knowledge for practice.
- CNSs design, implement, and evaluate programs of care and programs of research that address common problems for specialty populations.

1.4   Substantive Areas of CNS Practice

In the United States, the National Association of Clinical Nurse Specialists (NACNS) developed an organizing framework for core CNS competencies integrating three domains of practice (National Association of Clinical Nurse Specialists 2019). These domains are referred to as three spheres of impact: direct patient/family care, nurses/nursing practice, and organization/system (National Association of Clinical Nurse Specialists 2019). While CNS advanced competencies are integrated across the three spheres of impact, expert nursing practice in the patient/family sphere includes assessing, diagnosing, and treating illness. In addition, the CNS influences the practice of other nurses and healthcare personnel by supporting practice through advanced specialty clinical expertise, advocacy, consultation, collaboration, scholarship, and leadership (National Association of Clinical Nurse Specialists 2019). The CNS impacts outcomes by affecting decision-making at the system/organization level, removing barriers, and facilitating quality, safe, innovative, and evidence-based care.

In 2006, the NACNS commissioned Lewandowski and Ademle to examine CNS practice by conducting an extensive review of the literature evaluating reported CNS practice domains and related outcomes. Findings demonstrated that the substantive areas of CNS practice focuses in a specialty area of nursing to manage the care of complex and vulnerable populations, educate and support interdisciplinary staff, and facilitate change and innovation within healthcare systems (Lewandowski and Adamle 2009).

These substantive areas of CNS practice identified in the literature are consistent with and support the definitions in Canada, Finland, and the United States. These definitions are important because they differentiate the practice and role of a CNS from other APN roles. First, the CNS is educated and practices in a specialty area of nursing such as, but not limited to, critical care, palliative care, or oncology. Second, the definition delineates the types of patients the CNS cares for—the complex and vulnerable. Third, the definition clearly articulates the practice of a CNS extends beyond individual patient care to include education of interprofessional staff and facilitating change and innovations in healthcare systems since optimal care is delivered from an interprofessional perspective rather than in silos of disciplines. These activities are essential to also improve the healthcare system to help populations of patients to achieve their health goals.

The substantive areas of practice are similar in the countries highlighted in this book and are summarized in Table 1.2. CNS impact is primarily demonstrated in direct patient care. Most counties explain the underpinning of CNS practice is caring for the complex vulnerable patient populations. While consulting on the complex vulnerable patients, the CNS coaches and develops the staff nurses. The role of the CNS expands further into leadership. Some authors mention CNS-run clinics, while other authors explain CNS impact on implementation of evidence-based practice, improving safety and quality, and making policy decisions.

Table 1.2 Description of CNS role by country

Country	RN preparation Required	Post-generalist specialty education	Title	Domains of practice
Australia	Yes	Some states require postgraduate qualifications; other states recommend, but do not mandate postgraduate qualifications	Clinical Nurse Specialist Clinical Nurse Consultant	Direct and comprehensive care Support of systems Education Research and quality Professional leadership
Canada	Yes	Master's preparation, but lack title protection, so some nurses using the term CNS may not be master's prepared	Clinical Nurse Specialist	Patient/client Nurses/interprofessional teams Organizations/systems
China	Yes	Education and training beyond Master's of Nursing Specialist offered	Specialty Nurse Clinical Nurse Specialist	Direct patient care Nurses/education Research/clinical leader
Finland	Yes	Master's or doctoral preparation	Clinical Nurse Specialist	Direct patient care Nursing Organization/ scholarship Role domains: advanced clinical practice and practice development, consultation and staff education, transformational leadership, and scholarship activities
France	Yes A least 3 years of experience as RN to be registered as APN	Master's level Certification domain specified	Advanced practice nurse (Infirmière de pratique avancée) Protected title	Since 2018 • Patients living with chronic disease • Hematology and oncology • Renal disease, dialysis, renal transplant Since 2019 • Psychiatry and mental health
Germany	Yes	Education and training beyond basic nursing	Advanced Practice Nurse	Direct patient care Nurses/healthcare staff Organization
Ireland	Yes	Formal recognized post-registration education	Clinical Nurse Specialist	Patient/client Staff Service/healthcare Core concepts: client focus; advocacy; education and training; audit and research; consultancy

Table 1.2 (continued)

Country	RN preparation Required	Post-generalist specialty education	Title	Domains of practice
Japan	Yes	Master's preparation	Certified Nurse Specialist	Individuals/families/groups Nurses/healthcare professionals Organization/education/research
New Zealand	Yes	Not required, but the Ministry of Health strongly advocates for postgraduate education	Clinical Nurse Specialist Nurse Specialist Specialty Clinical Nurse	Patient/family Nursing personnel/nursing standards System/organization
Nigeria	Yes	Hospital-based pathway – Advanced specialty education University-based pathway – Master's or PhD prepared Task shifting-based pathway – Advanced skills serving specialty populations	Clinical Nurse Specialist	Direct patient care Nurses Organization
Saudi Arabia	Yes	Master's preparation	Clinical Nurse Specialist Clinical Specialist	Direct patient care Nurses/staff Organization/clinic
Taiwan	Yes	Master's or doctoral preparation	Advanced Practice Nurse	Direct patient care Nurses/medical team System leadership
Turkey	Yes	Postgraduate education Master's and doctoral programs offered	Specialist Nurse	Direct patient care Nurses Organizations/institutions
UK	No	Not yet established, graduate degree recommended	Clinical Nurse Specialist	Patient/family Nursing staff
USA	Yes	Master's or doctoral preparation	Clinical Nurse Specialist Title protected	Patient/family Nurses/nursing System/organization

1.5   Expanded Nursing Practice to Meet Patient Needs

The practice and science of nursing is a dynamic and ever-changing profession. From the beginning of modern nursing by Florence Nightingale working in military hospitals during the Crimean War in the 1850s and the Henry Street Settlement Visiting Nurses in New York City in the 1890s, nurses have dedicated their work to underserved and vulnerable patients. Often, nurses cared for patients who could not afford to visit a physician. Therefore, nurses provided care to these populations by performing physical and health exams on patients, evaluating the living conditions of communities, diagnosing the causes of illness as well as common medical conditions, prescribing pharmacologic and non-pharmacologic therapeutic interventions, and creating plans of care. This early work emphasized the autonomous scope of nursing and the focus on a holistic approach that included environmental conditions, family and social influences, cultural considerations, as well as physical and disease-related problems. In these practices nurses collaborated with physicians to co-manage complex medical conditions, sometimes using physician-initiated "standing orders" for medications and treatment and sometimes without (Keeling 2007). Standing orders were endorsed by the local medical society, which could be used until a physician could attend the patient or when specific orders were not left by the attending physician (Foley 1913).

The expansion of disease diagnosis and prescription of therapeutic measures in nursing practice led to the establishment of advanced practice registered nurses, specifically the roles of the clinical nurse specialist (CNS) in the early 1960s and the nurse practitioner (NP) in 1965. Medical and nursing scopes of practice overlap in multiple areas of care including disease diagnosis, prescription, and setting an independent plan of care with patients and families. This care can be shared between the two professional roles, especially for advanced practice nurses (APNs).

Much of what is considered expanded nursing practice, or APN practice, is nursing reclaiming its historical roots for holistic care that can include disease diagnosis and prescription of pharmacologic and non-pharmacologic interventions.

Like other APNs, CNS practice does extend into the medicine domain as new competencies in direct patient care are acquired (Fig. 1.1). Some CNSs devote a significant amount of time focused on direct patient care, utilizing competencies of diagnosis and prescription. In the United States, 21% of surveyed CNSs have prescriptive privileges (National Association of Clinical Nurse Specialists 2017). However, CNS practice differentiates itself by developing competencies advancing and extending the nursing domain to meet the nursing profession's need for a clinical expert, as was originally described in the 1960s. As demonstrated in Fig. 1.1, the autonomous scope of nursing practice includes interventions within generalist RN license. Interdependent practice is an area where physicians and nurses share responsibility for care, such as when a physician prescribes an intravenous medication and the nurse makes autonomous decisions about the placement and insertion, type of equipment, and maintenance of the intravenous device. APNs, including CNSs, may extend into the medical domain and practice autonomously by obtaining authority to practice in an expanded scope, which generally involves diagnosing

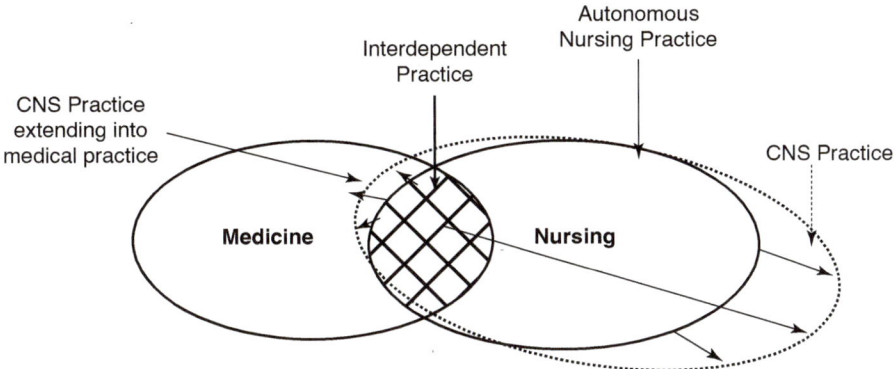

Fig. 1.1 Relationship between medical practice, nursing practice, and clinical nurse specialist practice (National Association of Clinical Nurse Specialists 2019)

disease, prescribing pharmacological agents, and ordering diagnostic tests. Consistent with the initial rationale for the CNS role, many CNSs practice by advancing the practice of nursing in the expanded autonomous domain and concentrate efforts on addressing care problems amenable to nursing's autonomous interventions.

Contemporary issues related to autonomous APN practice, such as the ability to independently evaluate and manage a patient's condition, prescriptive authority for therapeutic measures, clinical diagnosis of disease and illness, and obtaining hospital practice privileges to obtain authority to practice at the APN level, have taken different forms over the decades and continue to be areas of disagreement depending on the setting and country where the debate takes place (Schober 2016).

1.6   Regulatory Protection for the CNS Role

For CNSs to practice or for academic institutions to create CNS programs, a clear understanding of local or national laws, statutes, regulations, and the definition of nursing is essential. These legal mechanisms constitute the legal scope of practice for the CNS as an advanced practice nurse. A scope of practice is the legal framework that describes *who* is legally authorized to provide and be paid for *what* services [if payments are rendered], *for whom*, and *under what circumstances* (Schober 2016). Efforts by CNSs to establish or advance existing practice can start at the local level as demonstration projects. However, strategic efforts should be employed to advance at the regional or national level to establish practice authority and legitimacy (Schober 2017).

The authority to practice as a CNS is determined by professional and legal regulation. Professional regulation is determined by professional nursing and credentialing organizations. Professional nursing organizations establish scope and standards of practice at different levels of nursing, from the generalist RN to the APN. Nursing organizations develop competencies appropriate for the role and recommend education curricula to meet these competencies. Professional regulation for CNSs consists of rules and policies that recognize and officially certify/credential the CNS for practice. Various nursing organizations make recommendations for licensure, accreditation of CNS programs, certification, and education. Although these recommendations are taken seriously and used to standardize practice, nursing organizations do not have legal authority to determine practice.

Legal regulation occurs at the governmental level. Civil or government legislation determines the CNS's ability to practice, based on accepted policies addressing scope and standards of practice, licensure, title protection, educational preparation, and boundaries of practice. Legal regulation functions to legitimize the role, protect the public, and monitor the individual healthcare professional's practice and behavior (Schober 2016). Model language as found in Sect. 1.3 Definitions of advanced practice nurse and clinical nurse specialist can serve as scope of practice language countries can strive toward in obtaining legal recognition of CNS advanced practice.

1.7   Future of CNS Practice Globally

Advancing the CNS role globally requires nurse leaders to understand local and international standards, customs, and legal mechanisms that support or impede CNS education specifically and APN education and practice generally. Issues such as title protection, scope of practice, competencies, educational curriculum, professional certification, or governmental registration are different by country and even within jurisdictions in countries. Schober (Schober 2017) provides a variety of frameworks and tools for nurse leaders to consider when creating the APN role or advancing APN authority. Topics covered include strategic planning, theories of social and healthcare policy, evidence-based policy decisions, politics, and examples of effective changes in countries. Creating a strategic plan is essential in creating incremental and positive change.

It is also important to understand local or national understandings and potential tensions within nursing about the APN role where there is not universal understanding or acceptance of expansion of nursing practice. CNS practice encompasses responsibilities beyond direct care to individuals and families leaving open a debate about the appropriate emphasis for practice. Thoughtful dialogue leading to shared understanding of advanced practice nursing and the unique contributions of each APN role, including CNS role, is essential to moving nursing practice forward as a force for public health and well-being.

One tenet that remains true is that nurses are stronger when united rather than when they are divided in smaller groups. Creating an organization for all APNs, especially when the number of APNs in a country or region is small, can help create identity, share resources, and attain recognition as a group within the larger discipline of nursing. However, working in collaboration with other APNs, it is essential to recognize and honor the unique contributions of each APN role and avoid blending APN roles into one. Working within professional organizations to establish standards, guidelines, and strategy to advance the role of the CNS can create the sustainable energy necessary to serve patients, nurses, and healthcare institutions to improve the quality of care and outcomes for the people being served.

1.8 Conclusion

The CNS is one role under the inclusive term of advanced practice nurse and should be educationally prepared and practice according to the minimum requirements for all APNs. Core differentiators of the CNS role from other APN roles include a practice that is based on a specialty, focuses on complex and vulnerable patients and populations, educates and supports interprofessional staff, and creates change and innovation in healthcare systems. Depending on the local or regional healthcare needs of populations, clinical nurse specialist care is needed to improve the health outcomes of members of that community. Additionally, creating a clear understanding and a pathway of integration of the role within nursing and with the public is essential to the success of the CNS role.

References

Brown EL (1948) Nursing for the future. Russell Sage Foundation, New York, NY

Canadian Nurses Association (2014) Pan-Canadian core competencies for the clinical nurse specialist. https://www.cna-aiic.ca/-/media/cna/files/en/clinical_nurse_specialists_convention_handout_e. pdf?la=en&hash=E9DE6CADB7C0260D9CD969121DA79EB408B8466F. Accessed 29 July 2019

Foley E (1913) Department of visiting nursing and social welfare. Am J Nurs 13(6):451–455

International Council of Nurses (2020) International Council of Nurses Guidelines on advanced practice nursing 2020. International Council of Nurses, Geneva

International Council of Nurses (ICN) (2008) The scope of practice, standards and competencies of the advanced practice nurse, ICN regulation series. ICN, Geneva

Keeling AW (2007) Nursing and the privilege of prescription, 1893–2000. The Ohio State University Press, Columbus, OH

Lewandowski W, Adamle K (2009) Substantive areas of clinical nurse specialist practice. A comprehensive review of the literature. Clin Nurse Spec 23(2):73–90

National Association of Clinical Nurse Specialists (2017) 2016 clinical nurse specialists census. https://nacns.org/professional-resources/practice-and-cns-role/cns-census/. Accessed 2 July 2019

National Association of Clinical Nurse Specialists (2019) NACNS statement on clinical nurse specialist practice and education. 3rd edn

National Council of State Boards of Nursing (NCSBN) (2008) Consensus model for APRN regulation: Licensure, accreditation, certification & education. https://www.ncsbn.org/Consensus_Model_for_APRN_Regulation_July_2008.pdf. Accessed 25 July 2018

Peplau H (2003) Specialization in professional nursing. Clin Nurse Spec 17(1):3–9

Schober M (2016) Introduction to advanced nursing practice. An international focus. Springer International Publishing, Switzerland

Schober M (2017) Strategic planning for advanced nursing practice. Springer International Publishing, Switzerland

Conceptual Models for Clinical Nurse Specialist Role and Practice

2

Janet S. Fulton

Abstract

A model or framework is central to achieving clinical nurse specialist (CNS) role consistency and sustainability and in supporting evolution of CNS as a distinct and legitimate healthcare expert in the healthcare delivery system. Models can describe CNS practice, CNS role structure, or regulatory authority to practice as a CNS. A model explaining CNS role structure describes the elements and characteristics of the role and the relationships between and among those elements. A model for CNS practice is a process model demonstrating interrelationships among elements constituting practice including domains of practice, practice competencies, and desired outcomes. Process models explain the relationship between practice competencies and clinical outcomes. A regulatory model explains the authority to practice, including legal requirements and the associated scope of practice. Existing models explaining CNS role and practice are limited; many current models are developed to explain advanced practice nursing and are not role specific. Existing models and frameworks are discussed for their usefulness in explaining CNS role and practice. Multiple models are needed to provide deeper understanding of the unique characteristics of the CNS role and core CNS practice competencies. No one model is best; the best model is the one that explains the phenomenon of interest.

Keywords

Clinical nurse specialist · Advanced practice nurse · Conceptual model · Conceptual framework · Domains of practice · Practice competencies · Practice outcomes

J. S. Fulton (✉)
Indiana University School of Nursing, Indianapolis, IN, USA
e-mail: jasfulto@iu.edu

2.1   Introduction

The evolution of the clinical nurse specialist role has its roots in the mid-twentieth-century effort to move nursing education into academic institutions of higher learning and out of apprentice-based hospital training programs (Fulton 2014). University-based programs introduced theoretical and scientific knowledge into nursing curricula assuring that graduates used clinical reasoning and exercised sound judgment in the practice of nursing. Nursing education slowly shifted from a focus on performing tasks directed by others, primarily physicians, to autonomous decision-making grounded in scientific principles. This shift in focus caused nurse leaders to recognize a need for an advanced, clinically expert nurse who could provide direct care to patients and families while serving as a leader in the clinical setting promoting excellence in the practice of nursing. Frances Reiter (1966), the first dean of the Graduate School of Nursing at New York Medical College, described the expert nurse-clinician as a master practitioner for all dimensions of nursing practice. This expert clinician would provide clinical care while using judgment to assess problems, determine care priorities, and select the best nursing measures to achieve therapeutic objectives. In addition, the expert nurse would promote quality of care and remove system-level barriers to nursing care delivery (Reiter 1966). About this same time, the National League for Nursing (NLN) was developing the idea of a nurse with a clinical specialty to promote application of new knowledge and advanced clinical methods for the ever-evolving areas of specialty care (NLN 1958). Through these efforts, graduate education emerged in the United States, and the clinical nurse specialist (CNS) role was established. From the beginning, a CNS was defined as a graduate degree (postbaccalaureate)-prepared nurse with a deep knowledge of and clinical expertise in an area of specialty practice (Fulton 2014). Over the ensuing decades, hundreds of articles about the CNS role and practice have been published demonstrating remarkable consistency in the descriptions across many different specialty practices and varying health systems.

Clinical nurse specialist is one of several advanced clinical practice roles in nursing. Other commonly recognized advanced clinical practice roles include nurse practitioner, nurse-midwife, and nurse anesthetist, though the designation of advanced practice varies by country. Conceptualizations of the CNS role and practice have been published in the form of models and frameworks. This chapter explores models and frameworks for CNS practice and examines advanced clinical practice models applied to the CNS role as an advanced practice nurse. The objectives for this chapter are as follows:

1. Discuss the purpose of models and concepts central to CNS role and practice.
2. Examine selected models and frameworks of CNS practice and advanced clinical practice.
3. Discuss challenges, opportunities, and future directions for enhancing models for CNS role and practice.

The models discussed in this chapter were selected as representative of different types of models; this is not an exhaustive discussion of all published CNS or advanced practice models and frameworks. Readers are invited to consider other available models and frameworks for relevance in guiding CNS role development, education, practice, and regulation within the context of individual national healthcare systems.

2.2 Purpose of Conceptual Models

Concepts are abstract ideas existing in the mind as a representation, a mental construction of thoughts related to something generalized from particular instances. A conceptual model is a description of interrelated concepts in a rational scheme for structuring knowledge. The terms conceptual model and conceptual framework are used interchangeably. The concepts in a model can exist along a continuum from highly abstract to very concrete. Conceptual models are used to explain phenomenon of interest to a discipline. There is no one best conceptual model; multiple models of a same phenomenon provide alternative ways for explaining and examining a phenomenon.

A metaparadigm provides an overarching understanding of important concepts within a field of study. Nursing models should include the central concepts in the metaparadigm of nursing, which are humans, the environment, health, and nursing. The majority of scholarly work undertaken by nurses in the past four decades addresses these four concepts (Hicks 2014). Although there is no one best way to view a phenomenon such as clinical specialty nursing or advanced nursing, evolving conceptual models benefits patients, nurses, other providers, and stakeholders by ensuring consistency of practice and practice expectations. Models assist advanced nurses to articulate a professional role and practice, serve to organize knowledge about role competencies, and facilitate knowledge development about the role, practice, and associated outcomes. Models can demonstrate differentiation of advanced clinical roles (clinical nurse specialist, nurse practitioner, midwife, and nurse anesthetist), from other advanced or specialty roles (educator, administrator, and researcher). Models can also help differentiate one type of advanced clinical role from the other and distinguish advanced clinical roles from generalist staff nurses.

2.3 Definition of Clinical Nurse Specialist

The International Council of Nurses defines an advanced practice nurse as a "registered nurse who has acquired the expert knowledge base, complex decision-making skills and clinical competencies for expanded practice, the characteristics of which are shaped by the context and/or country in which s/he is credentialed to practice"

(ICN 2019). Other professional nursing organizations and governmental agencies also have published definitions and descriptions of the clinical nurse specialist that share similarities (American Nurses Association 2013; American Association of Critical-Care Nurse 2014; Canadian Nurses Association 2019; National Association of Clinical Nurse Specialists 2019; European Specialist Nurses Organizations 2015). A composite of existing definitions, practice expectations, and the associated characteristics of the CNS role is as follows.

The clinical nurse specialist (CNS) scope of practice extends beyond the generalist nurse in terms of expertise, role functions, mastery, and accountability and reflects a core body of nursing and health knowledge. In addition to providing expert specialty direct care to patients and their families, CNSs function as leaders in advancing nursing practice by teaching, mentoring, consulting, and ensuring nursing practice is evidence-based. CNSs interpret the public's need for nursing services by evaluating disease patterns, technological advances, environmental conditions, and political influences. CNSs help assure that the profession meets its social mandate to provide quality, cost-effective, cutting-edge nursing services to the public. The following characteristics delineate the CNS role and practice:

- CNSs are generalist-prepared professional nurses (registered nurses) with additional graduate-level (postbaccalaureate) preparation in a formal program of study (master's or doctoral degree).
- CNSs are expert clinicians providing direct clinical care in a specialized area of nursing practice. Specialty practice is influenced by scientific discovery and the public need for nursing services in delimited areas requiring in-depth knowledge and skill. Specialty areas of practice may be well established or emerging and can be categorized by developmental age or gender (e.g., pediatrics, geriatrics, women's health); clinical setting (e.g., critical care, emergency); a disease/pathophysiological state (e.g., oncology, diabetes); type of care (e.g., counseling, palliative, rehabilitation); or type of problem (e.g., pain, wound, incontinence).
- Clinical practice for a specialty population includes health promotion, risk reduction, and management of symptoms and functional problems related to disease and illness.
- CNSs provide direct care to patients and families, which may include diagnosis and treatment of disease.
- CNSs practice patient-/family-centered care that emphasizes strengths and wellness over disease and deficit.
- CNSs influence nursing practice outcomes by leading and supporting nurses to provide scientifically grounded, evidence-based care.
- CNSs implement improvements in the healthcare delivery system and translate high-quality research and other evidence into clinical practice to improve clinical and fiscal outcomes.
- CNSs participate in the conduct of research to generate knowledge for practice.
- CNSs design, implement, and evaluate programs of care and programs of research that address common problems for specialty populations.

- CNSs practice in a wide variety of healthcare settings, such as hospitals, community clinics, schools, mental health facilities, and occupational health clinics to name a few. CNSs practice in ways and in places that meet the needs of the public.

2.4   Building Blocks of Models and Frameworks

A model or framework is central to achieving CNS role consistency and sustainability and in supporting evolution of CNS as a distinct and legitimate healthcare expert in the healthcare delivery system. Models should embrace the definition of the CNS role, provide explanations for the relationships between practice and outcomes, and reflect practice consistent with nursing's metaparadigm of humans, nursing, health, and environment. No one model can easily encompass all elements, and multiple frameworks have been proposed for describing both advanced practice roles in general and the CNS role in particular. Models can describe one or more central concepts of the CNS role, such as CNS practice, CNS role structure, or regulatory authority to practice. The distinct purpose of many existing models and frameworks is often not stated, and comprehensive models frequently lack clarity and focus by attempting to explain all characteristics and dimensions of the CNS role.

Separate models and frameworks are needed to explain CNS role structure, CNS practice, and regulatory authority to practice. A model explaining CNS role *structure* describes the elements and characteristics of the role and the relationships between and among those elements. A model for CNS *practice* is a process model demonstrating interrelationships among elements constituting practice including domains of practice, practice competencies, and desired outcomes. Process models demonstrate the relationship between practice competencies and clinical outcomes. A *regulatory* model explains the legal requirements for practice and the associated scope of practice. Multiple models will provide deeper understanding of the CNS role and practice. No one model is best; the best model is the one that explains the phenomenon of interest.

Understanding the difference between CNS as an advanced practice *role* and CNS *practice* is a prerequisite for developing useful models and frameworks. A *role* is a unique set of functions for which the necessary knowledge and skills are obtained through education, training, or other requirements. For the CNS role, a prerequisite is formal education beyond the basic generalist nursing registered nurse education. Graduate nursing education includes common content for all advanced practice roles; however, each role (CNS, nurse practitioner, midwife, nurse anesthetist) has a unique curriculum designed to prepare graduates to function in that particular role.

Practice is the act of applying role-based knowledge and skills in the provision of care to patients, families, groups, or communities for the purpose of achieving designated outcomes. Competencies are statements of expected actions representing the application of role-specific knowledge and skill. Practice involves implementing the nursing process—assessment, diagnosis, planning, intervention, and evaluation—using the unique competencies of the role. A model for CNS practice should demonstrate linkages between the competencies of practice and the outcomes of practice.

A *regulatory model* describes the relationships between and among credentials necessary for practice, authority within a scope of practice, and other prerequisite or continuing requirements for practice. Credentials are mechanisms for validating achievement of competency in a role and may include academic degree, professional certification, clinical training verification, specialty training, or other documentation that serves to validate competency consistent with a role. A regulatory model should stipulate both the required credentials and the scope of authority in which the person holding the credentials has authority to practice. Where a license is issued by a governmental agency or body, the license is a mechanism for designating a scope of practice.

Multiple models and frameworks have been developed over the years to explain CNS and advanced practice nursing (Spross 2015; Arslanian-Engoren 2019). Models are often organized by *domains*, which are areas of similar concepts, knowledge, activities, or outcomes. Domains differentiate generalized areas of content. CNS practice has been conceptualized as occurring in three distinct, interacting domains—patient (direct care), nurses/nursing practice, and systems/organizations (NACNS 2019). The knowledge, skill, and activities within each of the domains are similar and related. In other models, the competencies have been organized by domains. Seven core competencies of advanced practice nursing, described by Hamric and Tracy (2019), are direct clinical practice, guidance and coaching, consultation, evidence-based practice, leadership, collaboration, and ethical decision-making. Each competency domain captures similar knowledge, skills, and activities.

Substantive areas of practice have also been used to describe CNS domains of practice. Three substantive areas of CNS, derived from Lewandowski and Adamle's (2009) review of the literature, were managing the care of complex and vulnerable populations, educating and supporting interdisciplinary staff, and facilitating change and innovation within healthcare systems. Substantive areas of practice are similar to the domains of practice and used interchangeably; however, the substantive areas of practice may be more precise and communicate more specificity.

Competencies are demonstrated in actual performance of a skill in a defined context and involve the application of critical thinking, knowledge, and technical and interpersonal skill. Professional organizations develop competencies for role and specialty practice. Professional competency statements guide curriculum development and student educational experiences. Having competence implies both the ability and capability to perform in a functional role and to achieve desired outcomes (Cowan et al. 2005).

A *scope of practice* is legal authority to act independently—use judgment and determine actions—within legally recognized boundaries. A scope of practice is granted by governmental body and regulated using a legal mechanism such as licensure. CNSs, like all advanced practice nurses, are first registered nurses holding a license to practice in an autonomous scope of nursing using independent judgment to diagnose and treat problems amenable to nursing interventions. An advanced practice nursing license extends the boundaries of practice beyond the registered nurse license. Legislative bodies determine a scope of practice in statute (law) and regulate the practice within the law using a licensing mechanism.

2.5   Critiquing APRN Models: Two Exemplars

To better understand the distinct purposes of models and the various uses of domains and competencies within models and frameworks, two models for advanced practice nursing are discussed. Hamric's model of advanced practice nursing, initially developed to explain the CNS role (Hamric and Spross 1989), has been expanded over the years to explain all advanced practice roles (Hamric and Tracy 2019). Graphically designed as four large concentric circles, the model is primarily a structural model that includes the criteria for authority to practice. In Fig. 2.1, the left side of the diagram is a graphic representation of Hamric's model. The model's first, innermost circle represents the primary criteria for an advanced practice nursing role and includes graduate education, professional certification, and practice focused on patient/family. The second and third circles of the model are competencies. The second circle, the central competency, is direct clinical practice. The third circle contains core competencies and includes guidance and coaching, consultation, evidence-based practice, leadership, collaboration, and ethical decision-making skills. In total, the model includes seven competency domains. The fourth and outermost circle in the model represents a fluid boundary between the profession and environmental elements affecting advanced practice nursing, including regulatory and

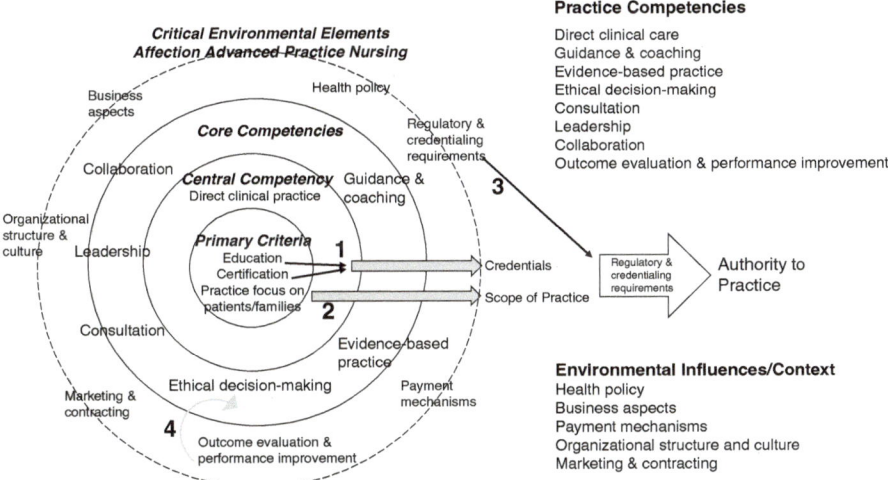

Fig. 2.1 Critique of Hamric's model (Hamric and Tracy 2019) for advanced practice nursing (Copyright © J.S. Fulton 2019)

credential requirements, business aspects, health policy, payment mechanisms, marketing and contracting, organizational structure and culture, and outcome evaluation and performance improvement. These environmental elements create a milieu, shape advanced practice, and must be managed as part of maintaining practice (Hamric and Tracy 2019).

Critique of Hamric's model. The innermost circle, identified as *primary criteria* for an advanced practice nursing role, includes credentials required for practice, education and certification, and a scope of practice that is patient and family centered. Credentials and scope of practice are elements of *authority to practice* model. In addition, the outer circle, environmental elements affecting practice, includes regulatory and credentialing requirements. All elements aligned with regulatory requirements could be placed in a separate, authority to practice model, which could be expanded to offer a clearer explanation (see #1, #2, and #3 in Fig. 2.1).

The profession is charged with meeting society's needs for nursing services. Perhaps public need for nursing should be the primary or central element. Identifying authority to practice as the primary criteria places regulatory authority as the central tenant of advanced practice, which diminishes the profession's responsibility to our social mandate. The profession first identifies needs and then advocates for governmental authority to practice in a scope so as to meet the public need. Authority to practice shaped by the public need is the last step in expanding nursing. More aptly the order of progress should be (1) public need, (2) education and training programs preparing nurses, and (3) regulatory authority to deliver the needed services.

While the innermost circle represents authority to practice, the second and third circles of the model define domains of *competencies.* With the exception of direct clinical practice being central, the competency domains are not weighted and are broad enough for each advanced practice role to create competency statements within the domains consistent with a functional role. Indeed, these competency domains can be found in many advanced practice nursing professional competency standards created by professional nursing organizations and government statements (American Nurses Association 2013; American Association of Critical-Care Nurse 2014; Canadian Nurses Association 2019; National Association of Clinical Nurse Specialists 2019; European Specialist Nurses Organizations 2015; United Kingdom, Department of Health 2015).

The fluid outer boundary between the profession and environment includes elements affecting and shaping advanced practice. The difference between an external element and a practice competency is not clear. Outcome evaluation and performance improvement is arguably an essential competency of advanced practice (see #4 in Fig. 1.2). Likewise it can be debated how many and to what extent the other external elements can be considered core competencies of advanced practice. Managing reimbursement and payment mechanisms, marketing and contracting services, and engaging in shaping health policy are arguably important competencies for advanced practice nurses. Hamric's model, revised over years, is based on considered thought but limited research. Primarily a structural model, it pulls together elements of advanced practice nursing. It has expanded over time to explain all advanced practice roles while also limiting its ability to explain any one role.

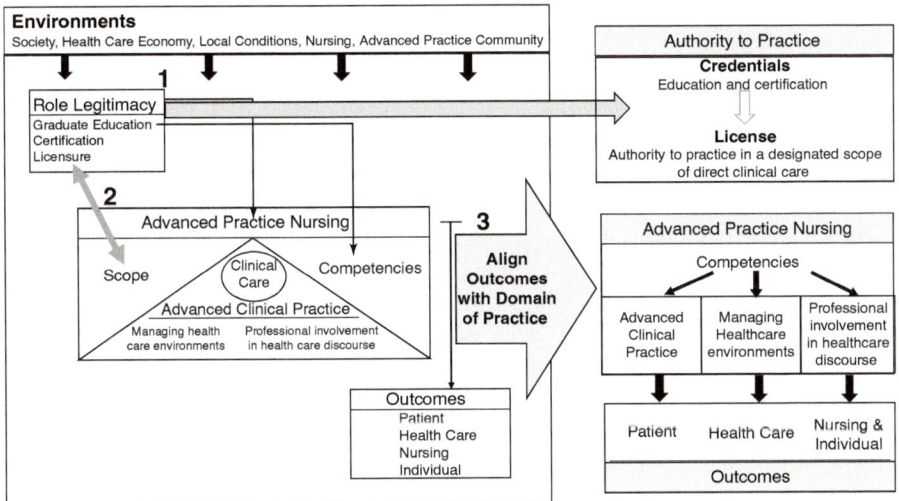

Fig. 2.2 Critique of Brown's (Brown 1998) framework for advanced practice nursing (Copyright © J.S. Fulton 2019)

Unlike Hamric's structural model, Brown's (1998) framework is a process model linking practice competencies with outcomes. Brown described the model as a broad, comprehensive framework of advanced practice nursing including four main elements: role legitimacy, advanced practice nursing, outcomes, and the environment in which practice occurs (Brown 1998). In Fig. 2.2, the left side depicts the original Brown model. Role legitimacy includes graduate education, certification, and licensure. A line depicts the linkage between graduate education and acquisition of clinical competencies; another line depicts the necessity of role legitimacy as prerequisite for advanced practice. Within the authority to practice box, the elements are graduate education, certification, and license. Within the advanced practice box, scope and competencies are balanced alongside the three domains of practice—advanced clinical practice, managing healthcare environments, and professional involvement in healthcare discourse. Outcomes are defined as the consequences of practice in the three domains. Patient outcomes are health outcomes for individuals. Healthcare environment outcomes include improved accessibility to care, availability of diverse healthcare services, and lower cost. Professional nursing outcomes reflect career enhancement opportunities for the individual advanced practice nurse. The framework links practice to clinical outcomes. In addition, the model depicts advanced practice nursing within the context of the larger environmental influences of society, healthcare economy, local conditions, and the advanced nursing community.

Critique of Brown's Framework. Brown's framework, like Hamric's model, includes authority to practice in the model, represented as role legitimacy. The model also includes scope of practice as an element of advanced practice. Scope is defined as specialization, expansion, autonomy, and accountability. Every license

includes a scope of legal authority in which the license holder practices autonomously and is held accountable. Role legitimacy elements would best be placed in
a separate authority to practice model with graduate education and certification as
credentials leading to a license to practice in a designated scope. Figure 2.2 demonstrates moving the role legitimacy and scope to a separate model, demonstrated on
the right side of the figure (see arrows #1 and #2 in Fig. 2.2).

Competencies, in Brown's Framework, include both core and role. Core competencies are expert guidance and counseling of patients and families; research critique, utilization, and conduct skills; and skills in working cooperatively with others.
Role competencies include clinical, diagnostic, and management experiences in
specialty areas and differing areas of expertise in organizational management.
Competencies practiced in the three domains of clinical care—clinical practice,
healthcare environments, and professional involvement—lead to outcomes in four
domains. As a practice model, the outcomes could be better aligned with their
respective domains of practice, as demonstrated in Fig. 2.2, arrow #3. Like Hamric's
model, Brown's framework represents considered thought but lacks empiric support. Brown has not updated or revised the model since it was originally published.

Reviewing and critiquing these two models demonstrates the importance of differentiating among models explaining structure, practice, and regulatory authority
and between domains of practice and domains of practice competencies. Both models included regulatory authority to practice that could best be explained in a separate model. Research is needed to demonstrate the value of CNS and other advanced
practice roles. Models linking practice competencies to clinical outcomes are
needed. Identifying and validating practice outcomes would make clear the expectations to the public and therefore the rationale for authority to practice.

2.6 Conceptual Models and Frameworks for CNS Role and Practice

Frameworks explaining structure of the CNS role describe the elements, characteristics, and domains of the CNS role. An example of a structural model is seen in
Fig. 2.3. This model, adopted by the NACNS (2004), demonstrates the structure of
the CNS role as three interacting practice domains imbedded in specialty practice
knowledge, skills, and standards of practice. Direct care is the central domain; two
additional domains, nurses/nursing practice standards and systems/organizations,
overlap inside the direct care domain. The three domains, called *spheres of influence*, became the organizing frame for CNS practice competencies (NACNS 2004).
Each of the three spheres of influence included practice competency statements
organized by assessment, diagnosis, outcome identification, and planning, interventions, and evaluation. Each sphere included outcomes aligned with the practice
competencies.

The model was revised by NACNS (2019) to include the larger context of CNS
practice represented by an outer boundary and included healthcare environment,
societal needs, healthcare policy, and interprofessional collaboration. The name of

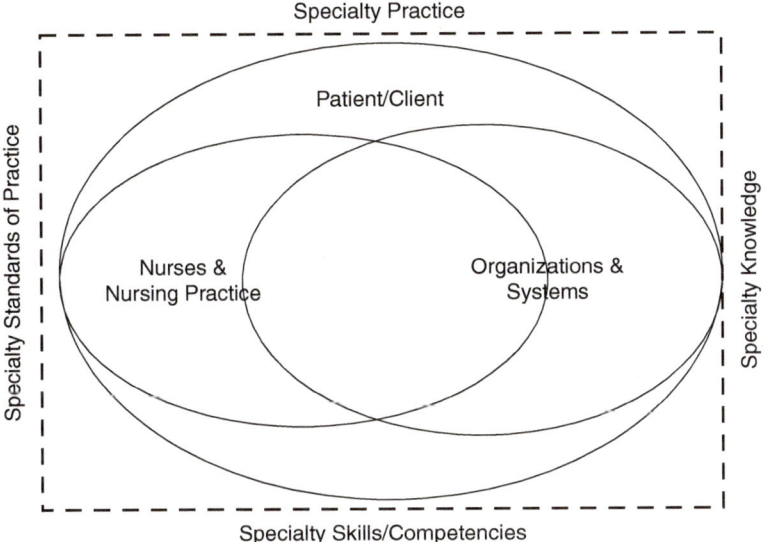

Fig. 2.3 Clinical nurse specialist practice conceptualized as core practice competencies in three interacting spheres of influence and guided by specialty knowledge, skills, and standards (Copyright © J.S. Fulton 2003)

the domains of practice were changed to *spheres of impact* from spheres of influence while retaining direct care as central with the two additional interacting spheres. Practice in one domain interacts with the other domains such that CNS practice in each domain is synergistic for the full practice actualization (NACNS 2019). As a model, it defines the domains of practice that explain role performance, the relationship of the domains to each other, and the contextual elements in which the domains are located. As a structural model, it does not explain the process of practice or link practice to outcomes. The revised model, seen in Fig. 2.4, depicts CNS competencies outside the domains; however, the accompanying explanation retains the structure of competencies organized by domain and existing within the spheres of impact, not external, and includes associated outcomes (NACNS 2019). Placing the competencies outside the spheres is an inaccurate representation of the narrative explanation.

Frameworks explaining practice describe the relationship between practice competencies and practice outcomes. These models incorporate processes and interactions by which practice competencies take place and make possible an intervention, therapy, or change. Practice models explain the linkages between practice competencies and practice outcomes in the designated domains of practice and across the scope of practice.

A model depicting the relationship between CNS practice competencies and outcomes was developed by Boyle (1996). Boyle's model recognizes both direct and indirect practice in three domains, including direct care, nursing staff, and healthcare

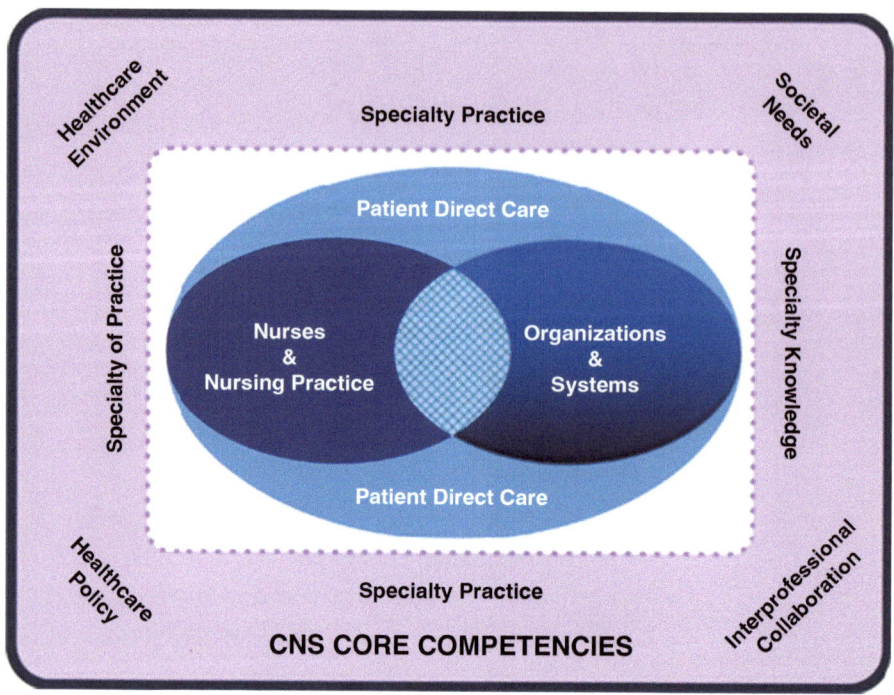

Fig. 2.4 Clinical nurse specialist practice conceptualized as practice in three interacting spheres actualized in specialty knowledge and standards occurring in a larger environment influenced by societal needs, health policy, healthcare environment, and interprofessional collaboration (NACNS 2019)

team/system. Direct care is defined as the provision of CNS services delivered directly to patients and families within a specialty consistent with specialty practice standards. The model also recognized the direct and indirect influence of CNS practice on personnel in the health system and identified indirect influence as an outcome of CNS practice because of a CNS's ability to improve outcomes through system-level interventions. Figure 2.5 is an adaptation of Boyle's model depicting relationships among CNS practice competencies in all three spheres and the culminating impact on patient and family outcomes within a given healthcare context or setting.

The new model links practice competencies and practice outcomes with sufficient specificity that it could be used to support research about the CNS role and practice, though neither the original Boyle's model nor the revised model has been empirically validated. The NACNS practice competencies and their related outcomes have been validated (Baldwin et al. 2007, 2009; Fulton et al. 2015) providing a measure of validity to the structure of the CNS role.

Frameworks explaining authority to practice are based in a social contract acknowledging professional rights and responsibilities of nurses and include a mechanism for public accountability. These frameworks describe the interrelationships of

Fig. 2.5 Clinical nurse specialist practice model demonstrating direct and indirect practice competencies and outcomes in three domains and occurring within a healthcare system (Copyright © J.S. Fulton 2019)

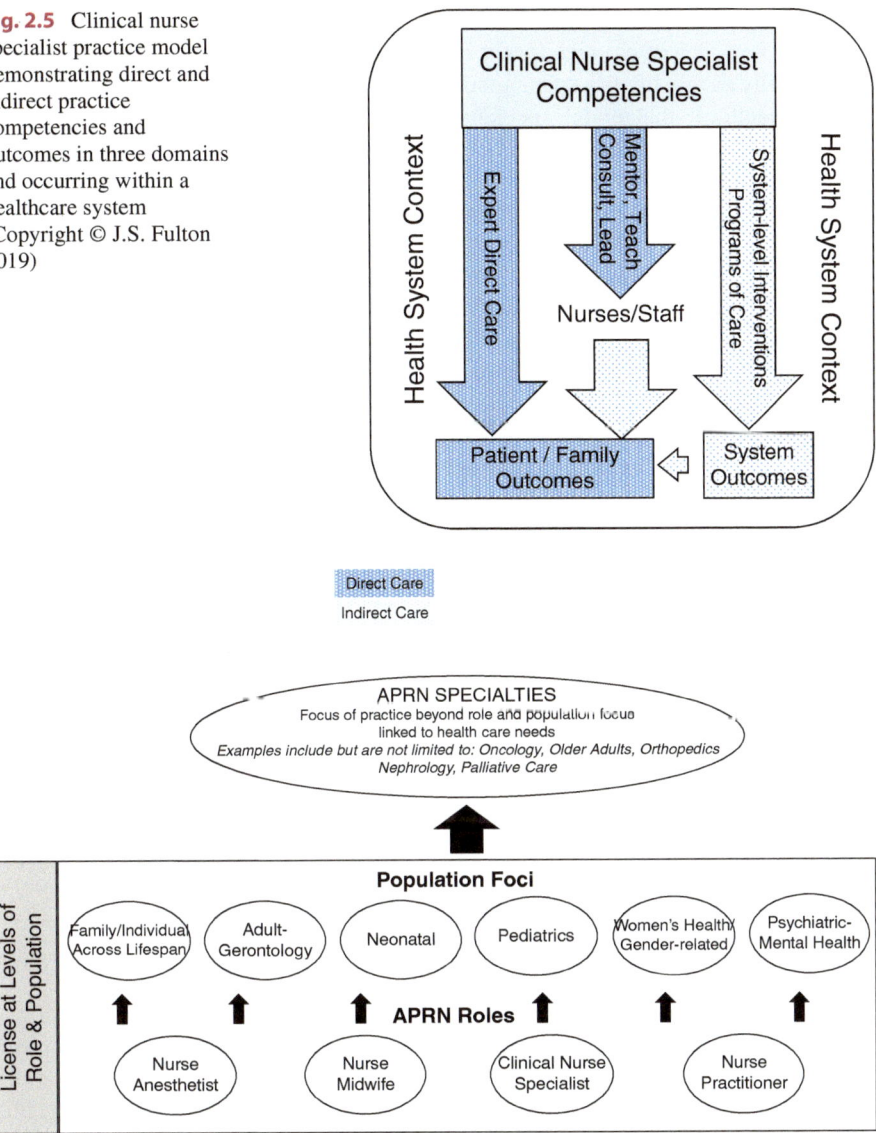

Fig. 2.6 Advanced practice registered nurse (APRN) regulatory model

the requirements for practice and an associated scope of practice. In the United States, the APRN Consensus Model (2008), depicted in Fig. 2.6, is a framework explaining authority to practice. The framework, developed by representatives from national nursing community, addresses variability in advanced practice nurse recognition and authority to practice by identifying both the roles eligible for advanced practice authority and the associated scope of practice. Advanced practice roles eligible for recognition are CNS, nurse practitioner, nurse-midwife, and nurse anesthetist. The scope of practice for the roles may be neonate, pediatric, adult/gerontology, family across the life span, gender health (men's or women's), and psychiatric/mental health. In this model, specialty practice beyond a population is not regulated, resulting in a decoupling of specialty education from graduate creating challenges for specialty education in CNS curricula.

In the United States, nursing practice is regulated at the state level, and the model proposes one approach to advanced practice recognition for all 50 states, each with different rules and requirements. The model stipulates requirements for educational preparation, accreditation of educational programs, professional nursing certification, and regulatory titling. For CNSs, the most significant gain was universal recognition of the CNS role as advanced practice. As could be anticipated, such a sweeping effort across the 50 states has, to date, met with varying success. One significant downside to the model is that specialty populations, which are limited to only six, exclude other, arguably equal specialty patient populations.

Two specialty populations not recognized in the model are oncology and critical care, both specialties representing complex, vulnerable populations and having a robust body of scientific evidence supporting practice. These specialties, with their individual knowledge and skill base, could easily support graduate education and prepare advanced nurses for a scope of practice in the specialty populations. The model also excludes the maternal-infant specialty population, which has led to a decline in advanced practice nurses caring for this vulnerable population. Thus the model, while affording some clarity to regulation across the 50 states, has been criticized for being too narrow and prescriptive. A challenge for any regulatory model is to find the right balance between prerequisite requirements and a scope of practice that enables nursing to respond to society's existing and changing needs for nursing services (Fulton 2019).

2.7 Differentiating CNS Practice

A shortcoming of many early CNS structural models was the failure to level competency domains for CNS advanced practice resulting in little distinction between generalist nursing and advanced practice nursing. Initially called "sub-roles," Hamric's early work (1989) identified CNS practice competency domains as clinician, educator, consultant, and researcher, which are not unique to CNS practice. All nurses are expected to practice as clinicians, educators, consultants, and researchers. The depth, scope, and related outcomes of practice in these areas depend on functional role and corresponding academic preparation and clinical training. For example, bachelor's-prepared nurses engage in research activities, as do master's-, practice doctorate (DNP)-, and research doctorate (PhD)-prepared nurses albeit not at the same level and with different expected outcomes.

Differentiating advanced practice from expert generalist practice was the purpose of Culkin's (1984) model, which was grounded in the definition of nursing as the diagnosis and treatment of human responses to actual or potential health problems. Assuming the possibility of human responses exists as a normal distribution, the model suggests that generalist nurses are prepared to deal with a more narrow range of the human response than an advanced practice nurse. Expert generalist nurses may excel at interventions for a wider range of responses when compared to more novice nurses, but would not be able to intervene across the wider range covered by an advanced practice role – a wider range of response due to graduate-level preparation in theory and science that supports problem-solving beyond expert experience. The model is theoretical, supported by examples for discussion, but lacks empiric verification.

An example of a research-based module that differentiated practice competencies for the advanced roles of CNS and nurse practitioner (NP) is Fenton and Brykczynski's (1993) adaptation of Benner's (1984) domains of practice. Benner's (1984) original work described seven domains of practice and identified practice competency within the domains as a continuum proceeding from novice to new clinician to expert in an area of practice. Benner's work resulted from interviews with generalist nurses, and while it included expert practice, it did not describe advanced practice. Fenton (1985) conducted an ethnographic study examining CNSs and their work. When comparing the findings to Benner's domains, Fenton identified several additional CNS-specific advanced competencies to existing domains, and one new domain, consultation, was added as a CNS practice domain. Similarly, Brykczynski (1989) conducted a naturalistic study to provide a contextual account of experienced nurse practitioners and suggested modifications to Benner's domains and competencies to reflect nurse practitioner practice. Comparing the results of the independent studies, Fenton and Brykczynski (1993) created a model that distinguished CNS practice from NP practice and distinguished both from expert generalist practice.

By comparing findings from independent studies, Fenton and Brykczynski's collaboration demonstrated that advanced practice can be multidimensional with both overlapping and distinct role competencies. NP practice has greater emphasis on management of patient health and illness status in the primary care setting compared to CNS practice with greater emphasis on consulting with staff around patient advocacy, interpreting nursing responsibilities to others, and role modeling nursing practice. Bryant-Lukosius (Fig. 2.7) further clarifies the essential distinctions between the two roles with an advanced practice continuum model, emphasizing how CNS practice focuses more on supporting clinical excellence through professional development, clinical leadership, education, and research while NP practice focuses more on direct patient care. Also indicated in the model is a point on the continuum of expansion where NP practice expands beyond the scope of the initial registered nurse license and needs additional authority to practice.

CNS practice is largely in a field historically viewed as nursing, and in extending the boundaries of traditional nursing, there has been little emphasis on additional authority to practice. In contrast, other advanced practice roles, including NPs, have been expanding nursing practice into areas historically identified with physician practice, often resulting in considerable pushback from physicians around regulatory authority to practice. Figure 2.8 depicts the different emphases of the CNS and

APN Continuum Model: Distinguishing NP from CNS Roles

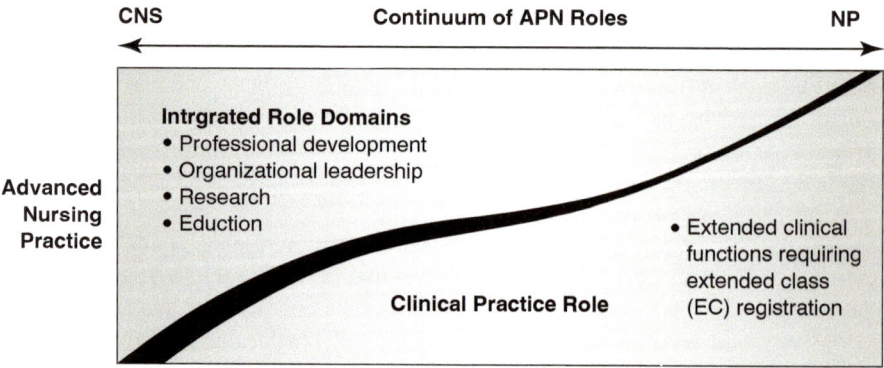

Source: Bryant-Lukosius, D. (2004 & 2008). *The continuum of advanced practice nursing roles.*
Unpublished document.

Fig. 2.7 The continuum of advanced practice nursing roles

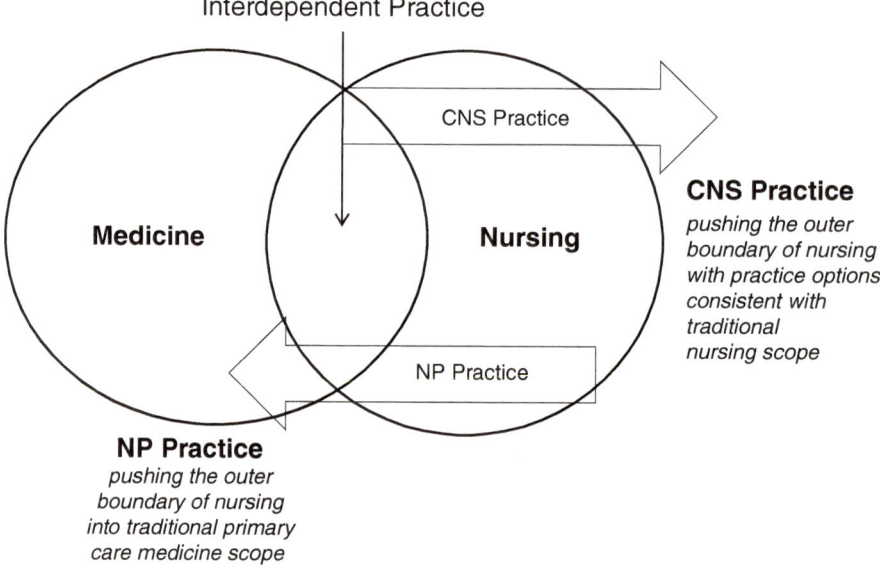

Fig. 2.8 Schema depicting clinical nurse specialist (CNS) and nurse practitioner (NP) practices expanding nursing practice in different directions, including area of interdependent practice (Copyright © Janet S. Fulton 2009)

NP roles, with the NP role expanding more into traditional medical practice. This figure also includes an overlapping area of practice identified as interdependent practice representing care that is interdependent on both providers for delivery of the total treatment. For example, insertion of an intravenous medical device may rest totally with a nurse's autonomous judgment for device selection and placement so that medically prescribed intravenous fluids and medications can be administered. As healthcare practices become more interprofessional, models are needed to distinguish nursing practice from medical and other practices.

CNS practice, existing predominantly in the traditional scope of nursing, allows for easier adaption of the role in differing countries and cultures. Whatever boundaries exist for nursing in a country, there is always a need to innovate and improve the care provided by nurses, to update standards of nursing practice, and to work within the healthcare system to facilitate best practices and remove barriers to care. The CNS role can support nurses in providing safe, high-quality, innovative care within the context of any setting, system, or culture.

2.8   Challenges and Opportunities

Over the years science has changed the precision of diagnostic techniques, led to the development of many more pharmaceutical agents, and made routine and complicated surgical procedures infection-free, restorative therapies. Nursing practice has changed too, to keep up with the scientific discoveries and specialized treatments. Yet it remains as true now as ever that wherever nursing is practiced, there will be a need for a nursing care expert to provide care to patients and families, identify the needs of populations, and lead others in promoting excellence in nursing practice. The CNS role was created by the nursing profession to fill the gap.

One ongoing challenge for CNSs is visibility. CNS practice is largely in the area of traditional nursing practice. Much about generalist nursing practice is poorly articulated to the public and outcomes are inadequately documented. In contrast to NP's higher public profile in delivering primary care, CNS practice is, like nursing practice in general, often invisible. Nursing practiced in what has been traditionally considered medicine, and, to a lesser extent, nursing practiced in the interdependent area, has a higher profile than the more traditional nursing interventions promoting care and comfort. Nurses teaching diabetic self-care may be invisible to other providers and the larger health system. A CNS expert in diabetes care supporting the nurses by designing evidence-based teaching guidelines and culturally appropriate resource materials is even more invisible (Fulton et al. 2019). Explaining that CNS practice is nursing practiced at an advanced level when nursing practice itself is invisible is quite a challenge. There is an urgent need for models that can be used to support research for documenting CNS practice outcomes.

Existing models and frameworks for CNS role and practice lack empiric support. Many models were developed by thought leaders and have served to guide the development of the roles and practice. However, research has often codified the language of the models without challenging the validity of the model itself. Researchers would often ask CNSs to identify or quantify activities in each of the old "sub-roles" while not considering the appropriate level of these activities for CNS practice or linking activities to outcomes. In addition, models used to describe all advanced practice roles fail to capture the nuances of each role and practice. Generalized models lack the specificity to capture the rich, detailed data needed to demonstrate CNS and nursing outcomes.

Additional conceptual work is needed to differentiate the CNS role and practice from other advanced practice roles. Understanding the unique knowledge, skill, and contributions of each role will help promote greater collaboration and cooperation among advanced practice nurses. The result will be a stronger profession better equipped to lead globally for the improvement of the health and well-being of the public. Our conceptual perception of ourselves becomes our reality. To that end the greatest opportunity is to more clearly define the CNS role and practice.

References

American Association of Critical-Care Nurses (2014) AACN scope and standards for acute care clinical nurse specialist practice. American Association of Critical-Care Nurses, Aliso Viejo, CA

American Nurses Association (2013) Nursing scope and standards of practice, 3rd edn. American Nurses Association, Silver Spring, MD

Arslanian-Engoren C (2019) Chapter 2. Conceptualizations of advanced practice nursing. In: Tracy MF, O'Grady ET (eds) Advanced practice nursing: an integrative approach. Elsevier, St. Louis, MO, pp 25–60

Baldwin KM, Lyon BL, Clark AP, Fulton JS, Davidson S, Dayhoff N (2007) Developing clinical nurse specialist practice competencies. Clin Nurse Spec 21(6):297–302

Baldwin KM, Clark AP, Fulton JS, Mayo A (2009) Validation of the NACNS clinical nurse specialist core competencies through a national survey. J Nurs Scholar 41(2):193–201

Benner P (1984) From novice to expert: excellence and power in clinical nursing practice. Addison-Wesley, Menlo Park, CA

Boyle DM (1996) Chapter 14. The clinical nurse specialist. In: Hamric AB, Spross JA, Hanson CM (eds) Advanced nursing practice: an integrative approach. W.B. Saunders, Philadelphia, PA, pp 299–336

Brown SJ (1998) A framework for advanced practice nursing. J Prof Nurs 14(3):157–164

Brykczynski KA (1989) An interpretive study describing the clinical judgment of nurse practitioners. Sch Inq Nurs Pract 3:75–104

Canadian Nurses Association (2019) Clinical nurse specialists. https://www.cna-aiic.ca/en/nursing-practice/the-practice-of-nursing/advanced-nursing-practice/clinical-nurse-specialists. Accessed 16 Dec 2019

Consensus Model for APRN Regulation: Licensure, Accreditation, Certification & Education. 2008. https://www.ncsbn.org/Consensus_Model_for_APRN_Regulation_July_2008.pdf. Accessed 16 Dec 2019

Cowan DT, Norman I, Coopamah VP (2005) Competence in nursing practice: a controversial concept—a focused review of the literature. Nurse Educ Today 25(5):355–362

Culkin JD (1984) A model for advanced nursing practice. J Nurs Adm 14(1):24–30

European Specialist Nurses Organizations (2015) Competences of the clinical nurse specialist (CNS): common plinth of competences for the common training framework of each specialty. http://www.esno.org/assets/harmonise-common_training_framework.pdf. Accessed 17 Dec 2019

Fenton MV (1985) Identifying competencies of clinical nurse specialists. J Nurs Adm 15(12):31–37

Fenton MV, Brykczynski KA (1993) Qualitative distinctions and similarities in the practice of clinical nurse specialits and nurse practitioners. J Prof Nurs 9(6):313–326

Fulton JS (2014) Chapter 1. Evolution of the clinical nurse specialist role and practice in the United States. In: Fulton JS, Lyon BL, Goudreau KA (eds) Foundations of clinical nurse specialist practice. Springer Company, New York, NY, pp 1–15

Fulton JS (2019) Fulfilling our social mandate. Clin Nurse Spec 33(2):61–62

Fulton JS, Mayo A, Walker J, Urden L (2015) Core practice outcomes for clinical nurse specialists: a revalidation study. J Prof Nurs 32(4):271–282

Fulton JS, Mayo A, Walker J, Urden LD (2019) Description of work processes used by clinical nurse specialists to improve patient outcomes. Nurs Outlook 67(5):511–522

Hamric AB, Spross JA (1989) The clinical nurse specialist in theory and practice, 2nd edn. W.B. Saunders Co., Philadelphia, PA

Hamric AB, Tracy MF (2019) Chapter 3. A definition of advanced practice nursing. In: Tracy MF, O'Grady ET (eds) Advanced practice nursing: an integrative approach. Elsevier, St. Louis, MO, pp 61–79

Hicks FD (2014) Chapter 3. Philosophical underpinnings of advanced nursing practice: a synthesizing framework for clinical nurse specialist practice. In: Fulton JS, Lyon BL, Goudreau KA (eds) Foundations of clinical nurse specialist practice. Springer Company, New York, NY, pp 33–39

International Council of Nurses (ICN) Nurse Practitioner: Advanced Practice Nurse Network (2019) Definition and characteristics of the role. https://international.aanp.org/Practice/APNRoles. Accessed 16 Dec 2019

Lewandowski W, Adamle K (2009) Substantive areas of clinical nurse specialist practice. A comprehensive review of the literature. Clin Nurse Spec 23(2):73–90

National Association of Clinical Nurse Specialists (2004) Statement on clinical nurse specialist practice and education, 2nd edn. Author, Harrisburg, PA

National Association of Clinical Nurse Specialists (2019) Statement on clinical nurse specialist practice and education, 3rd edn. Author, Reston, VA

National League for Nursing (NLN) (1958) Report of the National Working Conference: education of the clinical specialist in psychiatric nursing. Author, New York, NY

Reiter F (1966) The nurse-clinician. Am J Nurs 66:274–280

Spross JA (2015) Chapter 2. Conceptualizations of advanced practice nursing. In: Hamirc AB, Hanson CM, Tracy MF, O'Grady ET (eds) Advanced practice nursing: An integrative approach. Elsevier, St. Louis, MO, pp 27–66

Core Clinical Nurse Specialist Practice Competencies

3

Jane A. Walker

Abstract

Professional practice standards and competencies have been created by a variety of international organizations for the purpose of guiding clinical nurse specialist (CNS) practice, education, and credentialing. Competencies also address knowledge, skills, abilities, and judgment required to safely carry out one's profession. The focus of this chapter included a review and examination of definitions and purposes of competencies, use of competencies in nursing practice, evolution of competencies with respect to CNS practice, similarities and differences in international conceptualizations of CNS practice with respect to advanced practice nursing, comparison of published CNS competencies, and examination of the relationship of research-based themes of CNS practice to published competencies. Much consistency in international competency domains of CNS practice existed regardless of the methods used to develop them. Common core competency domains included direct care, research and evidence-based practice, quality improvement, education and teaching, communication, consultation, collaboration, leadership, and policy. Published research reports supported the existence of these competency domains. Although international variability is present regarding whether or not CNSs are considered to be advanced practice nurses, competencies and domains of practice are actually stable and can be used internationally to articulate the CNS role with clarity and consistency.

Keywords

Clinical nurse specialist · Competencies · Practice competencies · CNS practice · Credentialing · Certification

J. A. Walker (✉)
Purdue University Northwest College of Nursing, Hammond, IN, USA
e-mail: walker1@pnw.edu

3.1   Introduction

In 1953, the International Council of Nurses (ICN) published its first document outlining a code of ethics, with the most recent edition, published in 2012, addressing several aspects of competency and standards (International Council of Nurses 2012). Specifically, the ICN outlined the need for professional nurses to be responsible for maintaining personal competence; consider competency of self and others when assuming responsibility or delegating duties to others; and assume "the major role in determining and implementing acceptable standards of…practice…and education" (ICN 2012: 3). Therefore, it is a professional responsibility for nurses to be involved in the process of determining practice standards and related competencies.

During the past several decades, various international nursing organizations and government agencies have written and published professional standards and competencies. These documents have guided nursing practice across levels of education and nursing practice roles, including advanced practice nursing (APN) (Canadian Nurses Association 2019; International Council of Nurses 2019; National Association of Clinical Nurse Specialists 2019; Royal College of Nursing 2018a). These competency statements can be useful for standardizing scope of practice, knowledge, and skills across advanced practice nursing roles, including CNS practice.

In addition to standardizing practice, published competency statements can provide a framework for understanding similarities and differences in CNS practice across the world. This understanding can also provide contextual clarity when reading publications or publishing manuscripts related to CNS practice. Similarly, an understanding of competency statements may be useful for organizations that are in the process of developing or revising CNS competencies.

However, in spite of the presence of competency statements, CNS role confusion continues to exist due to international variability in definitions, education requirements, scope of practice, and classification of CNS practice as advanced practice nursing or not (Dury et al. 2014; ICN 2019; King et al. 2017; Stasa et al. 2014). The purpose of this chapter will be to explore definitions and purposes of competencies, describe how competencies are used in nursing practice, review the evolution of competencies with respect to CNS practice, examine similarities and differences in international conceptualizations of CNS practice with respect to advanced practice nursing, compare published CNS competencies, and relate research-based themes of CNS practice to published competencies.

3.2   Definitions

Internationally, definitions of competence and competency are very similar. For example, the American Nurses Association (ANA) (2015) defined competency as "…an expected level of performance that integrates knowledge, skills, abilities, and judgement" (p. 44). Similarly, the ICN (2009) defined competence as "the effective application of a combination of knowledge, skill and judgement demonstrated by an individual in daily practice or job performance" (p. 6).

Published competencies are used for a variety of purposes. One purpose is to clearly articulate professional role and scope of practice. Written competencies describe the knowledge and skills that correspond with respective nursing roles, thus delineating role expectations. When role expectations are clearly defined, licensure bodies can then use published competencies as a basis for practice regulation (APRN Consensus Work Group 2008; ICN 2019). Finally, competencies are used as a guide for developing curricula in nursing education and to assess attainment of education outcomes (Fulton 2009). For example, international and US-based national nursing education accreditors require programs to demonstrate the extent to which program graduates achieve program-specific competencies upon graduation (ACEN 2017; CCNE 2018; ICN 2019).

3.3   Evolution of CNS Competencies

Clinical nurse specialist competency domains began appearing in the literature in the 1960s (Fulton 2014). According to these early publications, role/competency domains focused on practice based on synthesis of the biobehavioral sciences; role modeling; quality improvement; consultation; staff and patient teaching; group dynamics; interpersonal communication skills; interprofessional teamwork/collaboration; change agency; research and inquiry; and improvement of patient outcomes through creative practice (Fulton 2014). Over the following 10 years, various authors continued to publish papers describing the CNS role and competencies. Interestingly, as noted by Fulton (2014), the CNS role remained similar throughout this time period.

In 1998, the National Association of Clinical Nurse Specialists based in the United States published the first document of CNS competencies written by a nursing association (Fulton 2014; NACNS 1998). These competencies integrated earlier conceptualizations of CNS practice using a three spheres of influence framework consisting of patient/client, nurses and nursing practice, and organizations and systems (Fulton 2014). By organizing the competencies in the spheres of influence framework, it was possible to describe competencies in their respective contexts as opposed to discrete skills. Thus, a more wholistic conceptualization of CNS practice competencies was possible while retaining enough detail to describe practice expectations (Fulton 2014; NACNS 1998). It is also important to note that the 1998 NACNS competencies and subsequent updates focused on core competencies independent from specialty. Fulton (2014) noted that it was important to separate the concept of role from specialty, because specialty focuses on specialty knowledge and specialties in healthcare continually evolve. By being able to focus on role, it was possible to write core competencies that cross specialty boundaries and apply to CNS practice irrespective of specialty or context (Fulton 2014).

Since that time, the 1998 NACNS competencies have been updated several times (NACNS 2004, 2019), and other international organizations have also published CNS-specific competencies (Canadian Nurses Association 2019; European Specialist Nurses Organisations 2015; ICN 2019). Work is ongoing internationally to define the CNS role and subsequent competencies (ICN 2019; Jokiniemi et al. 2018).

3.4   Clinical Nurse Specialists and Advanced Practice Nursing

Before addressing similarities and differences among international CNS competency statements, the question of whether CNS practice represents advanced practice nursing will be discussed. Note that this discussion represents an international sample and is not meant to be exhaustive. The ICN (2019) recently published guidelines on advanced practice nursing. In this document, the ICN defined the advanced practice nurse as "…a generalist or specialized nurse who has acquired, through additional graduate education (minimum of a master's degree), the expert knowledge base, complex decision-making skills and clinical competencies for advanced nursing practice…" (p. 4). The ICN also recognized CNSs and nurse practitioners as the most commonly identified advanced practice nurses (2019). In the United States, CNSs, along with nurse practitioners, certified nurse anesthetists, and certified nurse-midwives, are all recognized as advanced practice nurses (APRN Consensus Workgroup 2008). Similarly, in Canada, CNSs and nurse practitioners are recognized as advanced practice (Canadian Nurses Association 2019). Finally, CNS practice has been considered to be advanced practice in Europe (European Specialist Nurses Organisations 2015), Japan (Kondo 2013), and the Republic of Ireland (ICN 2019).

Alternative conceptualizations of advanced nursing practice and the CNS role exist in Australia and the United Kingdom. For example, the Nursing and Midwifery Board of Australia (NMBA) recognizes, for regulatory purposes, two categories of advanced practice: "advanced nursing practice" and "advanced practice nursing." Advanced nursing practice refers to registered nurses, or nurse practitioners who practice at an advanced generalist or specialist level. Therefore, advanced nursing practice is not considered to be role based, but refers instead to a level of practice (NMBA 2016). Advanced practice nursing refers solely to nurse practitioner practice (NMBA 2016).

Ongoing work to delineate nursing roles has been taking place in Australia. For example, Gardner et al. (2017) carried out a large national cross-sectional study of nursing practice and used cluster analysis to identify seven separate clusters of nursing. Their analysis revealed a cluster focused on nurse practitioner that was characterized by a significant level of advanced practice. The analysis also revealed an advanced practice nurse cluster comprised of several advanced nursing titles, including the clinical nurse specialist (Gardner et al. 2017).

The use of non-role-based umbrella terms of "advanced level nursing practice" is also occurring in the United Kingdom with agreement by the health departments of England, Northern Ireland, Scotland, and Wales (RCN 2018a). For example, the Royal College of Nursing defined advanced practice as "a level of practice rather than a type of practice" (RCN 2018b: 6). The RCN recognized various advanced nursing roles that are developing, including clinical nurse specialists, with a focus on education at the master's level with skill and expertise in the advanced practice pillars of practice: clinical/direct care; leadership and collaborative practice; improving quality and developing practice; and developing self and others (RCN 2018b). Therefore, nurses practicing at an advanced level would practice according to the four pillars regardless of their role. Note that the names of the four pillars may vary somewhat among the four UK countries but are conceptually similar.

Of interest, an effort is underway in England to conceptualize advanced clinical practice with respect to multiple types of healthcare providers (NHS Health Education England 2017). Within this framework, the focus is on advancing practice within practice pillars that apply to multiple professions. Clinical nurse specialists would then practice within this multi-professional umbrella.

Based on the preceding discussion, it can be seen that international differences in terminology and conceptualizations of CNS practice as advanced practice exist. Additionally, differences in defining advanced practice by role, as opposed to defining advanced practice as advanced knowledge, skills, and expertise, may lead to misconceptions about CNS practice and about advanced practice nursing in general.

3.5   Clinical Nurse Specialist Competencies

A comparison of international CNS competencies is important to understand how CNS work is similar and different around the world. Published comparisons of CNS competencies from an international perspective are limited. However, Sastre-Fullana et al. (2014) published a literature review of competency frameworks used in advanced practice nursing. In addition to reviewing competency models, the authors reviewed competency assessment tools and focused on mapping and standards of practice (Sastre-Fullana et al. 2014). The authors used a systematic search strategy to select 119 documents from the literature in addition to 97 documents from gray literature. The authors analyzed the selected documents using a content analysis process. As a result of this analysis, the authors extracted 17 common competency domains of advanced practice nursing represented by 29 countries (Sastre-Fullana et al. 2014). The most common domains, accounting for approximately 44% of the competency dimensions across countries, included research, clinical and professional leadership, mentoring and coaching, and expert clinical judgment (Sastre-Fullana et al. 2014). The four domains with the least amount of commonality across countries included communication, cultural competencies, advocacy, and change management (Sastre-Fullana et al. 2014).

The review carried out by Sastre-Fullana et al. (2014) was extensive and included competencies of all advanced nursing practice roles. In this chapter, competencies focused on CNS practice are described. When competencies were published as advanced-level competencies and included CNS practice, they were included. Also included were intermediate-level nurse specialist competencies requiring education beyond that required for entry-level nursing practice.

To locate published competencies, a search of scientific databases was performed in addition to searching for competencies from country-specific and international nursing organizations. Lists of potential countries with CNS competencies were located through publications by Sastre-Fullana et al. (2014) and by Schober and Green (2018). It is possible, however, that all published competency statements were not located. A description of CNS and advanced-level competencies can be found in Table 3.1.

A review of the domains of competencies listed in Table 3.1 demonstrated much similarity in CNS and advanced-level competencies existing across the world. All organizations addressed competencies related to direct practice. Within the domain of direct practice, common competencies related to clinical management, expert assessment, teaching, decision-making, and diagnosing. All organizations included competencies related to education and teaching.

As mentioned under the direct practice domain, patient teaching was commonly mentioned, but teaching also included competencies related to staff education and ongoing personal continuing education. Research and evidence-based practice was another domain addressed by all competency sets. Research-specific competencies included skills of appraisal, utilization, research participation, and dissemination. Similarly competencies addressed the application and translation of evidence into practice.

Competencies in managing quality and skills specific to audit and practice monitoring were frequently included in the competency domains. Common competency domains related to mentoring, communicating, consulting, and interacting with staff and other professionals existed. Finally, competencies focused on leadership, interprofessional collaboration, and teamwork based on foundations of ethical practice were included.

In addition to competency statements, several published papers focused on CNS role perception in a number of countries that are in the process of formalizing the CNS role. In Finland, Nieminen et al. (2011) performed focus group interviews with selected CNSs and APN students to examine perceptions of role competencies and their relationship to practice. The researchers completed content analysis of interview transcripts, and themes relating to five competency domains emerged. The domains included "assessment of patients' caring needs and nursing care activities," "caring relationship," "multi-professional teamwork," "development of competence and nursing care," and "leadership in a learning and caring culture" (Nieminen et al. 2011: 664). Supporting categories included concepts such as independence, education, teaching, research, and cooperation. The authors concluded that clinical competency at the advanced practice level represented more than advanced skills and included quality relationships with patients and collaboration with other healthcare providers (Nieminen et al. 2011).

Table 3.1 Core CNS/advanced-level competencies/practice themes

Statement author	Underlying framework	Competency domains
Canadian Nurses Association (2019)	Pan-Canadian Framework: *Focus of competencies; advanced practice nursing. CNS-specific competencies also exist (see below) and are compatible with the 2019 advanced practice nursing competencies*	• Direct care: Includes clinical expertise, client-family-centered care, and interprofessional collaboration in the context of specialty. Also includes managing complex patients, measuring outcomes, and disseminating knowledge • Health systems: Includes advocacy, innovation, policy, cost-effectiveness, consultation, quality improvement, and change • Education: Includes providing education to clients/families, all healthcare providers, and students. Also includes precepting, mentoring, and promoting continuous learning and professional development • Research: Includes applying and generating evidence. Also includes evaluating outcomes of care and evidence-based practice • Leadership: Includes change agency, program evaluation, innovation, and advocacy • Consultation and collaboration
Canadian Nurses Association (2014)	Three areas of influence including client, practice settings, and organization/ systems	• Clinical care • Systems leadership • Advancement of nursing practice • Evaluation and research
European Specialist Nurses Organisations (2015)	European Qualifications Framework *Focus of competencies: CNS practice*	• Clinical role • Patient relationship • Patient teaching/coaching • Mentoring • Research • Organization and management • Communication and teamwork • Ethics and decision-making • Leadership and policy making • Public health

(continued)

Table 3.1 (continued)

Statement author	Underlying framework	Competency domains
National Association of Clinical Nurse Specialists (2019)	Spheres of impact: Patient direct care, nurses and nursing practice, organization/system *Focus of competencies: CNS practice*	• Patient direct care: Includes direct interaction with patients, families, or groups of patients; advanced nursing management of health, illness, and disease; relationship-building and communication, education, consultation, and ethical practice • Nurses and nursing practice: Includes all aspects of EBP; health work environment; relationships and communication; quality improvement; mentorship; staff education; change; fiscal management; and leadership and policy • Organization/system: Includes professional advocacy, quality, and all aspects of EBP, interprofessional consultation and communication, research and dissemination, fiscal responsibility, leadership, and ethical practice
National Council for the Professional Development of Nursing and Midwifery Ireland (2008)	Scope of Nursing and Midwifery Practice Framework *Focus of competencies: CNS practice which is considered to be advanced nursing practice and different from nurse practitioner practice. The more recently published Nursing and Midwifery Board of Ireland's 2017 document of advanced practice nursing standards does not apply to CNS practice*	• Clinical focus, either direct or indirect • Patient client advocate involving communication and collaboration • Education and training involving staff development, patient education, and personal continuing education • Audit and research, including EBP • Consultancy, including inter- and intradisciplinary consultation
National Health Service Health Education England (2017)	Multi-professional Advanced Clinical Practice framework *Focus of capabilities: Advanced clinical practice (note not specific to nursing or CNS practice)*	• Clinical/direct care practice: Includes autonomous practice, partnerships, communication skills, complex decision-making, managing complex and unpredictable situations, collaboration • Leadership and management: Includes relationship/team focus, role modeling, practice evaluation, peer review, leadership, professional boundary management • Education: Includes developing self and others, shared decision-making, health literacy, interprofessional learning, mentoring others • Research: Includes research engagement, quality monitoring, critical appraisal and synthesis, EBP, dissemination, facilitating linkages between practice and academia

Table 3.1 (continued)

Statement author	Underlying framework	Competency domains
National Health Service Wales (2010)	Pillars of Advanced Practice. *Focus of competencies: Advanced practice*	• Direct clinical practice: Includes autonomous practice, clinical judgment, diagnosing, patient-centered care • Leadership and collaborative practice: Includes stakeholder engagement, negotiation, evidence synthesis, and implementation • Education and learning: Includes continuing education; educating, supervising and mentoring other nurses, audit, and practice evaluation • Research and evidence-based practice: Includes participation in research activities to improve healthcare quality, research appraisal, evidence-based practice, dissemination, application of research methods
Northern Ireland Practice and Education Council for Nursing and Midwifery (2016)	Northern Ireland's Advanced Nursing Practice Framework. *Focus of competencies: Advanced nursing practice*	• Direct clinical practice: Includes autonomous practice, expertise re: diagnosis and patient management, clinical judgment, patient-centered care, and quality monitoring • Leadership and collaborative practice: Includes development of partnerships, stakeholder engagement, resilience, and evidence synthesis and implementation • Education and learning: Includes continuing education; educating, supervising, and mentoring; audit; and practice evaluation • Research and evidence-based practice: Includes participation in research activities to improve healthcare quality; research application; evidence-based practice; dissemination; application of research methods
Royal College of Nursing (2018a)	Pillars of Advanced Level Nursing Practice. *Focus of competencies: Advanced level nursing practice*	• Clinical/direct care: Includes autonomy, diagnosis and management, health promotion, professional judgment, technology, boundary management • Leadership and collaborative practice: Includes demonstrating value of advanced level nursing, consultancy, leadership, stakeholder engagement, partnership development and maintenance, change management • Improving quality and developing practice: Includes quality improvement activities and ongoing monitoring, research appraisal dissemination and application, knowledge generation, cost management • Developing self and others: Includes peer review, education, evidence-based practice, collaboration, organizational culture, and communication

(continued)

Table 3.1 (continued)

Statement author	Underlying framework	Competency domains
Scottish Government (2010)	NHS Education for Scotland (NES) Advanced Nursing Practice Themes *Focus of competencies: Advanced nursing practice*	• Clinical/professional leadership: Includes governance, ethical decision-making, negotiation, teamwork • Facilitating learning: Includes teaching/learning for staff and patients, mentorship, and coaching • Research and development: Includes accessing research, appraisal, audit, using research in practice, dissemination • Advanced clinical practice: Includes decision-making, critical thinking, managing complexity and risk, prescribing (depending on context), outcome improvement, communication skills
Singapore Nursing Board (2018)	Not specified *Note that CNSs are not specifically named by the Board. Competencies apply to nurses in specialty practice*	• Professional, legal, and ethical nursing practice: Includes understanding of regulation and legal aspects of practice, ethical practice, cultural sensitivity • Management of care: Includes clinical skills, diagnostic reasoning, communication skills, knowledge, professionalism • Leadership and management: Includes consultancy, interprofessional collaboration, quality improvement, research, and EBP • Professional development: Includes self-development, research, and EBP

In one of several follow-up studies, also conducted in Finland, Jokiniemi et al. (2018) determined construct validity of CNS core competencies. The researchers reported work that took place over several years and involved a series of studies. Multiple methods were used including a Delphi study, cross-mapping of CNS competencies under development in Finland with international competencies, and two phases of content validity assessment (Jokiniemi et al. 2018). As a result of this work, the authors decreased the number of potential competencies from 75 to 50 with a content validity index of 0.94. The four resulting competency domains included patient, nursing, organization, and scholarship (Jokiniemi et al. 2018).

While not focused specifically on competencies, Onishi and Kanda (2010) conducted a study to examine managers' perspectives of certified nurse specialist (CNS) roles in Japan. The CNS role in Japan is focused on nursing practice, consultation, care coordination, ethical care, education, and research (Japanese Nurses Association 2016). Whereas CNSs are educated at the master's level, there also exists a certified nurse (CN) who completes 6 months of education beyond entry level. Role expectations for the CN include "practice, teaching and consultation" (Onishi and Kanda 2010: 312). The researchers completed focus group interviews with nurse administrators to explore their expectations regarding roles of the CNS/CN as well as their perceptions about managing CNSs and CNs. Analysis of the interviews revealed three themes of expectations focusing on staff education, quality improvement, and role development. The administrators identified that communication skills and negotiating skills were necessary for the role to be effective (Onishi and Kanda 2010).

The role dimensions and themes that emerged from the primary studies mirrored the competencies listed in Table 3.1. As can be seen from a review of these studies and competency statements, much international similarity in the core role of the CNS exists. Core CNS competency domains also aligned well with the common advanced practice domains identified by Sastre-Fullana et al. (2014). The primary difference was that communication competencies appeared to be more commonly addressed in the CNS competencies than in the common advanced practice competencies.

3.6 Discussion

In this review of competency statements and research, much similarity in international CNS practice exists. Common domains of CNS competencies related to direct care; education and teaching; research and evidence-based practice; quality improvement; communication, consultation and mentoring; leadership, interprofessional collaboration, and ethics. Several competency statements addressed CNS competencies related to working with nurses and positively influencing work setting culture. Clinical nurse specialist competencies also focused on dissemination.

It is interesting that such a high level of international agreement on CNS competencies exists when one considers the variety of ways that competencies developed over the years. The original, 1998 NACNS competencies were developed inductively through a job analysis process (Baldwin et al. 2007). An expert panel consisting of practicing CNSs and educators reviewed over 80 job descriptions representing a wide geographic area in the United States and representing a variety of specialties. The panel extracted themes from the job descriptions and then reviewed published work that related to core CNS practice. Through these analyses, the three themes of patient/client, nurses and nursing personnel, and organization/system emerged. A series of internal and external reviews of draft and revised competency statements followed the competency development process (Baldwin et al. 2007). A 2004 update of the NACNS competencies followed a similar process of extensive internal and external feedback (Baldwin et al. 2007). A new edition of NACNS competencies was released in 2019 (NACNS 2019).

The Canadian Nurses Association approach to developing the pan-Canadian CNS competencies (2014) differed from that used by NACNS. The Canadian Nurses Association used a five-phase process including a review of current CNS practice and competency frameworks; development of a competency profile by CNSs from across the country; review and input by a competency development steering committee; stakeholder review and validation using a snowball survey approach; and final revisions by the steering committee incorporating stakeholder feedback.

In the United Kingdom, the RNC published in 2018 updated competencies (RCN 2018a) that represent a collaboration among the four countries: England, Northern Ireland, Scotland, and Wales. Each country uses a pillar of practice approach to designate practice domains, although the pillars of practice have evolved somewhat differently in each country (RCN 2018a).

It can be seen that some of the methods used to create CNS/ANP competencies were similar, but there also existed a mix of inductive and deductive processes. These different processes have converged, resulting in very similar international CNS competencies and role patterns. This convergence confirms the validity of CNS competencies on a worldwide basis.

3.7   Future Directions

It is expected that existing CNS competency statements will continue to be revised over time. Based on recent activity focused on competency creation, we can also expect that additional countries and regions of the world will continue to create, promote, and institutionalize CNS competencies (European Specialist Nurses Organisations 2019; Jokiniemi et al. 2018).

It is unclear to what extent CNS competencies will change over the next 10–20 years. In the United States, NACNS has recommended requiring the Doctor of Nursing Practice (DNP) degree in the future for entry into CNS practice (NACNS 2015). However the master's degree is still considered to be the degree required for entry to advanced practice, including CNS practice (ICN 2019). Additionally, NACNS's 2019 competencies were written to be applicable for master's as well as

DNP entry into practice. Competency domains have therefore remained fairly stable and universal for a number of years and will likely continue to be appropriate as a framework for CNS practice.

Another question is how the role of competencies will evolve in the future. O'Connell et al. (2014) questioned the usefulness of competencies to address the complexities surrounding advanced nursing practice. They indicated that competencies can be helpful when describing needed knowledge and skills in stable situations, but might not fully ensure that providers will be competent when faced with a complex, dynamic problem or situation (O'Connell et al. 2014). To address this gap, O'Connell and colleagues recommended adopting a capability framework to replace the use of competencies as a guide for advanced practice. O'Connell et al. (2014), citing the Australian Capability Network, defined capability as "the combination of skills, knowledge, values and self-esteem which enables individuals to handle change" (p. 2731). They further indicated that specialist expertise depends on capability and that specialists who are capable continue to build their skills during their career (O'Connell et al. 2014).

There is evidence that several countries are using a capability as opposed to competency approach for conceptualizing advanced practice. For example, England's multi-professional framework for advanced clinical practice uses capabilities as opposed to competencies (NHS Health Education England 2017). Similarly, (NHS Education for Scotland has published a number of capability framework documents, including a document addressing nurses, specialists, and carers of individuals with cancer 2008). It will be interesting to see how these ideas evolve over time.

3.8 Conclusions

In summary, CNS and advanced nursing practice competencies have been used to guide practice for approximately 20 years. Many similarities exist among published competency statements and domains of CNS practice regardless of the methods used to develop them. This consistency provides insights into the universality of the CNS role. Although international variability is present regarding the titles used to describe CNS practice, competencies and domains of practice are actually stable and can be used internationally to articulate the CNS role with clarity and consistency.

References

Accreditation Commission for Education in Nursing (2017) ACEN accreditation manual section III 2017 standards and criteria. http://www.acenursing.net/manuals/SC2017.pdf. Accessed 13 Feb 2020

American Nurses Association (2015) Nursing scope and standards of practice, 3rd edn. American Nurses Association, Silver Spring, MD

APRN Consensus Work Group & the National Council of State Boards of Nursing APRN Advisory Committee (2008) Consensus model for APRN regulation: licensure, accreditation, certification, & education. https://www.ncsbn.org/Consensus_Model_for_APRN_Regulation_July_2008.pdf. Accessed 13 Feb 2020

Baldwin KM, Lyon BL, Clark AP, Fulton J, Dayhoff N (2007) Developing clinical nurse specialist practice competencies. Clin Nurse Spec 21:297–303

Canadian Nurses Association (2014) Pan-Canadian core competencies for the clinical nurse specialist. https://cna-aiic.ca/~/media/cna/files/en/clinical_nurse_specialists_convention_handout_e.pdf. Accessed 13 Feb 2020

Canadian Nurses Association (2019) Advanced practice nursing. A Pan-Canadian framework. https://www.cna-aiic.ca/-/media/cna/page-content/pdf-en/apn-a-pan-canadian-framework.pdf. Accessed 13 Feb 2020

Commission on Collegiate Nursing Education (2018) Standards for accreditation of baccalaureate and graduate nursing programs. https://www.aacnnursing.org/Portals/42/CCNE/PDF/Standards-Final-2018.pdf. Accessed 13 Feb 2020

Dury C, Hall C, Danan JL, Aguiar Barbieri-Figueiredo MC, Costa MAM, Debout C (2014) Specialist nurse in Europe: education, regulation and role. Int Nurs Rev 61:454–462

European Specialist Nurses Organisations (2015) Competences of the clinical nurse specialist (CNS): common plinth of competences for the common training framework of each specialty. http://www.esno.org/assets/harmonise-common_training_framework.pdf. Accessed 13 Feb 2020

European Specialist Nurses Organisations (2019) Position statement. The specialist nurses in European healthcare towards 2030. https://www.esno.org/assets/esno_position_statement_april_2019_final.pdf. Accessed 13 Feb 2020

Fulton JS (2009) Practice competencies front and center. Clin Nurse Spec 23:121–122

Fulton JS (2014) Evolution of the clinical nurse specialist role and practice in the United States. In: Fulton JS, Lyon BL, Goudreau KA (eds) Foundations of clinical nurse specialist practice, 2nd edn. Springer, New York, NY, pp 1–15

Gardner G, Duffield C, Doubrovsky A, Bui UT, Adams M (2017) The structure of nursing: a national examination of titles and practice profiles. Int Nurs Rev 64:233–241. https://doi.org/10.1111/inr.12364

International Council of Nurses (2009) ICN framework of competencies for the nurse specialist. https://siga-fsia.ch/files/user_upload/08_ICN_Framework_for_the_nurse_specialist.pdf. Accessed 14 Feb 2020

International Council of Nurses (2012) The ICN code of ethics for nurses. https://www.icn.ch/sites/default/files/inline-files/2012_ICN_Codeofethicsfornurses_%20eng.pdf. Accessed 13 Feb 2020

International Council of Nurses (2019) Guidelines on advanced practice nursing. International Council of Nurses, Geneva

Japanese Nurses Association (2016) Nursing in Japan. https://www.nurse.or.jp/jna/english/pdf/nursing-in-japan2016.pdf. Accessed 13 Feb 2020

Jokiniemi K, Meretoja R, Pietilä AM (2018) Constructing content validity of clinical nurse specialist core competencies: exploratory sequential mixed-method study. Scand J Caring Sci 32:1428–1436. https://doi.org/10.1111/scs.12588

King A, Boyd ML, Dagley L, Raphael DL (2017) Implementation of a gerontology nurse specialist role in primary health care: health professional and older adult perspectives. J Clin Nurs 27:807–818. https://doi.org/10.1111/jocn.14110

Kondo A (2013) Advanced practice nurses in Japan: education and related issues. J Nurs Care S5:004. https://doi.org/10.4172/2167-1168.S5-004

National Association of Clinical Nurse Specialists (1998) Statement on clinical nurse specialist practice and education. National Association of Clinical Nurse Specialists, Glenview, IL

National Association of Clinical Nurse Specialists (2004) Statement on clinical nurse specialist practice and education, 2nd edn. National Association of Clinical Nurse Specialists, Harrisburg, PA

National Association of Clinical Nurse Specialists (2015) NACNS position statement on the Doctor of Nursing Practice. http://www.nacns.org/wp-content/uploads/2016/12/DNP-Statement1507. pdf. Accessed 15 May 2018

National Association of Clinical Nurse Specialists (2019) Statement on clinical nurse specialist practice and education, 3rd edn. National Association of Clinical Nurse Specialists, Reston, VA

National Council for the Professional Development of Nursing and Midwifery (2008) Framework for the establishment of clinical nurse/midwife specialist posts. 4th edn. https://www.lenus.ie/bitstream/handle/10147/565741/CNSCMSFrameworkNCNM2008. pdf?sequence=1&isAllowed=y. Accessed 17 Feb 2020

National Health Service Education for Scotland (2008) Working with individuals with cancer, their families and carers. Professional development framework for nurses, specialist and advanced levels. https://www.nes.scot.nhs.uk/media/268259/working_with_individuals_with_cancer_their_families_and_carers_aug_2008.pdf. Accessed 17 Feb 2020

National Health Service Health Education England (2017) Multi-professional framework for advanced clinical practice in England. https://www.hee.nhs.uk/sites/default/files/documents/ Multi-professional%20framework%20for%20advanced%20clinical%20practice%20in%20 England.pdf. Accessed 13 Feb 2020

National Health Service Wales (2010) Framework for advanced nursing, midwifery and allied health professional practice in Wales. http://www.wales.nhs.uk/sitesplus/documents/829/ NLIAH%20Advanced%20Practice%20Framework.pdf. Accessed 16 Feb 2020

Nieminen AL, Mannevaara B, Fagerström L (2011) Advanced practice nurses' scope of practice: a qualitative study of advanced clinical competencies. Scand J Caring Sci 25:661–670. https:// doi.org/10.1111/j.1471-6712.2011.00876.x

Northern Ireland Practice and Education Council for Nursing and Midwifery (2016) Advanced nursing practice framework. https://www.health-ni.gov.uk/sites/default/files/publications/ health/advanced-nursing-practice-framework.pdf. Accessed 13 Feb 2020

Nursing and Midwifery Board of Australia (2016) Fact sheet: advanced nursing practice and specialty areas within nursing. https://www.nursingmidwiferyboard.gov.au/documents/default.asp x?record=WD16%2f21634&dbid=AP&chksum=sLK71ybpoWvK3dj7SXUpWA%3d%3d. Accessed 13 Feb 2020

Nursing and Midwifery Board of Ireland (2017) Advanced practice (nursing) standards and requirements. https://www.nmbi.ie/NMBI/media/NMBI/Advanced-Practice-Nursing-Standards-and-Requirements-2017.pdf?ext=.pdf. Accessed 13 Feb 2020

O'Connell J, Gardner G, Coyer F (2014) Beyond competencies: using a capability framework in developing practice standards for advanced practice nursing. J Adv Nurs 70:2728–2735. https://doi.org/10.1111/jan.12475

Onishi M, Kanda K (2010) Expected roles and utilization of specialist nurses in Japan: the nurse administrators' perspective. J Nurs Manag 18:311–318. https://doi. org/10.1111/j.1365-2834.2010.01070.x

Royal College of Nursing (2018a) Section 2: advanced level nursing practice competencies. https://www.rcn.org.uk/-/media/royal-college-of-nursing/documents/publications/2018/july/ pdf-006896.pdf?la=en. Accessed 13 Feb 2020

Royal College of Nursing (2018b) Section 1: the registered nurse working at an advanced level of practice. https://www.rcn.org.uk/-/media/royal-college-of-nursing/documents/publica-tions/2018/july/pdf-006895.pdf?la=en. Accessed 13 Feb 2020

Sastre-Fullana P, Pedro-Gómez JE, Bennasar-Veny M, Serrano-Gallardo P, Morales-Asencio JM (2014) Competency frameworks for advanced practice nursing: a literature review. Int Nurs Rev 61:534–542

Schober M, Green A (2018) Global perspectives on advanced nursing practice. In: Joel LA (ed) Advanced practice nursing. Essentials for role development, 4th edn. F.A. Davis Company, Philadelphia, PA, pp 54–89

Scottish Government (2010) Advanced nursing practice roles. Guidance for NHS boards. http://
  www.advancedpractice.scot.nhs.uk/media/614/sg-advanced-practice-guidance-mar10.pdf.
  Accessed 13 Feb 2020
Singapore Nursing Board (2018) Core competencies of advanced practice nurse. https://www.
  healthprofessionals.gov.sg/docs/librariesprovider4/publications/core-competencies-of-apn_
  snb_jan-2018.pdf. Accessed 13 Feb 2020
Stasa H, Cashin A, Buckley T, Donoghue J (2014) Advancing advanced practice—clarifying the conceptual confusion. Nurs Educ Today 34:356–361. https://doi.org/10.1016/j.
  nedt.2013.07.012

Educational Considerations

4

Ann Mayo, Linda D. Urden, and Janet S. Fulton

Abstract

Clinical nurse specialists (CNSs) are advanced practice nurses and are prepared in graduate nursing programs with curriculum specifically designed to prepare CNSs. This chapter discusses educational standards for use in developing a CNS program curriculum. The discussion includes foundational standards underpinning graduate nursing education, standards and recommendations for preparing nurses in advanced clinically focused functional roles, and standards and competencies for preparing clinical nurse specialists. Criteria for evaluating and accrediting CNS programs are also discussed. By using the standards and guidelines discussed in this chapter or others, CNS faculty will have the tools necessary to create a robust curriculum for preparing CNSs for expert specialty practice in a variety of clinical settings.

Keywords

Clinical nurse specialist (CNS) · Clinical nurse specialist education · Education standards · Graduate nursing programs · CNS curriculum · CNS competencies

A. Mayo (✉) · L. D. Urden
University of San Diego Hahn School of Nursing, San Diego, CA, USA
e-mail: amayo@sandiego.edu; urden@sandiego.edu

J. S. Fulton
Indiana University School of Nursing, Indianapolis, IN, USA
e-mail: jasfulto@iu.edu

© Springer Nature Switzerland AG 2021
J. S. Fulton, V. W. Holly (eds.), *Clinical Nurse Specialist Role and Practice*,
Advanced Practice in Nursing, https://doi.org/10.1007/978-3-319-97103-2_4

4.1 Introduction

Clinical nurse specialists (CNSs) are advanced practice nurses, and the educational preparation of CNSs should follow the recommendations for all advanced practice nurses (APN). The International Council of Nurses (ICN) recommends APN be prepared (1) at an advanced level and (2) in a formal education program (accredited or other approval mechanism) and (3) recognized by a formal system for credentialing graduates for entry into advanced practice (licensure, registration, certification) (ICN 2019). Advanced-level education is best achieved through graduate education programs designed on the assumption that students first completed an undergraduate bachelor's degree. A master's degree or practice doctoral degree are the two options for formal, graduate-level advanced educational preparation. However, advanced nursing practice is continuing to evolve, and many countries and educational systems do not offer graduate degree options for nurses. At minimum, advanced education should be formal education beyond basic, generalist preparation and recognized by certificate or other mechanism denoting formal preparation at an advanced level.

This chapter examines standards and guidelines for designing, implementing, and evaluating clinical nurse specialist educational programs at the graduate level. The recommendations are intended to assist faculty interested in developing a CNS education program that prepares graduates to practice in the CNS role. CNS practice is shaped by both professional standards and local needs for CNS leadership and services in the community.

4.2 Education Standards

Nursing education leaders and faculty have an obligation to graduate highly competent clinical nurse specialists prepared to safely practice nursing at an advanced level. One way to assure well-prepared graduates is to use professional, national or international standards to guide curriculum development, implementation, and evaluation.

Education standards are goal-directed systems of instruction designed to guide the mastery of knowledge and skills of learners (Great Schools Partnership 2017). Using standards to guide curriculum helps assure that students achieve the required knowledge and expected performance competencies. Standards can also be used by external bodies to evaluate the scope and quality of the academic program and to accredit the program as having met established standards. In designing a CNS curriculum, a standards-based approach is recommended.

Educational standards may be developed by external organizations, such as professional nursing organizations, or may be developed internally by faculty as part of designing an academic program. Externally developed standards may be adopted completely or may be adapted to meet local needs, resources, and circumstances. Internally developed curricula should reflect a systematic approach using a framework for the design and implementation of curriculum and evaluation of student learning.

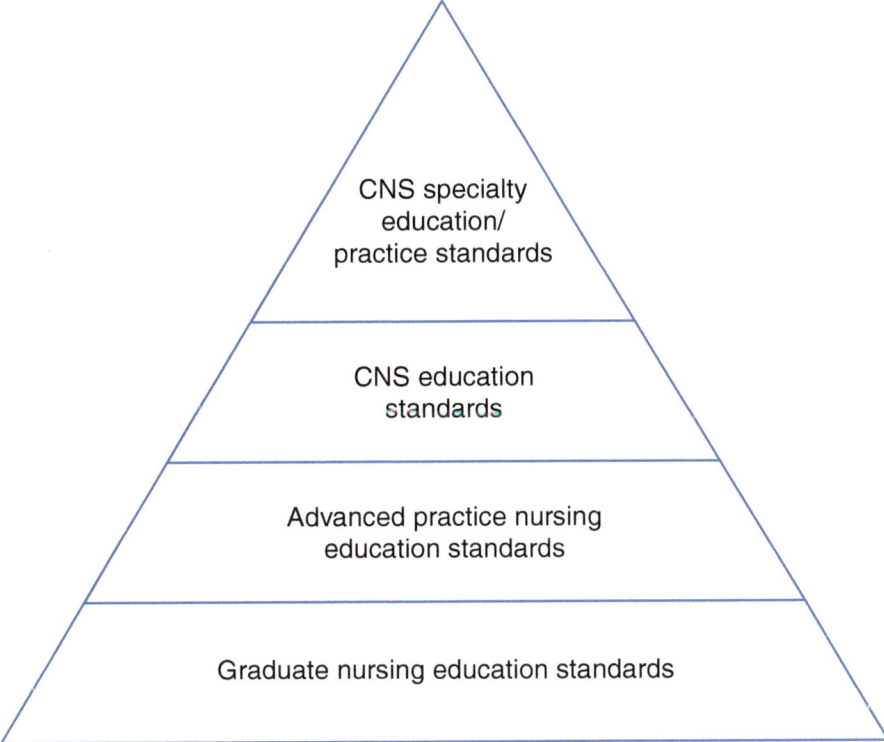

Fig. 4.1 Educational standards building blocks for graduate-level clinical nurse specialist education

Faculty prepared and experienced in the advanced practice role that the curriculum is being designed to prepare should lead curriculum development. Accordingly, faculty prepared as CNSs should lead the design and implementation of curriculum for CNS programs. Experienced CNS faculty should be consulted when a school is beginning a new CNS program and lacks CNS faculty.

The standards to be considered in developing a CNS curriculum should include (a) graduate-level nursing education standards, (b) advanced practice nursing education standards, (c) CNS-specific nursing education standards, and (d) CNS specialty practice standards. See Fig. 4.1.

4.3 Graduate Nursing Education Standards

Standards for graduate nursing education are foundational to developing a CNS graduate curriculum. Graduate education standards are built on the expectation that students enter the graduate program with an undergraduate degree in nursing prepared to practice as generalists. Graduate education in nursing is designed to prepare students to practice in advanced, differentiated functional roles. Clinical nurse specialist is a functional role. Examples of other advanced functional roles are nurse administrator, educator, informaticist, nurse practitioner, or midwife. Some advanced functional roles focus on indirect care practices, such as nurse administrator or informaticist. Other advanced functional roles are focused on direct care. In the United States, four advanced direct care functional roles are recognized—clinical nurse specialist, nurse practitioner, nurse anesthetist, and nurse-midwife. Not all countries recognize these four functional roles as advanced practice, while other roles are recognized as advanced practice. In many countries clinical nurse specialists have different titles, such as nurse consultant. Regardless of the advanced role, all advanced nurse graduates should be prepared with similar foundational content. This content typically includes nursing theory/theoretical underpinnings of practice, research and evidence-based practice, statistical analysis, leadership theory and principles, and health policy and advocacy.

One widely used standard for graduate nursing education is the American Association of Colleges of Nursing's *The Essentials of Master's Education in Nursing* (AACN 2011). This standard includes recommendations for nine content areas that are foundational for all graduate education in nursing. Also, the Canadian Association of Schools of Nursing (CASN) has developed a framework and standards for undergraduate, master's, and doctoral education. The framework includes six domains applicable to all nursing programs, which are (1) knowledge; (2) research, methodologies, critical inquiry skills, and evidence-based practice; (3) nursing practice; (4) communication and collaboration; (5) professionalism; and (6) leadership. Guiding principles are included for each domain (CASN 2015).

The International Council of Nurses recommends a master's degree for entry-level education for an advanced nursing role (ICN 2019); however, nursing has not yet achieved the goal of universal baccalaureate degree for entry into practice. Associate degree and hospital-based diploma programs prepare basic, generalist nurses. Graduates of these non-baccalaureate programs need additional coursework or degrees prior to entering a graduate program. Faculty can use undergraduate educational standards to identify gaps in academic content and build learning bridges (courses or degrees) to move associate degree and diploma-prepared nurses into graduate-level nursing programs. To identify gaps faculty should conduct a gap analysis between non-baccalaureate programs and baccalaureate programs using established standards for undergraduate education such as the American Association of Colleges of Nursing *Essentials of Baccalaureate Education* (AACN 2008) or the Canadian Association of Schools of Nursing's National Nursing Education Framework (CASN 2015).

4.4   Advanced Practice Nursing Standards

Standards specific to advanced practice nursing are the next level of more specific educational criteria after the foundational standards (Fig. 4.1). Advanced practice nursing functional roles, with practices focused on direct care, share a common core of knowledge for practice. The only known standards for advanced nursing practice curriculum regardless of the functional role are *The Essentials of Doctoral Education for Advanced Nursing Practice* (AACN 2006), which were specifically developed for preparing advanced nurses with a practice doctorate (Doctor of Nursing Practice, DNP). Practice doctorates have only recently been introduced in the United States. Advanced practice nurses continue to be largely prepared at the master's level.

Standards and guidelines for preparing advanced practice nurses have been developed by professional nursing organizations. In the United States, Advanced Practice Registered Nurses (APRN) Consensus Work Group and National Council of State Boards of Nursing APRN Advisory Committee's *Consensus Model for APRN Regulation: Licensure, Accreditation, Certification & Education* (2008) recommends three separate graduate-level *advanced* core courses, one each in physiology/pathophysiology, pharmacology, and health assessment. In addition, a minimum of 500 supervised clinical practice hours are recommended be included in the master's curriculum for all advanced practice functional roles.

Other professional organizations recommend core advanced practice competencies that should be considered in planning a CNS curriculum. The Canadian Nurses Association's *Advanced Nursing Practice: A National Framework* (CNA 2008) describes common elements of graduate nursing education required for students to achieve proficiencies in clinical practice competencies in all advanced functional roles. The United Kingdom's *Advanced Level Nursing: A Position Statement* (2010) describes the level of practice expected of nurses working at advanced level providing direct care to patients. These and other documents, country-specific guidelines and standards describing overall competency expectations for advanced practice, can be helpful in developing a curriculum that supports students in meeting advanced practice expectations.

4.5   Clinical Nurse Specialist Core Education Standards

The International Council of Nurses (ICN) defines a nurse specialist as a nurse holding advanced education and expertise in a defined area of nursing and requiring (1) a formal recognized program of study built upon education initially required for recognition to practice as a nurse (registered/licensed) and (2) preparation and authorization consistent with the scope of practice, education, and regulatory requirements for post-basic education (ICN 2009). ICN does not provide curriculum standards for advanced specialty preparation; however, it does provide a competencies framework (ICN 2009). This framework follows the domains for generalist nursing practice building on the knowledge and practice competencies of the registered nurse. The domains of the framework are (1) professional, ethical, and legal practice; (2) care provision and management, and (3) professional, personal, and quality development (see Table 4.1).

Developing professional competence in students is the goal of educational programs. Professional practice competency is demonstrated in the actual performance of a skill in a defined context and consistent with institutional policies. Competent performance involves the application of knowledge, judgment, technical ability, and

Table 4.1 International Council of Nurses' competencies framework (reference: ICN Framework of Competencies for the Nurse Specialist 2009)

Domain: Professional, ethical, legal practice	
Elements	Accountability
	Legal practice
	Ethical principles
Domain: Care provision and management	
Elements	Key principles of care
	Therapeutic communication and relationships
	Health promotion
	Assessment
	Planning
	Implementation
	Evaluation
	Leadership and management
	Interprofessional health care
	Delegation and supervision
	Safe environment
Domain: Professional, personal, and quality development	
Elements	Enhancement of the profession
	Quality improvement
	Continuing education

interpersonal skills directed at achieving a desired outcome (Cowan et al. 2005). Competency frameworks and competency standards are developed by professional nursing organizations and should be used to inform educational program preparing clinical nurse specialists and other advanced practice nurses.

In addition to the ICN competency framework, two professional organizations have published clinical competencies for clinical nurse specialists that are organized into domains of practice such that they can provide a framework for organizing educational content—the Canadian Nurses Association (CNA) and the National Association of Clinical Nurse Specialists (NACNS) in the United States. The two sets of practice competencies are similar in content. The Pan-Canadian Core Competencies for the Clinical Nurse Specialist (CNA 2014) organize the competencies into four domains of practice: (1) clinical care; (2) systems leadership; (3) advancement of nursing practice; and (4) evaluation and research. The NACNS competencies are organized into three domains of practice: (1) patient care; (2) nurses and nursing practice; and (3) organizations and systems (NACNS 2019). The NACNS *Statement on Clinical Nurse Specialist Practice and Education* (2019) includes recommendations for CNS education specifically designed to achieve the NACNS core CNS practice competencies. See Table 4.2.

4.6   CNS Specialty Practice Education Standards

Central to CNS practice is advanced clinical expertise in diagnosis and intervention to prevent, remediate, or alleviate illness and promote health with a defined specialty population – be that specialty broad or narrow, well established, or emerging

Table 4.2 Summary of essential core content areas for developing clinical nurse specialist competencies

1. **Theoretical and empirical foundations for CNS practice**
Content: Theories, conceptual models, scientific principles, research, and other evidence related to advanced, specialty practice

2. **Phenomena of concern**
Content: Phenomenon of concern for nursing including health promotion, risk reduction, symptom management, functional status, health-related quality of life, and self-management

3. **Design, implement, and evaluate innovative nursing interventions**
Content: Assessment and environmental scanning; designing, implementing, and evaluating evidence-based interventions and programs of care addressing needs of specialty populations

4. **Clinical inquiry/critical thinking/clinical judgment**
Content: Apply critical thinking and clinical judgment to the process of clinical inquiry for solving problems and exploring possibilities. Examine innovative care options with improved clinical and fiscal outcomes

5. **Healthcare technology, products, and devices**
Content: Select, use, and evaluate technology, products, and devices to support nursing practice and improved outcomes. Explore the development of new technology, products, and devices

6. **Teaching and coaching**
Content: Theories and evidence related to health behaviors, teaching, and coaching of learners including patients/families, nurses, and other healthcare professionals

7. **Influencing change**
Content: Theory and evidence-based approaches to implementing change in the practice setting

8. **Systems thinking**
Content: System theory, organizational behaviors, change theory, using influence and power, health policy and advocacy

9. **Leadership for interprofessional collaboration**
Content: Leadership theory and skills, collaboration, interprofessional practice, healthy work environments, care coordination, and transition management

10. **Consultation theory**
Content: Consultation theory, consultation methods and processes, application of consultation principles

11. **Quality improvement and safety**
Content: Theories and evidence related to quality improvement and safety, quality improvement methods, improving safety in practice setting

12. **Measurement and outcome evaluation methods**
Content: Principles of measurement and instrumentation; data collection, management, and analysis. Application of principles to clinical assessment and evaluation

13. **Evidence-based practice and knowledge translation**
Content: Evidence-based practice principles and methods, processes for knowledge translation, conducting analysis, developing practice guidelines

14. **Interpersonal communication and leadership**
Content: Communication and leadership theory and principles, conflict management, critical conversations, peer feedback, shared decision-making, and interprofessional practice

15. **Advocacy and ethical decision-making**
Content: Scope and standards of practice, ethics in nursing practice, application of ethics for decision-making and advocacy

Clinical practicum experiences

1. Emphasis is on learning the CNS role and practice competencies under the guidance of an experienced practicing CNS preceptor in a structured clinical practicum. Students have opportunities to integrate knowledge and skills and develop competencies in all practice domains

(continued)

Table 4.2 (continued)

2. Opportunities to individualize the program of study, develop areas of strength, meet personal career goals, develop competencies related to selected specialty population
3. Socialization into professional clinical and professional leadership, exploration of career options, establishment of a network of CNS colleagues for professional collaboration and continuing development

National Association of Clinical Nurse Specialists (NACNS), Statement on Clinical Nurse Specialist Practice and Education (2019). Reston, VA: Author

(NACNS 2019). Specialty practice evolves to meet the needs of the public for advanced nursing services. Examples of specialty practice areas include pediatrics, geriatrics, and women's health (population-based); critical care, emergency, and perioperative (setting-based); dementia, oncology, psychiatric, and diabetes (disease-based); behavioral health, and rehabilitation (care-based); or falls, wound, incontinence, and pain (problem-based). Schools of nursing offer educational programs organized by specialty, such as the University of Regina, Canada, which offers advanced specialty programs in mental health, geriatrics, indigenous studies, palliative care, maternity, medical-surgical, and pediatrics (University of Regina https://www.uregina.ca/nursing/programs/CNS/index.html. Accessed July 19, 2019).

Specialty organizations in nursing exist to address the unique needs of nurses caring for specialty populations. To serve the needs of their members, specialty organizations create standards of practice clinical care of the special population. Most often the specialty standards of practice are developed at the generalist level; however, a few organizations have prepared standards of practice for advanced practice nurses and/or clinical nurse specialists. Two professional nursing organizations that have developed advanced practice standards are the American Association of Critical-Care Nurses (AACN 2014) and the Gerontological Advanced Practice Nurses Association (GAPNA 2015). When available, advanced specialty standards should be incorporated into a curriculum that prepares CNSs to practice in that specialty. If advanced specialty standards of practice are not available for a specialty, then generalist standards should be considered in planning curriculum content.

4.7   Specialty-Specific Example of a Curriculum

A well-designed CNS curriculum incorporates standards for graduate nursing education, advanced practice nursing education, CNS education, and CNS specialty practice. An example is the Adult-Gerontology CNS curriculum at the University of San Diego. Table 4.3 lists the individual courses in the curriculum, the level of educational standard, and provides an example of an appropriate level standard that supported the course design. The specialty competencies for this example are the Adult-Gerontology Clinical Nurse Specialist Competencies (AACN 2010) collaboratively developed by the Hartford Institute for Geriatric Nursing at New York University and NACNS with funding from the John A. Hartford Foundation. The

Table 4.3 Adult/gerontology clinical nurse specialist curriculum example

Course title	Level of educational standards (see Fig. 4.1)	Example standard
Evidence-Based Practice: Role of Theory and Research	Graduate nursing education	AACN Essentials of Master's Education in Nursing (2011)
Influencing the Healthcare Environment: Policy and Systems	Graduate nursing education	AACN Essentials of Master's Education in Nursing (2011)
Introduction to Health Care Information Management	Graduate nursing education	AACN Essentials of Master's Education in Nursing (2011)
Advanced Pathophysiology	Advanced practice nursing education	APRN Consensus Model Curricular Recommendations (2008)
Advanced Physical Assessment and Diagnosis	Advanced practice nursing education	APRN Consensus Model Curricular Recommendations (2008)
Advanced Pharmacology	Advanced practice nursing education	APRN Consensus Model Curricular Recommendations (2008)
CNS Specialty Role and Practice Foundations	CNS education	CNS Education (NACNS 2019)
Adult Gerontology I: CNS Practice in Patient Sphere Course and Practicum	CNS education Specialty practice	CNS Education (NACNS 2019) Adult-Gerontology CNS Specialty Practice Competencies (AACN 2010)
Adult Gerontology II: CNS Practice in Nurse Sphere Course and Practicum	CNS education Specialty practice competencies	CNS Education (NACNS 2019) Adult-Gerontology CNS Specialty Practice Competencies (AACN 2010)
Adult Gerontology III: CNS Practice in Organizational/ Systems Sphere Course and Practicum	CNS education Specialty practice competencies	CNS Education (NACNS 2019) Adult-Gerontology CNS Specialty Practice Competencies (AACN 2010)
Adult Gerontology IV: CNS Advanced Practice Capstone Course and Practicum	CNS education Specialty practice competencies	CNS Education (NACNS 2019) Adult-Gerontology CNS Specialty Practice Competencies (AACN 2010)

specialty competencies are designed to be used with The Essentials of Master's Education in Nursing (AACN 2011). The example CNS program includes three courses with practicum that address the domains of practice described by NACNS (2019)—patient/direct care, nursing and nursing practice, and systems/organizations. The courses build upon standards as demonstrated in Fig. 4.1 from general graduate education standards to narrower, specialty population standards.

Supervised clinical practicum is included in the curriculum such that students complete 500 hours of practice within the specialty population. Clinical practicum experiences are designed to achieve the NACNS (2019) recommendations for CNS education by emphasizing learning the CNS role and practice competencies in all three domains, integrating knowledge and skills, developing personal areas of strength, meeting personal career goals, and developing expertise in care of a specialty population. In addition, clinical experiences provide socialization into the CNS role, strengthen leadership abilities, and assist students in establishing a network of CNS colleagues for professional collaboration and continuing development. Student clinical experiences are supervised by volunteer preceptors who are practicing CNSs guiding the application of knowledge to practice.

4.8   Accreditation and Evaluation of Programs

Schools of nursing should be accredited or recognized by appropriate regulatory bodies and professional organizations. In addition, CNS programs within schools should meet established criteria for CNS programs. The accreditation process and accrediting bodies for schools vary by country based on governmental and other regulations and requirements. Professional organizations that accredit schools should meet governmental and other standards for operating as accrediting bodies. For example, in the United States, accrediting bodies meet requirements set forth by the US Department of Education and are monitored for compliance by that department.

Each accrediting organization publishes criteria that schools must meet for academic program accreditation. The National League for Nursing (NLN) Commission for Nursing Education Accreditation (CNEA) (2016) and Commission on Collegiate Nursing Education (CCNE) (2018) both accredit graduate nursing programs. The CNEA accredits all levels of nursing education programs; the CCNE accredits only baccalaureate and higher education programs.

The CNEA Accreditation Standards for Nursing Education Programs include five standards:

- Culture of Excellence—Program Outcomes
- Culture of Integrity and Accountability—Mission, Governance, and Resources
- Culture of Excellence and Caring—Faculty
- Culture of Excellence and Caring—Students
- Culture of Learning and Diversity—Curriculum and Evaluation Processes

Each standard requires evidence of measurable outcome indicators. Outcomes related to each standard are reviewed by an evaluation team, and accreditation is granted based on the school having demonstrated successful achievement of the criteria. The NLN accreditation criteria and procedures are available at http://www. nln.org/docs/default-source/accreditation-services/cnea-standards-final-february-2 01613f2bf5c78366c709642ff00005f0421.pdf?sfvrsn=12 (Accessed July 19, 2019).

Similarly, the Commission on Collegiate Nursing Education (CCNE) has accreditation standards that schools must achieve. Accreditation is granted when a school presents evidence that it meets the published standards, available at https://www. aacnnursing.org/Portals/42/CCNE/PDF/Standards-Final-2018.pdf (Accessed July 19, 2019). The CCNE accreditation standards are:

- Standard I—Program Quality: Mission and Governance
- Standard II—Program Quality: Institutional Commitment and Resources
- Standard III—Program Quality: Curriculum and Teaching-Learning Practices
- Standard IV—Program Effectiveness: Assessment and Achievement

CNS programs within schools should also meet specific criteria for CNS programs. NACNS developed the only known criteria to date for evaluating the adequacy of CNS programs, organized by these five overarching standards: program organization and administration; program resources; student admission, progression, and graduation requirements; curriculum; and program evaluation (NACNS 2019). See Table 4.4.

Table 4.4 Summary of National Association of Clinical Nurse Specialists' (NACNS) CNS program evaluation criteria (NACNS 2019)

Criterion 1 Program organization and administration

1-1.	Program operates within or is affiliated with an institution of higher education; is accredited by a nursing accrediting body recognized by the US Department of Education
1-2.	Purpose of the program is clear; outcomes are aligned with the mission of the parent institution and mission/goals of the nursing unit
1-3.	The individual who has responsibility for the overall leadership or oversight of the CNS program has educational and/or experiential preparation for the CNS role

Criterion 2 CNS program resources: faculty, clinical, and institutional

2-1a.	Faculty teaching in the CNS program are appropriately credentialed to teach CNS students and were prepared as a CNS through a master's, postgraduate, or practice doctoral program.
2-2.	Faculty teaching in the CNS program maintain expertise in area of specialization and contribute scholarly work to the specialty field
2-3.	Faculty are adequate in number and expertise to teach content for CNS students, develop policies, advise students, conduct ongoing curriculum development and evaluation
2-4.	Enough faculty and clinical preceptors are available to ensure quality clinical experiences and provide adequate direct and indirect supervision and evaluation of students
2-5.	Faculty retain responsibility for evaluating student performance and the quality of the clinical experiences supervised by preceptors
2-6.	CNS prepared preceptors supervise students in clinical experiences through direct or virtual interactions; additional professionals may also precept for selected clinical experiences
2-7.	Preceptors who supervise CNS students in clinical settings are oriented to curriculum requirements, course objectives, and expectations regarding student supervision and evaluation
2-8.	Clinical facilities are adequate in quality and number to provide high-quality, comprehensive experiences for CNS students in all domains of practice
2-9.	Adequate resources support ongoing professional development, scholarly activities, and practice of faculty teaching in the CNS program
2-10.	Learning resources and support services ensure educational quality in the CNS program

(continued)

Table 4.4 (continued)

Criterion 3 Student admission, progression, and graduation requirements
3-1.   Program builds on baccalaureate-level nursing competencies and culminates in a
       master's degree, postgraduate certificate, or doctorate
3-2.   Faculty teaching in CNS programs participate in developing, approving, and revising
       the admission, progression, and graduation criteria for the program
3-3.   Students in the CNS program are a licensed RN before and throughout their
       enrollment in CNS clinical courses

Criterion 4 Curriculum
4-1.   The curriculum is congruent with state requirements, national standards for graduate
       APRN programs, and nationally recognized CNS competencies
4-2.   Program requires a minimum of 500 supervised clinical (clock) hours for master's and
       postgraduate preparation

Criterion 5 CNS program evaluation
5-1.   Program has a comprehensive evaluation plan addressing curriculum, faculty
       resources, student outcomes, clinical sites, preceptors, and program resources
5-2.   Program collects and analyzes data to evaluate achievement of program outcomes
5-3.   Faculty teaching in and students enrolled in program have input in the ongoing
       development and evaluation of the program
5-4.   The CNS curriculum is evaluated on an ongoing basis, using relevant data to inform
       revisions
5-5.   Faculty teaching are evaluated regularly, according to parent institution or nursing unit
       policies
5-6.   The clinical agencies and preceptors utilized for the CNS program are evaluated
       annually by faculty members and students
5-7.   Evaluation of students is cumulative and multi-method and incorporates clinical
       observation of performance by faculty and preceptors

4.9   Designing a Curriculum

The design of a CNS educational program is a strategic process and includes conducting a needs assessment to determine community need for CNS services and
specialties, designing a curriculum to address identified needs, recruiting qualified
faculty, obtaining necessary approval from academic and regulatory bodies, and
recruiting qualified students. In geographic areas and countries where few nurses
hold a bachelor's degree, it may be necessary to first start with academic bridge
programs to assure that students are prepared for graduate-level coursework. Where
graduate programs are not possible, faculty can apply the standards, guidelines, and
criteria to certificate and other post-generalist programs to achieve the high-quality
education for nurse specialists.

The program should be designed to meet any postgraduate requirements for
licensure, certification, or registration, which may require adapting standards and
guidelines to assure practice opportunities for graduates. Globally, nurses are working within existing governmental and education structures to promote opportunities
for advanced nursing education and to guarantee governmental and regulatory protections for a scope of practice for which the nurse is prepared. Faculty developing

a CNS program will need to advocate for the CNS role and scope of practice and will also need to include policy and advocacy in the curriculum to assure that students are well prepared to understand and advocate for the CNS role.

4.10 Conclusion

The CNS role and practice are well-suited to fit into any culture or country. At the core of CNS practice is the focus on advancing the practice of nursing to improve patient outcomes, to support nurses in providing the best possible, evidence-based nursing care, and to facilitate best-practice nursing within a health system by removing barriers and creating innovative programs of care. Regardless of how or where nursing is practiced, a CNS can support that practice—constantly striving for the best for patients, families, and communities. A CNS curriculum that incorporates national and international educational standards, prepares graduates to master advanced role competencies, and meets external accreditation and regulatory requirements will provide CNS students the knowledge and skills to advance nursing practice anywhere and everywhere!

References

American Association of Colleges of Nursing (2010) Adult-gerontology clinical nurse specialist competencies. Author, Washington, DC. http://nacns.org/wp-content/uploads/2016/11/adult-geroCNScomp.pdf. Accessed 20 July 2019

American Association of Colleges of Nursing (AACN) (2006) The essentials of doctoral education for advanced nursing practice. Author, Washington, DC

American Association of Colleges of Nursing (AACN) (f) The essentials of baccalaureate education in nursing. Author, Washington, DC

American Association of Colleges of Nursing (AACN) (2011) The essentials of master's education in nursing. Author, Washington, DC

American Association of Critical Care Nurses (2014) AACN scope and standards for acute care clinical nurse specialist practice. Author, Aliso Viejo, CA

Canadian Association of Schools of Nursing (CASN) (2015) National Nursing Education Framework. Canada Association of Schools of Nursing: Author, Ottawa. https://www.casn.ca/wp-content/uploads/2018/11/CASN-National-Education-Framwork-FINAL-2015.pdf. Accessed 20 July 2019

Canadian Nurses Association (CAN) (2008) Advanced nursing practice: a national framework. Author, Ottawa, ON. https://www.cna-aiic.ca/en/~/media/nurseone/page-content/pdf-en/anp_national_framework_e. Accessed 20 July 2019

Canadian Nurses Association (CAN) (2014) Pan-Canadian Core competencies for the clinical nurse specialist. Author, Ottawa, ON. https://cna-aiic.ca/~/media/cna/files/en/clinical_nurse_specialists_convention_handout_e.pdf. Accessed 20 July 2019

Commission on Collegiate Nursing Education (2018) Standards for accreditation of baccalaureate and graduate nursing programs. Author, Washington, DC. https://www.aacnnursing.org/Portals/42/CCNE/PDF/Standards-Final-2018.pdf. Accessed 20 July 2019

Cowan DT, Norman I, Coopamah VP (2005) Competence in nursing practice: a controversial concept—a focused review of the literature. Nurse Educ Today 25(5):355–362. https://doi.org/10.1016/j.nedt.2005.03.002

Department of Health United Kingdom (2010) Advanced level practice: a position statement. https://assets.publishing.service.gov.uk/government/uploads/system/uploads/attachment_data/file/215935/dh_121738.pdf. Accessed 20 July 2019

Gerontological Advanced Practice Nurses Association (GAPNA) (2015) GAPNA consensus statement on proficiencies for the APRN gerontological specialist. Author, Pitman, NJ

Great Schools Partnership (2017) The glossary of education reform. https://www.edglossary.org/standards-based/. Accessed 20 July 2019

http://cna-aiic.ca/~/media/cna/files/en/clinical_nurse_specialists_convention_handout_e.pdf

http://www.nln.org/docs/default-source/accreditation-services/cnea-standards-final-february-201613f2bf5c78366c709642ff00005f0421.pdf?sfvrsn=12. Accessed 19 July 2019

https://www.gapna.org/sites/default/files/documents/GAPNA_Consensus_Statement_on_Proficiencies_for_the_APRN_Gerontological_Specialist.pdf. Accessed 20 July 2019

International Council of Nurses (2009) Framework of competencies for the nurse specialist. Author, Geneva. https://siga-fsia.ch/files/user_upload/08_ICN_Framework_for_the_nurse_specialist.pdf. Accessed 20 July 2019

International Council of Nurses (2019) Nurse practitioner/advanced practice nurse: definition and characteristics. Author, Geneva. https://international.aanp.org/Practice/APNRoles. Accessed 14 July 2019

National Association of Clinical Nurse Specialists (NACNS) (2019) Statement on clinical nurse specialist practice and education, 3rd edn. Author, Reston, VA

National Council of State Boards of Nursing (NCSBN) (2008) Consensus model for APRN regulation: licensure, accreditation, certification & education. Author, Chicago, IL. https://www.ncsbn.org/Consensus_Model_for_APRN_Regulation_July_2008.pdf. Accessed 20 July 2019

National League for Nursing, Commission for Nursing Education Accreditation (2016) Accreditation standards for nursing education programs. Author, Washington, DC

University of Regina. https://www.uregina.ca/nursing/programs/CNS/index.html. Accessed 19 July 2019

Part II

North America

Clinical Nurse Specialist Role and Practice in the United States of America

5

Vincent W. Holly and Janet S. Fulton

Abstract

In the United States, the clinical nurse specialist (CNS) is an advanced practice nursing role. Emerging in the 1960s in response to a recognized need for clinical experts in nursing care, CNSs practice in three interrelated domains—called spheres of impact. In the direct care sphere, CNSs provide care to prevent, remediate, or alleviate illness and promote health with a defined specialty population. In the nursing/nursing practice sphere, CNSs teach, coach, mentor, and lead nurses and nursing personnel in the delivery of evidence-based care for specialty populations. In the system sphere, CNSs lead organizational-level change, coordinate specialized care, and implement programs of care for quality improvement, patient safety, and improved clinical and fiscal outcomes. The National Association of Clinical Nurse Specialists (NACNS), founded in 1995, developed a model of practice including core practice competencies and expected outcomes for each practice domain. NACNS created recommendations for essential content in CNS graduate curricula to assure students develop requisite knowledge and skill practice. CNS practice is regulated as an advanced practice nurse, and CNSs are expected to hold professional certification as a CNS in a specialty

This chapter has been written before the 2020 APN ICN guidelines were published and reflects the views of the authors.

V. W. Holly (✉)
Critical Care Services, Indiana University Health Bloomington Hospital,
Bloomington, IN, USA
e-mail: vholly@iuhealth.org

J. S. Fulton
Indiana University School of Nursing, Indianapolis, IN, USA
e-mail: jasfulto@iu.edu

© Springer Nature Switzerland AG 2021
J. S. Fulton, V. W. Holly (eds.), *Clinical Nurse Specialist Role and Practice*,
Advanced Practice in Nursing, https://doi.org/10.1007/978-3-319-97103-2_5

population. Each of the 50 states regulates CNS practice, though with some variability. National regulatory guidelines are available presenting both opportunity and challenges for CNSs.

Keywords
Clinical nurse specialist · Advanced practice registered nurse · National Association of Clinical Nurse Specialists (NACNS) · Advanced practice nurse · Core practice competencies

5.1   History of CNS Role and Practice

In the United States, the clinical nurse specialist (CNS) role was developed in response to a recognized need for an advanced clinical expert nurse at a time when nursing's emphasis was on preparing excellent educators and hospital supervisors. The landmark Brown Report (1948) called attention to the need to abandon hospital apprentice-type training and move to collegiate-based education. The report noted the need for nurses to make unique contributions to clinical care, improve and develop nursing skills, teach and mentor nurses and nursing personnel, and collaborate with other professions as peers in the design and delivery of care (Allen et al. 1948). Nursing education began slowly moving into university settings, and by the 1960s it was apparent that nursing needed a clinical expert to provide direct care to complex patients, to lead the design and implement nursing practice advancements and innovations, and to teach and mentor nurses at the bedside. The CNS role was developed by nurse leaders in education and practice to be that clinical expert. The role required graduate nursing preparation with specialty knowledge and skill that was to be imbedded in the graduate curriculum—specialty was foundational, not in addition to, clinical nursing expertise. The first CNS graduate program was the psychiatric/mental health CNS under the direction of Dr. Hildegard Peplau at Rutgers University (Fulton 2014).

The number of CNS programs continued to grow with the support of the US government nursing workforce development grants. Multiple specialty areas were developed to address the need for nurse experts in emerging and established areas of practice. The criterion for practicing as a CNS was a graduate degree in nursing from a program that prepared graduates as CNSs in a specialty area. Professional certification was optional, available for some specialties and considered a measure of excellence; 3 years of experience was required for certification eligibility. No agreed-upon curricular standards existed for graduate nursing programs preparing CNSs. However, four curricular content areas were considered central to academic preparation of CNSs including (1) psychopathology and pathophysiology related to the clinical specialty, (2) knowledge and skills in the clinical practice of the specialty including teaching and research, (3) behavioral sciences essential to leadership and systems thinking, and (4) knowledge of the social framework in which health care is delivered (Fulton 2014).

To further distinguish the CNS role and practice from other advanced practice roles, it became increasingly important to establish core practice competencies, develop educational standards, and create regulatory protections for CNSs. In 1995 the National Association of Clinical Nurse Specialists (NACNS) was founded, and in 1998 NACNS released the *Statement on Clinical Nurse Specialist Practice and Education*, which included core CNS practice competencies regardless of specialty and educational recommendations for achieving the core competencies (NACNS 1998). NACNS also advocated for regulatory protections for the CNS role recommending guidelines for governmental regulations. NACNS continues to advocate for CNS practice and education and, in 2019, released the third edition of the *Statement on Clinical Nurse Specialist Practice and Education* (NACNS 2019). Across the years, CNSs have been the clinical nursing expert for specialty care in three domains—direct care to patients and families, leadership for advancing nursing practice for nurses and nursing personnel, and system-level change agent for removing barriers and facilitating best practices. This tripartite practice maintains the original intent of the CNS to fill the need for an advanced clinical nursing expert by and for nursing practice.

5.2   Definition of Clinical Nurse Specialist

The clinical nurse specialist (CNS) role is one of the four advanced practice registered nurse (APRN) roles recognized in the United States. The other APRN roles are nurse practitioner, nurse-midwife, and nurse anesthetist. All APRN scopes of practice extend beyond the generalist nurse in terms of expertise, role functions, mastery, and accountability and reflect a core body of nursing and health knowledge.

Professional nursing organizations have similar definitions of the CNS. The American Nurses Association defines a CNS as an advanced practice nurse who diagnoses, treats, and provides ongoing management of patients; provides expertise and support to nurses caring for patients; helps drive practice changes throughout the organization; and ensures use of best practices and evidence-based care to achieve the best possible patient outcomes (ANA 2019). The American Association of Critical-Care Nurses defines an acute care CNS as an advanced practice nurse practicing within a defined specialty as an expert clinician and patient advocate, leader in advancing nursing practice, and leader in organizational and system change (AACN 2014). The NACNS defines a clinical nurse specialist as a clinical expert in a specialty area practicing in three interrelated domains—patient/family, nurses/nursing practice, and organizations/systems. CNSs provide direct patient care to prevent, remediate, or alleviate illness and promote health with a defined specialty population—be that specialty broad or narrow, well established, or emerging. CNSs teach, coach, mentor, and lead nurses and nursing personnel in the delivery of evidence-based care for specialty populations. CNSs lead change, coordinate specialized care, and implement evidence-based programs of care at the system level for quality improvement, patient safety, and improved clinical and fiscal outcomes (NACNS 2019).

Consistent with the International Council of Nurses (ICN) definition of an advanced nurse, a CNS is a registered nurse (RN) with preparation beyond the level of a generalist nurse, has an earned graduate degree in nursing (master's or doctorate), has been educationally prepared in the CNS role, has the requisite knowledge and skills for specialty care, and is authorized to practice as a CNS. ICN states that specialist practice includes clinical, teaching, administration, research, and consultant roles (ICN 2009). A CNS is a clinical practice role that incorporates elements of teaching, research, and consultation for the purpose of advancing the practice of nursing. The focus of the CNS role is clinical care.

In summary, a CNS is defined as an advanced practice nurse prepared with a graduate degree in nursing to evaluate disease patterns, technological advances, environmental conditions, and political influences so as to interpret nursing's responsibility to serve the public's need for nursing services. CNSs function as expert clinicians, leading the advancement of nursing practice. CNS practice may adapt to clinical needs and system priorities; however, the following characteristics delineate the CNS role and practice:

- CNSs are professional nurses with a graduate-level preparation.
- CNSs are expert clinicians providing direct clinical care in a specialized area of nursing practice.
- CNS practice within a specialty population includes health promotion, risk reduction, and management of symptoms and functional problems related to disease and illness.
- CNSs provide direct care to patients and families, which may include diagnosis and treatment of disease.
- CNSs provide patient-/family-centered care that emphasizes strengths and wellness over disease or deficit.
- CNSs influence nursing practice outcomes by leading and supporting nurses to provide scientifically grounded, evidence-based care.
- CNSs implement improvements in the healthcare delivery system and translate high-quality research and other evidence into clinical practice to improve clinical and fiscal outcomes.
- CNSs participate in the conduct of research to generate knowledge for practice.
- CNSs design, implement, and evaluate programs of care and programs of research that address common problems for specialty populations.
- CNSs practice in a wide variety of healthcare settings, such as hospitals, community clinics, schools, mental health facilities, and occupational health clinics.

5.3   A Model of CNS Practice

Clinical nurse specialist (CNS) practice occurs across three highly interactive domains. Initial conceptualizations of the CNS role and practice were organized as "sub-roles," including but not limited to expert clinician, educator, researcher, change agent, and consultant. These sub-roles were not clearly defined and alternatingly represented skill sets, practice activities, and practice outcomes (Hamric and

Spross 1989; Sparacino et al. 1990; Gawlinski and Kern 1994). Portioning CNS practice into discrete units of skills or activities belied the integrated nature of CNS practice while simultaneously failing to identify unique practice competencies and associated outcomes. Additionally, the knowledge and skills associated with the sub-roles as skills represent practice expectations for all nurses. For example, all nurses teach, but the level of skill and expected outcomes varies by specialty role and academic preparation. The sub-roles conceptualization of the CNS contributed greatly to confusion about the CNS role. A role is a unique set of functions achieved thorough academic preparation. Practice is the act of applying knowledge and skills in a competent manner within the scope of the functional role. A role is a unified whole. While the skills and activities imbedded in the sub-roles model are germane to CNS practice, the sub-roles conceptualization of CNS role has been abandoned in favor of a more explanatory model of CNS practice.

CNS practice is better explained by three distinct yet interrelated domains of practice each with designated core practice competencies and outcome expectations (NACNS 1998, 2004). The model was developed using a systematic process including a comprehensive literature review, review of a national sample of CNS job descriptions, and expert panel review by nurse leaders (Baldwin et al. 2007). The model includes three domains of CNS practice—direct patient care, nurses/nursing practice, and organization/system. A subsequent comprehensive review of literature identified substantive areas of CNS practice that closely aligned with the three domains (Lewandowski and Adamle 2009). The substantive areas of practice identified were (a) managing the care of complex and/or vulnerable populations of patients and families through expert direct care, care coordination, and collaboration with the interdisciplinary team; (b) educating and supporting the interdisciplinary team through education, consultation, and collaboration; and (c) facilitating change and innovation within healthcare systems through change agency. NACNS has continued to develop the model and update the core practice competencies and outcomes organized by the three domains of practice. The practice competencies and outcomes have been independently validated by researchers (Baldwin et al. 2009; Fulton et al. 2015).

The NACNS model for CNS practice assumes (1) CNS practice is highly integrated across three domains, (2) expert advanced clinical care is central to CNS practice, (3) practice occurs within specialty with specialty knowledge and skill, and (4) practice occurs in the larger context of society and the healthcare environment. The domains and concepts in the model are interactive and are enacted through practice within a scope unique to the CNS role (NACNS 2019). In the updated 2019 model, the names of the domains were changed to *spheres of impact* from the previous name *spheres of influence* (NACNS 2019) (Fig. 5.1).

5.4   Practice Competencies

Core CNS practice competencies are foundational to defining CNS practice in today's complex and evolving healthcare system. The core competencies are comprehensive, entry-level competencies expected of graduates of all nursing programs

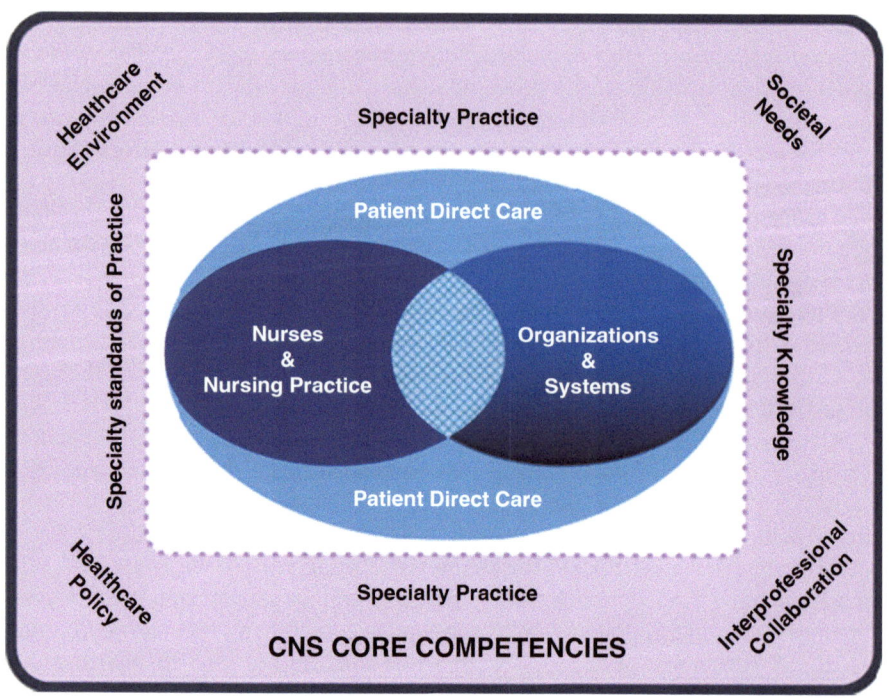

CNS CORE COMPETENCIES

Fig. 5.1 CNS practice conceptualized as core competencies in three interacting spheres actualized in specialty practice and guided by specialty knowledge, skills/competencies, and practice competencies within the context of the ever-changing healthcare environment, healthcare policy, interprofessional collaboration, and societal needs (NACNS 2019). (Used with permission)

preparing CNSs. Due to the wide range of specialties in which CNSs practice, these competencies are core for CNS practicing in any specialty (NACNS 2019). In 2019, NACNS revised the competencies originally written in 1998 and revised in 2004 and 2010. The earlier versions of the core CNS competencies have been validated by expert panel and research (Baldwin et al. 2007, 2009), and the 2019 competencies were validated by an invitational panel representing 20 nursing organizations providing structured partner input to the current, updated competencies (NACNS 2019). The NACNS core CNS practice competencies are summarized in Table 5.1.

5.5   Outcome Measures and Evaluation

With greater focus on healthcare reporting of quality measures, CNSs are called to make measurement, evaluation, and dissemination of CNS outcomes a priority. One ongoing challenge to CNS outcome measurement and evaluation is the lack of standardized metrics for CNS outcomes. Unlike other advanced practice roles that use many of the metrics established for medical care, CNS practice across three domains lacks established measures for many outcomes.

Table 5.1 NACNS core CNS practice competencies (NACNS 2019) (*Published with permission*)

Competencies: Patient direct care sphere

P.1	Uses relationship-building communication to promote health and wellness, healing, self-care, and peaceful end of life
P.2	Conducts a comprehensive health assessment in diverse care settings including psychosocial, functional, physical, and environmental factors
P.3	Synthesizes assessment findings using advanced knowledge, expertise, critical thinking, and clinical judgment to formulate differential diagnoses
P.4	Designs evidence-based, cost-effective interventions, including advanced nursing therapies, to meet the multifaceted needs of complex patients
P.5	Implements customized evidence-based advanced nursing interventions, including the provision of direct care
P.6	Prescribes medications, therapeutics, diagnostic studies, equipment, and procedures to manage the health issues of patients
P.7	Designs and employs educational strategies that consider readiness to learn, individual preferences, and other social determinants of health
P.8	Uses advanced communication skills in complex situations and difficult conversations
P.9	Provides expert consultation based on a broad range of theories and evidence for patients with complex healthcare needs
P.10	Provides education and coaching to patients with complex learning needs and atypical responses
P.11	Evaluates impact of nursing interventions on patients' aggregate outcomes using a scientific approach
P.12	Leads and facilitates coordinated care and transitions in collaboration with the patient and interprofessional team
P.13	Facilitates patient and family understanding of the risks, benefits, and outcomes of proposed healthcare regimens to promote informed, shared decision-making
P.14	Facilitates resolution of ethical conflicts in complex patient care situations
P.15	Analyzes the ethical impact of scientific advances, including cost and clinical effectiveness, on patient and family values and preferences
P.16	Advocates for patient's preferences and rights

Nurses and nursing practice sphere

N.1	Provides expert specialty consultation to nurses related to complex patient care needs
N.2	Promotes interventions that prevent the impact of implicit bias on relationship building and outcomes
N.3	Advocates for nurses to practice to the full extent of their role in the delivery of health care
N.4	Leads efforts to resolve ethical conflict and moral distress experienced by nurses and nursing staff
N.5	Fosters a healthy work environment by exhibiting positive regard, conveying mutual respect, and acknowledging the contributions of others
N.6	Employs conflict management and negotiation skills to promote a healthy work environment
N.7	Assesses the nursing practice environment and processes for improvement opportunities
N.8	Uses evidence-based knowledge as a foundation for nursing practice to achieve optimal nurse-sensitive outcomes
N.9	Mentors nurses and nursing staff in using evidence-based practice principles
N.10	Leads nurses in the process of planning, implementing, and evaluating change considering intended and unintended consequences
N.11	Evaluates the outcomes of nursing practice using methods that provide valid data
N.12	Facilitates opportunities for nurses, students, and other staff to acquire knowledge and skills that foster professional development

(continued)

Table 5.1 (continued)

N.13 Engages nurses in reflective practice activities that promote self-awareness and invite peer feedback to improve the practice of nursing

N.14 Mentors nurses to analyze legislative, regulatory, and fiscal policies that affect nursing practice and patient outcomes

Organization/system sphere

O.1 Cultivates a practice environment in which mutual respect, communication, and collaboration contribute to safe, quality outcomes

O.2 Uses leadership, team building, negotiation, collaboration, and conflict resolution skills to build partnerships within and across systems and/or communities

O.3 Consults with healthcare team members to integrate the needs, preferences, and strengths of a population into the healthcare plan, to optimize health outcomes and patient experience within a healthcare system

O.4 Leads and participates in systematic quality improvement and safety initiatives based on precise problem/etiology identification, gap analysis, and process evaluation

O.5 Provides leadership for the interprofessional team in identifying, developing, implementing, and evaluating evidence-based practices and research opportunities

O.6 Partners with research-focused, doctorally prepared (e.g., PhD) colleagues to translate, conduct, and disseminate research that addresses gaps and improves clinical knowledge and practice

O.7 Leads and participates in the process of selecting, integrating, managing, and evaluating technology and products to promote safety, quality, efficiency, and optimal health outcomes

O.8 Leads and facilitates change in response to organizational and community needs in a dynamic healthcare environment

O.9 Evaluates system-level interventions, programs, and outcomes based on the analysis of information from relevant sources

O.10 Demonstrates stewardship of human and fiscal resources in decision-making

O.11 Disseminates CNS practice and fiscal outcomes to internal stakeholders and to the public

O.12 Promotes nursing's unique contributions to advancing health to stakeholders (such as the organization, the community, the public, and policy-makers)

O.13 Advocates for equitable health care by participating in professional organizations and public policy activities

O.14 Advocates for ethical principles in protecting the dignity, uniqueness, and safety of all

Measuring CNS outcomes and evaluating the impact requires determining outcomes associated with and sensitive to CNS practice. Doran et al. (2014) conducted a literature review to identify evidence of CNS impact on patient-focused and organization-focused outcomes. The review included 25 articles published between 1989 and 2006, including 12 randomized controlled trials. Patient-focused outcomes demonstrating sensitivity to CNS practice included (a) disease-/condition-specific outcomes; (b) physical and psychosocial symptom outcomes; (c) early identification and prevention of complications; (d) self-management and adherence to treatment; and (e) patient satisfaction. Organization-focused outcomes sensitive to CNS practice included (a) unit/hospital length of stay and (b) total health-care costs.

A systematic review conducted by Newhouse et al. (2011) compared processes and outcomes of care delivered by APRNs to a comparison provider group, most often physicians. The review included studies published between 1990 and 2008 with findings from 11 studies of CNS outcomes, including 4 randomized controlled trials. Findings demonstrated that CNS practice had a high impact on length of stay (seven studies) and cost of care (four studies) and a moderate impact on physical complications (three studies). CNS impact on patient satisfaction (three studies) was similar to comparison groups. The Doran et al. (2014) and Newhouse et al. (2011) reviews were conducted for different purposes, yet the years of the literature overlapped. Only 4 studies were included in both reviews suggesting the difficulty in accurately locating research related to CNS outcomes and the quality of the reports.

In an international review of CNS practice outcomes including 24 articles covering 2012 to 2018, Bryant-Lukosius and Kietkoetter (2021) identified outcomes of CNS practice by sphere of impact. CNS-sensitive outcomes in the patient sphere included (1) prevention, alleviation, or reduction of disease- or treatment-related symptoms, functional problems, or risk behavior; prevention of complications or error prevention; and (2) improved quality of life and functional abilities. Examples of specific outcomes include improved comfort, increased patient satisfaction, improved patient/family knowledge, increased patient/family involvement in care and decision-making, increased rates of smoking cessation, reduced hospital readmission, reduced patient safety risks, and rapid response to deteriorating physiologic conditions.

CNS outcomes in the nurses/nursing practice sphere included improved implementation of best practices; increased number of nurses achieving required competencies; increased number of nurse-led evidence-based practice projects; sustained integration of practice changes; improved interprofessional team communication; increased staff satisfaction; cost saving through reduction in labor costs; increased nurse engagement; and empowerment. Outcomes related to engaging nurses in research included successful completion of studies, improved climate of inquiry, and nurse satisfaction in study participation. In addition, the outcomes in this sphere were also found to be relevant to other health professional consistent with CNS's initiatives working with interprofessional teams.

In the organization/system sphere, CNS outcomes demonstrated innovative care delivery models across the continuum of care, staff compliance with regulatory requirements and standards, and changes to policies and protocols to improve patient care. Specific examples of CNS outcomes include organizational achievement of Magnet; sustained integration of policy/practice change; strengthened organizational culture of inquiry; increased nurse use of patient education plans; increased organizational involvement in national initiatives; reduced hospital staffing costs (reduced nurse overtime and turnover); reduced 30-day readmission; reduced infection rates; reduced pressure ulcer rates; reduced catheter-associated urinary tract infection rates; and improved quality of care for ventilated patients with fewer intensive care readmissions and reduced length of stay.

CNS-sensitive outcomes were developed by the NACNS to correspond with core practice competencies. In a study to validate the practice outcomes, a national sample of CNSs rated the outcomes as highly important and reported the outcomes frequently were incorporated in employer job descriptions. When the CNS participants were not held accountable for the outcomes by others in the workplace, they nonetheless reported using the outcomes to guide practice priorities and initiatives

(Fulton et al. 2015). Although there was high agreement on outcome accountability and perceived importance, fewer CNSs indicated that they always monitor outcomes, suggesting a need to create standards and methods for collecting, analyzing, and reporting outcomes of CNS practice (Fulton et al. 2015). Reporting formats using templates and technology could facilitate linking outcomes to job responsibilities and job performance. The ability to aggregate data from multiple CNS specialty practices is needed to demonstrate the contributions of CNSs to patients, nursing practice, and the healthcare system. The NACNS CNS practice outcomes are listed in Table 5.2.

Table 5.2 NACNS practice outcomes by sphere of impact (NACNS 2019) (*Published with permission*)

Outcomes: Patient direct care sphere	
PO.1	Phenomena of concern requiring nursing interventions are identified
PO.2	Diagnoses are accurately aligned with assessment data and etiologies
PO.3	Plans of care are appropriate for meeting patient needs with available resources, reflecting patient/family treatment preferences and shared decision-making
PO.4	Nursing interventions target specified etiologies
PO.5	Programs of care are designed for specific populations (e.g., oncology, specific ethnic groups, end of life)
PO.6	Prevention, alleviation, and reduction of symptoms, functional problems, or risk behaviors are achieved
PO.7	Nursing interventions, in combination with interventions by members of other disciplines, result in synergistic patient outcomes
PO.8	Unintended consequences and errors are prevented
PO.9	Predicted and measurable nurse-sensitive patient outcomes are attained through evidence-based practice
PO.10	Interventions have measurable outcomes that are incorporated into guidelines for practice with deletion of inappropriate interventions
PO.11	Collaboration with patients/families, nursing staff, physicians, and other healthcare professionals occurs as appropriate
PO.12	Desired measurable patient outcomes are achieved (Desired outcomes of care may include improved clinical status, quality of life, functional status, alleviation or remediation of symptoms, patient/family satisfaction, and cost-effective care)
PO.13	Innovative educational programs for patients, families, and groups are developed, implemented, and evaluated
PO.14	Transitions of patients are fully integrated across the continuum of care to decrease fragmentation
PO.15	Reports of new clinical phenomena and/or interventions are disseminated through presentations and publications
PO.16	Interventions that are effective in achieving nurse-sensitive outcomes are incorporated into guidelines and policies
Outcomes: Nurses and nursing practice sphere	
NO.1	Knowledge and skill development needs of nurses are delineated
NO.2	Evidence-based practices are used by nurses
NO.3	The research and scientific base for innovations is articulated, understandable, and accessible
NO.4	Nurses can articulate their unique contributions to patient care and nurse-sensitive outcomes
NO.5	Nurses are empowered to solve patient care problems at the point of service

Table 5.2 (continued)

NO.6	Desired patient outcomes are achieved through the synergistic effects of collaborative practice
NO.7	Nurses' career enhancement programs are ongoing, accessible, innovative, and effective
NO.8	Nurses experience job satisfaction
NO.9	Nurses engage in learning experiences to advance or maintain competence
NO.10	Nurses use resources judiciously to reduce overall costs of care and enhance the quality of patient care
NO.11	Competent nursing personnel are retained because of increased job satisfaction and career enhancement
NO.12	The impact of implicit bias on relationships and outcomes is recognized and minimized
NO.13	Educational programs that advance the practice of nursing are developed, implemented, evaluated, and linked to evidence-based practice and effects on clinical and fiscal outcomes
NO.14	Nurses have an effective voice in decision-making about patient care
Outcomes: Organization/system sphere	
OO.1	Clinical problems are articulated in the context of the organization/system structure, mission, culture, policies, and resources
OO.2	Patient care processes reflect continuous improvements that benefit the system
OO.3	Change strategies are integrated throughout the system
OO.4	Policies enhance the practice of nurses individually as members of multidisciplinary teams
OO.5	Innovative models of practice are developed, piloted, evaluated, and incorporated across the continuum of care
OO.6	Evidence-based, best practice models are developed and implemented
OO.7	Nursing care and outcomes are articulated at organizational/system decision-making levels
OO.8	Stakeholders (nurses, other healthcare professionals, and management) share a common vision of practice outcomes
OO.9	Decision-makers within the institution are informed about practice problems, factors contributing to the problems, and the significance of those problems with respect to outcomes and costs
OO.10	Patient care initiatives reflect knowledge of cost management and revenue enhancement strategies
OO.11	Patient care programs are aligned with the organization's strategic imperatives, mission, vision, philosophy, and values
OO.12	Staff comply with policies, protocols, and standards of care that reflect regulatory requirements and standards
OO.13	Policy-making bodies are influenced to develop regulations/procedures to improve patient care and health services

5.6   CNS Education

CNSs are educated with a graduate degree in nursing at the master's or doctoral level. CNS curricula are built on foundational content for all graduate programs, recommendations for advanced practice nurses, recommendations for CNS content, and finally specialty practice (Fig. 5.2). The foundational content for master's-level education is the American Association of Colleges of Nursing's *The Essentials of Master's Education in Nursing* (AACN 2011), which includes nine foundational

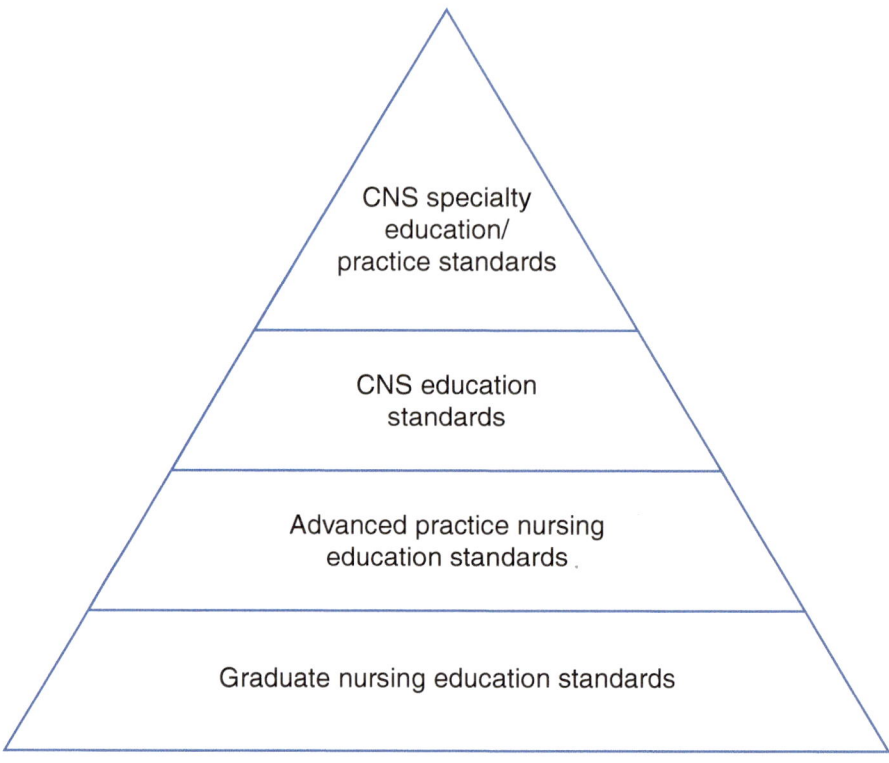

Fig. 5.2 Educational standards building blocks for graduate-level clinical nurse specialist education

content areas recommended for all graduate nursing education. A summary of the master's Essentials is in Table 5.3.

Advanced practice nursing functional roles, with practices focused on direct care, share a common core of knowledge for practice. Standards specific to advanced practice nursing are the next educational criteria build upon the foundational standards. The only known standards for advanced nursing practice curriculum regardless of the functional role are *The Essentials of Doctoral Education for Advanced Nursing Practice* (AACN 2006) developed for preparing advanced nurses with a practice doctorate (Doctor of Nursing Practice, DNP). Practice doctorates have only recently been introduced in the United States. The master's degree continues to be the dominant degree option for entry into practice as a CNS or advanced practice nurse. NACNS has called for the DNP to be the entry into practice degree for CNSs by 2030 (NACNS 2015).

The *Advanced Practice Registered Nurses (APRN) Consensus Model* was developed by the nursing community and includes APRN educational recommendations for three separate graduate-level courses. Educational programs preparing APRNs,

Table 5.3 Essentials of master's nursing education (AACN 2011)

Essential I	**Background for practice from sciences and humanities** Recognizes that the master's-prepared nurse integrates scientific findings from nursing, biopsychosocial fields, genetics, public health, quality improvement, and organizational sciences for the continual improvement of nursing care across diverse settings
Essential II	**Organizational and systems leadership** Recognizes that organizational and systems leadership are critical to the promotion of high-quality and safe patient care. Leadership skills are needed that emphasize ethical and critical decision-making, effective working relationships, and a systems perspective
Essential III	**Quality improvement and safety** Recognizes that a master's-prepared nurse must be articulate in the methods, tools, performance measures, and standards related to quality, as well as prepared to apply quality principles within an organization
Essential IV	**Translating and integrating scholarship into practice** Recognizes that the master's-prepared nurse applies research outcomes within the practice setting, resolves practice problems, works as a change agent, and disseminates results
Essential V	**Informatics and healthcare technologies** Recognizes that the master's-prepared nurse uses patient-care technologies to deliver and enhance care and uses communication technologies to integrate and coordinate care
Essential VI	**Health policy and advocacy** Recognizes that the master's-prepared nurse is able to intervene at the system level through the policy development process and to employ advocacy strategies to influence health and health care
Essential VII	**Interprofessional collaboration for improving patient and population health outcomes** Recognizes that the master's-prepared nurse, as a member and leader of interprofessional teams, communicates, collaborates, and consults with other health professionals to manage and coordinate care
Essential VIII	**Clinical prevention and population health for improving health** Recognizes that the master's-prepared nurse applies and integrates broad, organizational, client-centered, and culturally appropriate concepts in the planning, delivery, management, and evaluation of evidence-based clinical prevention and population care and services to individuals, families, and aggregates/identified populations
Essential IX	**Master's-level nursing practice** Recognizes that nursing practice, at the master's level, is broadly defined as any form of nursing intervention that influences healthcare outcomes for individuals, populations, or systems. Master's-level nursing graduates must have an advanced level of understanding of nursing and relevant sciences as well as the ability to integrate this knowledge into practice. Nursing practice interventions include both direct and indirect care components

regardless of role, should include one course each in physiology/pathophysiology, pharmacology, and health assessment. In addition, a minimum of 500 supervised clinical practice hours are recommended be included in the master's curriculum for all advanced practice functional roles (National Council of State Boards of Nursing 2008).

The NACNS *Statement on Clinical Nurse Specialist Practice and Education* (2019) includes recommendations for CNS education specifically designed to achieve the NACNS core CNS practice competencies. Specialty knowledge and skills are the last layer of content to be included in the curricula. A summary of the NACNS curricular recommendations is in Chap. 4, Table 4.2. Professional specialty organizations publish standards for specialty practice that should be incorporated in the curriculum as part of specialty graduate education. NACNS also publishes criteria for evaluating CNS graduate programs. These criteria are summarized in Chap. 4, Table 4.4.

Schools of nursing preparing CNSs must be accredited by a professional accrediting organization approved and monitored for ongoing quality by the US Department of Education. The National League for Nursing (NLN) Commission for Nursing Education Accreditation (CNEA) and Commission on Collegiate Nursing Education (CCNE) are two professional organizations that accredit graduate nursing programs. Each accrediting organization publishes criteria that schools must meet in order to achieve academic program accreditation (Commission on Collegiate Nursing Education 2018; National League for Nursing 2016).

5.7 Credentialing

Credentialing of CNSs occurs through legal entities, such as state governments, and professional nursing organizations. Authority to practice within a legally designated scope is granted by a state legislature through statutory code (law), usually referred to as the Nurse Practice Act. The rules for obtaining authorized practice within a designated legal scope are stipulated in corresponding regulations developed to guide implementation of the statute. Under delegated authority from the legislature, a state board of nursing (or board of health professions) establishes and implements regulations. Though similar across the country, in the United States, each of the 50 states has separate laws and regulations for granting practice authority to nurses, including CNSs. Authority to practice as a CNS must be obtained from each state in which a CNS practices with a few exceptions. Nurses practicing in federal health systems, such as the Veterans Administration or a branch of the US military, can practice with authority from any of the 50 states. An interstate compact has been designed to allow nurses authorized/licensed to practice in one state to likewise practice in another state, provided both states are members of the compact. To date very few states are participating in the advanced practice interstate compact.

Professional credentialing involves certification by professional organizations. Certification represents professional validation of competencies in a circumscribed specialty area of practice. The American Nurses Association (2017) defines a specialty as encompassing a specified area of discrete study, research, and practice as defined and recognized by the profession. Specialists are those who elect to focus their professional practice to their identified specialty. A specialty includes, among other criteria, a well-derived knowledge base particular to the practice of the nursing specialty; existing mechanisms to develop, support, review, disseminate, and integrate research into practice; competencies for the area of specialty nursing practice; and defined educational criteria for specialty preparation or graduate degree.

Whereas certification was initially designed as a measure of excellence, it has since become a measure of entry-level competency. Each certification body has eligibility requirements including evidence of graduation for a CNS graduate program; submission of a transcript demonstrating three separate courses in advanced pathophysiology, pharmacology, and physical assessment; and school attestation that the curriculum included 500 clock hours of supervised clinical experiences in the CNS role.

To address variability in requirements to practice as an advanced practice registered nurse (APRN), the nursing community collaborated on guidelines to align educational requirements, educational program accreditation, professional certification, and legal authority to practice. This effort resulted in the creation of the *Consensus Model for APRN Regulation: Licensure, Accreditation, Certification and Education* (National Council of State Boards of Nursing 2008). The model specifies that all APRNs must hold a graduate degree from an accredited graduate program that prepared graduates in one of the four recognized APRN roles (CNS, nurse practitioner, nurse-midwife, nurse anesthetist) and be certified by a professional organization. The model delineates only six specialty populations—neonatal, pediatrics, adult/gerontology, women's/men's health, family across the life span, and psychiatric/mental health across the life span. Specialty practice is in addition to population focus. A major shortcoming of the model is the limitations on specialty practice. Currently, CNSs do not have certification options in all specialties or for all populations.

CNSs obtain practice privileges from their respective states through an application process and are granted a license or other recognition to practice. When available, CNSs should be certified in a specialty area of practice, though not all states require certification for authority to practice as a CNS. Legal authority to practice as a CNS includes the autonomous authority to assess, diagnose, and initiate orders for treatment and therapy to include prescriptive authority for pharmacologic and non-pharmacologic therapies (National Council of State Boards of Nursing 2008).

5.8 Moving Forward: Challenges and Opportunities

For over 50 years, the CNS role has existed in the United States. In 1998, the NACNS created a model of CNS practice linking core practice competencies to expected outcomes. The model has been refined over the years with the latest version published in 2019. As a model *of* practice, it explains *how* CNSs practice—as an interactive process across three domains called spheres of impact that are linked to outcomes. As with any model, it needs continual theoretical and empiric support to remain a valid explanation of contemporary CNS practice. Additional research to validate the model, competencies, and outcomes is needed.

Measuring outcomes of CNS practice is a continuing challenge for CNSs. Comprehensive literature reviews of CNS practice outcomes provide strong evidence of the value of CNS practice (Lewandowski and Adamle 2009; Doran et al. 2014; Newhouse et al. 2011; Bryant-Lukosius and Kietkoetter 2021). Continued efforts are needed to establish measures evaluating CNS practice competencies and outcomes. The delivery of health care has been undergoing many changes in the United States. Measurement of CNS practice outcomes should reflect priorities of patients, healthcare systems, and insurance and government agencies as payers.

While hundreds of existing publications provide a consistent core representation of the CNS role and practice, it is curious that so often publications include commentary noting CNS role ambiguity. Understanding the CNS role and practice is inextricably tied to the ability to articulate the value of nursing, suggesting that continuing assertions about CNS role ambiguity reflects a lack of clarity about nursing and nursing practice. As a profession, nursing frequently lacks the ability to define its value to the public health and well-being, making it even more challenging to describe CNS practice as nursing practiced at an advanced level.

The *APRN Consensus Model* as a guide for education, certification, and regulation presents challenges for CNSs. Limited to only six designated specialty populations limits CNS's ability to lead nursing practice in new and emerging areas of specialty need compromising nursing's responsibility to a social mandate (Fulton 2019). As designed, the *APRN Consensus Model* is unnecessarily prescriptive and restrictive.

As the premier organization representing CNSs in the United States, the NACNS needs greater outreach and interaction with CNSs globally. Improving the ability of CNSs to network and engage with ICN, other national CNS organizations/groups, universities, and other education and research institutions will strengthen the global value of the CNS as an advanced practice nurse.

5.9   Exemplar of Clinical Nurse Specialist Practice: Critical Care CNS

Patients with complex, life-threatening disease and injury are treated in critical care units. These critically ill patients are at risk for developing physical and cognitive problems related to their underlying disease, medical treatments, and the restrictive, high-tech intensive care environment. A crucial care CNS leads nursing and interprofessional teams in preventing or minimizing risk for problems such as deconditioning, delirium, and pressure ulcers. One intervention known to reduce risks for critical care patients is early progressive mobility, which can reduce the number of days on mechanical ventilation, decrease length of intensive care unit stay, minimize physical deconditioning, and prevent delirium (Lai et al. 2017; Inouye et al. 1999; Connolly et al. 2016). CNSs assess patients and develop mobility plans that incorporate baseline functioning and goals of medical treatment. Individualized mobility plans address barriers such as oversedation, untreated pain, and devices that restrict mobility such as urinary catheters and intravenous lines. The CNS leads the interprofessional team in collaborating to safely and successfully mobilize patients. For example, a CNS collaborates with respiratory therapists to identify ways to monitor the endotracheal tube and oxygenation, physical therapists to direct the team in proper body mechanics and safe patient movement, and nurses and nursing assistants to support safe mobility and prevent falls. A CNS is essential in directing the team of professionals to enable mobilization, promote positive outcomes, eliminate fear of falling, and reinforce to the interprofessional team the importance of early mobility of critically ill patients.

In addition to individual patient care interventions, a CNS works at the system level to change practice by leading the development, implementation, and evaluation of evidence-based protocols for early mobility of critical care patients. A CNS bridges the gap between what is known and what is practiced by creating provider order sets, policies setting mobility as an expectation, and interprofessional educational programs for staff and employees. CNSs develop audit tools to measure and evaluate clinical and fiscal outcomes. A CNS is the content expert and consultant in each step of the process of designing a progressive mobility protocol.

Along with other CNSs in a multi-facility hospital system, the critical care CNS designed and implemented a progressive mobility protocol. Protocol implementation involved an interprofessional team, led by the CNSs. After implementation, the hospital's critical care unit experienced a 26% decrease in ventilator days, 36% reduction in hospital-acquired pressure injuries, and a 50% reduction in falls.

References

Allen RB, Koos EL, Bradley FR, Wolf LK (1948) The Brown report. Am J Nurs 48(12):736–742

American Association of Colleges of Nursing (AACN) (2006) The essentials of doctoral education for advanced nursing practice. Author, Washington, DC

American Association of Colleges of Nursing (AACN) (2011) The essentials of master's education in nursing. Author, Washington, DC

American Association of Critical-Care Nurses (2014) AACN scope and standards for acute care clinical nurse specialist practice. American Association of Critical-Care Nurses, Aliso Viejo, CA

American Nurses Association (2017) Recognition of a nursing specialty, approval of a nursing specialty nursing scope of practice statement, acknowledgement of specialty nursing standards of practice, and affirmation of focused practice competencies. https://www.nursingworld.org/~4989de/globalassets/practiceandpolicy/scope-of-practice/3sc-booklet-final-2017-08-17.pdf. Accessed 11 Nov 2019

American Nurses Association (2019) Advanced practice registered nurse (APRN) specialty roles. [cited 2019 July 29]. https://www.nursingworld.org/practice-policy/workforce/what-is-nursing/aprn/

Baldwin KM, Lyon BL, Clark AP, Fulton JS, Davidson S, Dayhoff N (2007) Developing clinical nurse specialist practice competencies. Clin Nurse Spec 21(6):297–302

Baldwin KM, Clark AP, Fulton JS, Mayo A (2009) Validation of the NACNS clinical nurse specialist core competencies through a national survey. J Nurs Scholar 41(2):193–201

Brown EL (1948) Nursing for the future. Russell Sage Foundation, New York, NY

Bryant-Lukosius D, Kietkoetter S (2021) Nurse sensitive outcomes. In: Fulton JS, Goudreau KA, Swartzell K (eds) Foundations of clinical nurse specialist practice, 3rd edn. Springer Company, New York, NY

Commission on Collegiate Nursing Education (2018) Standards for accreditation of baccalaureate and graduate nursing education. https://www.aacnnursing.org/CCNE-Accreditation/Accreditation-Resources/Standards-Procedures-Guidelines. Accessed 25 Nov 2019

Connolly B, O'Neill B, Salisbury L, Blackwood B (2016) Physical rehabilitation interventions for adult patients during critical illness: an overview of systematic reviews. Thorax 71(10):881–890

Doran DM, Sidani S, DiPietro T (2014) Nurse-sensitive outcomes. In: Fulton JS, Lyon BL, Goudreau KA (eds) Foundations of clinical nurse specialist practice. Springer, New York

Fulton JS (2014) Evolution of the clinical nurse specialist role and practice. In: Fulton JS, Lyon BL, Goudreau KA (eds) Foundations of clinical nurse specialist practice. Springer, New York

Fulton JS (2019) Fulfilling our social mandate. Clin Nurse Spec 33(2):61–62

Fulton JS, Mayo A, Walker J, Urden L (2015) Core practice outcomes for clinical nurse specialists: a revalidation study. J Prof Nurs 32(4):271–282

Gawlinski A, Kern LS (1994) The clinical nurse specialist role in critical care. W. B. Saunders, Philadelphia, PA

Hamric AB, Spross JA (1989) The clinical nurse specialist in theory and practice, 2nd edn. WB Saunders, Philadelphia

Inouye SK, Bogardus ST, Charpentier PA, Leo-Summers L, Acampora D, Holford TR et al (1999) A multicomponent intervention to prevent delirium in hospitalized older patients. N Engl J Med 340(9):669–677

International Council of Nurses (2009) ICN framework of competencies for the nurse specialist, ICN regulation series. ICN, Geneva

Lai CC, Chou W, Chan KS, Cheng KC, Yuan KS, Chao CM, Chen CM (2017) Early mobilization reduces duration of mechanical ventilation and intensive care unit stay in patients with acute respiratory failure. Arch Phys Med Rehabil 98(5):931–939

Lewandowski W, Adamle K (2009) Substantive areas of clinical nurse specialist practice. A comprehensive review of the literature. Clin Nurse Spec 23(2):73–90

National Association of Clinical Nurse Specialists (1998) Statement on clinical nurse specialist practice and education. Author, Harrisburg, PA

National Association of Clinical Nurse Specialists (2004) NACNS statement on clinical nurse specialist practice and education, 2nd edn. National Association of Clinical Nurse Specialists, Harrisburg, PA

National Association of Clinical Nurse Specialists (2015) Position statement on the doctor of nursing practice. NACNS archived documents

National Association of Clinical Nurse Specialists (2019) NACNS statement on clinical nurse specialist practice and education, 3rd edn. National Association of Clinical Nurse Specialists, Reston, VA

National Council of State Boards of Nursing (NCSBN) (2008) Consensus model for APRN regulation: licensure, accreditation, certification & education. [cited 2019 July 30]. https://www.ncsbn.org/Consensus_Model_for_APRN_Regulation_July_2008.pdf

National League for Nursing, Commission for Nursing Education Accreditation (2016) Accreditation standards for nursing education programs. http://www.nln.org/docs/default-source/accreditation-services/cnea-standards-final-february-201613f2bf5c78366c709642ff00005f0421.pdf?sfvrsn=12. Accessed 25 Nov 2019

Newhouse RP, Stanik-Hutt J, White KM, Johantgen M, Bass EB, Zangaro G, Wilson RF, Fountain L, Steinwachs DM, Heindel L, Weiner JP (2011) Advanced practice nurse outcomes 1990-2008: a systematic review. Nurs Econ 29(5):230–250

Sparacino PAS, Cooper DM, Minarik PA (1990) The clinical nurse specialist: implementation and impact. Appleton & Lange, Norwalk, CT

Clinical Nurse Specialist Role and Practice in Canada

6

Denise Bryant-Lukosius

Abstract

In Canada, the clinical nurse specialist (CNS) role is recognized as an advanced practice nursing role focused on improving nursing practice and patient, population, and health system outcomes. The CNS role is multidimensional in nature involving the integration of knowledge, skills, and expertise in clinical care, leadership, consultation, collaboration, education, and research. The competencies for CNS practice have been organized into four main categories related to clinical practice, systems leadership, advancement of nursing practice, and evaluation and research. While recent progress has been made, full integration and optimal use of the CNS role within the Canadian healthcare system remains elusive. Pan-Canadian strategies to clarify and communicate the role to key stakeholders, develop national credentialing mechanisms, increase access to CNS-specific education, and create healthcare policies and funding mechanisms

This chapter has been written before the 2020 APN ICN guidelines were published and reflects the views of the authors.

D. Bryant-Lukosius (✉)
School of Nursing and Department of Oncology, McMaster University, Hamilton, ON, Canada

Canadian Centre for Advanced Practice Nursing Research (CCAPNR), McMaster University, Hamilton, ON, Canada

Canadian Centre of Excellence in Oncology Advanced Practice Nursing (OAPN) Juravinski Hospital and Cancer Centre at Hamilton Health Sciences, Hamilton, ON, Canada

Escarpment Cancer Research Institute, Faculty of Health Sciences, McMaster University, Hamilton, ON, Canada
e-mail: bryantl@mcmaster.ca

© Springer Nature Switzerland AG 2021
J. S. Fulton, V. W. Holly (eds.), *Clinical Nurse Specialist Role and Practice*,
Advanced Practice in Nursing, https://doi.org/10.1007/978-3-319-97103-2_6

to support utilization of the role are required. Research to evaluate the outcomes and impact of the CNS role within the context of the Canadian healthcare system is also needed.

Keywords
Clinical nurse specialist · Advanced practice nurse · Role implementation · Competencies · Outcomes

The CNS is a strategically important role for addressing the health and health system needs of Canadians. It is one of two types of advanced practice nursing roles recognized in Canada, with the other being the nurse practitioner (NP) role. The early evolution of the CNS role dates back to the 1960s when it was introduced in acute care hospitals to provide specialized nursing expertise. Advances in medical treatment and technology and subsequent increases in patient acuity and the complexity of care resulted in the need for nurses with advanced specialized knowledge and skills to support nurses at the bedside and to improve the quality of nursing care (Bryant-Lukosius et al. 2010; Canadian Nurses Association 2018).

6.1 Definition of the CNS

The Canadian Nurses Association defines the CNS as a "registered nurse who holds a graduate degree in nursing and has a high level of expertise in a clinical specialty" (Canadian Nurses Association 2014: 1). The CNS role is a multidimensional clinical role focused on improving patient, population, and health system outcomes through the integration of knowledge, skills, and expertise in clinical care, leadership, consultation, collaboration, education, and research. Similar to the view of CNSs in the United States (National CNS Competency Task Force, National Association of Clinical Nurse Specialists 2010), the CNS role in Canada is felt to positively impact at three levels: the patient or client, nurses and interprofessional teams within practice settings, and organization/systems. CNSs work in a variety of specialty areas that may be defined by the type of illness (e.g., cancer), patient health needs (e.g., pain management), type of care (e.g., critical care), or the age of patient populations served (e.g., pediatrics, geriatrics) (Bryant-Lukosius et al. 2010).

6.2 Current Status and Deployment

Development and integration of the CNS role within the Canadian health system has fluctuated over the years due to the influence of several factors including geography, demographics, the economy, and healthcare policies (Bryant-Lukosius et al. 2018). Geographically, Canada is the second largest country in the world but also one of the most sparsely populated countries with a population of 35 million people (Wikipedia 2018). Over 82% of Canadians live in urban centers in the southern regions of the country, and as a result healthcare resources are concentrated in these areas with disparate services in rural, northern, and remote communities (Statistics Canada 2017a). Healthcare legislation, funding, and policies at the federal level and regionally across 13 provinces and territories also impact on how nursing and healthcare services are organized and delivered.

Perhaps the peak development of CNS roles occurred in the late 1990s. Although there were no specific CNS education programs, the introduction of graduate nursing programs in most provinces in the 1970s and 1980s stimulated the development of nursing in general and also the CNS role. In the 1980s, the Canadian Clinical Nurse Specialist Interest Group was established to support the national development of the role by creating practice standards, hosting national conferences, and disseminating regular newsletters (Bryant-Lukosius et al. 2010). In 1992, this interest group evolved to become the Canadian Association of Advanced Practice Nurses as the national voice for CNSs and also NPs, whose roles were also progressing (Easson-Bruno n.d.). By 2000, many CNS leaders in Canada had transitioned to become acute care NPs, especially in the largest province of Ontario, where a master's program specifically for this role had been introduced. The enhanced scope of practice and autonomy associated with the acute care NP role may have influenced these transitions. Job security may have also been a factor as the number of CNS positions was declining due to a downturn in the economy and financial constraints within the healthcare system (Bryant-Lukosius et al. 2010).

The actual numbers of master's prepared CNSs in Canada are difficult to determine because the role is not title protected and there are no regulatory or credentialing systems in place to identify and monitor nurses working in these roles. Only self-identified CNSs can be captured through provincial/territorial nurse regulating bodies. Best estimates from current data suggest that the number of CNS in Canada continues to decline. From 2000 to 2016, the number of self-identified CNSs decreased from 2624 (with and without a master's degree) to 550 (with a master's degree) (Canadian Nurses Association 2006; Canadian Institute for Health Information 2017). If the current number is accurate, CNSs make up less than 0.02% of the registered nurse workforce, compared to NPs who account for 1.6%. A national study indicated that more than 33% of self-identified CNSs were working in positions that were akin to but not titled as a CNS role (Jokiniemi et al. 2018). Thus, it is possible that the actual number of CNSs is underestimated with additional nurses working in CNS-type roles, but because the job title is not CNS, they do not identify as such. Lack of consistent reporting about which CNSs are master's prepared also makes it difficult to accurately assess deployment trends of CNSs who meet international criteria for advanced practice.

Recent studies demonstrate that 80–90% of CNSs work in urban communities (Jokiniemi et al. 2018; Kilpatrick et al. 2013). There is also evidence of increased health system integration with over 40% of CNSs now working outside of hospitals in diverse practice settings including the community, home care, primary care, long-term care, hospice, government agencies, and correctional institutions. The majority (68%) of CNSs report working these five specialty areas: gerontology-rehabilitation, medical-surgical, emergency-critical care, psychiatry-mental health, and community health (Kilpatrick et al. 2013).

6.3   Models of CNS Practice

CNS practice is highly variable as the roles are shaped to address the unique contexts of the practice settings in which CNSs work and the patient populations they serve. As a result, there is no one common model of CNS practice. In a national survey of CNSs, almost 40% reported they were not involved in the direct provision of patient care, 30% worked in a consultative role, and 28% provided direct care to a broad range of patients or those with specific needs related to risk factors, chronic conditions, case management, or acute episodic illness (Kilpatrick et al. 2013).

The paucity of publications about CNS roles in Canada limits current understanding about the scope and impact of various models of CNS practice. One area for which there are several publications relates to geriatric care as new models of CNS practice have evolved to address the health needs of a rapidly aging Canadian population (Statistics Canada 2017b). One model is the geriatric emergency nurse where the CNS screens for high-risk patients, conducts comprehensive assessments, and facilitates care planning and care coordination (Asomaning and Van Den Broek 2011). Another proactive model with a strong focus on health promotion and illness prevention involves the CNS providing expert coaching and guidance, consultation, leadership, and collaboration to provide care to older adults in long-term care facilities in rural communities (Smith Higuchi et al. 2006). New models of CNS practice in oncology and palliative care emphasize triage and patient navigation as important aspects of the role requiring in-depth knowledge and comprehensive assessment, interprofessional collaboration, and care coordination skills (Desrochers et al. 2016; Stilos and Daines 2013; Marchand 2010). Several publications highlight the essential leadership role CNSs play to improve patient safety and quality of care by designing and implementing innovative evidence-based services, practices, and policies related to breast cancer screening and assessment (Marchand 2010), geriatric care (McDonald 2012; Smith Higuchi et al. 2006), pain management in long-term care (Kaasalainen et al. 2015), a search protocol in psychiatric inpatient units (Abela-Dimech et al. 2017), wound care (Canadian Nurses Association 2012a), and pediatric vascular access devices (Gordon and Kenny 2017). A frequently reported theme in the literature is that CNSs are focused on addressing complex patient care needs and clinical situations and that their activities extend beyond practice settings to impact on the health of populations and communities and the regional delivery of healthcare services (Canadian Nurses Association 2012a; Marchand 2010; McDonald 2012; Smith Higuchi et al. 2006.

6.4 Outcome Measures and Evaluation

Although CNSs have existed in Canada for over 50 years, evidence about their effectiveness and impact is largely anecdotal. Systematic reviews of CNS roles document the absence of randomized controlled trials or comparative studies conducted in Canada (Bryant-Lukosius et al. 2015a, b; Donald et al. 2013; Kilpatrick et al. 2014a, 2015). Capacity to evaluate the impact of CNS roles is constrained by the ad hoc nature and short timeline in which the roles are introduced, limited access to research and role evaluation expertise, insufficient electronic documentation systems to track CNS activities and outcomes, and health services research funding priorities that are not aligned with needs for research focused on nursing roles. In a national study, CNSs were asked to report on the frequency (scale 1 (seldom) to 4 (constantly)) in which they achieved specific outcomes (Kilpatrick et al. 2013). Highest mean scores (2.5 to 2.91) related to improvements in patient outcomes including knowledge, satisfaction, comfort level, quality of life, anxiety, and self-care ability. CNSs also perceived they positively impacted on family outcomes related to knowledge, satisfaction, and anxiety (mean scores 2.8 to 2.89). CNSs felt that they had less frequent impact on system outcomes related to health care or treatment costs (mean scores 2.05 to 2.12). Narrative reports by CNSs and their key stakeholders (e.g., patients, nurses) indicate that CNSs contribute to improved system outcomes such as timely access to care and patient referrals to appropriate community services (Desrochers et al. 2016; Marchand 2010; McDonald 2012; Canadian Nurses Association 2012a), reduced emergency department visits (Canadian Nurses Association 2012a) and hospital admissions (Smith Higuchi et al. 2006), better quality of care (McDonald 2012), fewer patient safety incidents (Abela-Dimech et al. 2017), increased team efficiency (Stilos and Daines 2013), and the delivery of tailored, individualized, and patient-centered care (Desrochers et al. 2016).

6.5 CNS Competencies

In 2014, new pan-Canadian competencies for the CNS were established (Canadian Nurses Association 2014). These competencies build on a national framework for advanced nursing practice (Canadian Nurses Association n.d.). There were several aims for developing these competencies including to promote CNS role clarity, increase awareness and understanding of the CNS role for improving health and healthcare services, inform the development of CNS education programs, support CNSs to implement their roles, and guide employers who are introducing CNS roles in their organizations. A total of 65 competencies are organized into 4 categories related to clinical care, systems leadership, advancement of nursing practice, and evaluation and research. In a recent role delineation study, Canadian CNSs reported spending some or a great extent of their work time enacting most of the competencies (Jokiniemi et al. 2018). No competencies were not enacted. While there was a high degree of variability in time spent, these finding suggests that the new competencies reflect CNS practice.

6.6   CNS Education

A major barrier to the development of CNS roles in Canada is limited access to CNS-specific graduate nursing education programs and specialty-based education. Canada's geographic size and small population base make it difficult to recruit sufficient numbers of CNS students for any one university, and most universities do not have faculty resources or expertise to offer specialty education (Martin-Misener et al. 2010). It is only recently that a few universities have offered a graduate program stream specific to CNSs. As a result, most CNSs graduate from generic master's programs and may not have a good understanding of the role or the knowledge, skills, and confidence to successfully implement the role (Bryant-Lukosius et al. 2010). The lack of CNS education programs has also resulted in a shortage of CNSs in areas of identified need.

6.7   Credentialing: Regulatory, Legal, and Certification Requirements

In Canada, the regulation of nurses occurs at the provincial/territorial level and is governed by a nursing college or association. In most provinces, the CNS has the same scope of practice as a registered nurse, and as such, the role is not regulated or title protected. In Quebec, title protection exists for CNSs in infection prevention and control (Ordre des infirmières et infirmiers du Québec 2011), and work is in progress to establish CNS regulation and graduation education (Ordre des infirmières et infirmiers du Québec 2016). In Alberta, the "specialist" title is protected for registered nurses who have relevant graduate nursing education and 3 or more years of experience in a specialty area (College and Association of Registered Nurses of Alberta n.d.). However, the specialist title is not specific to the CNS role. Except for Quebec, there are no provincial credentialing systems in place to ensure that nurses have the minimum requirements to be a CNS related to education, specialty certification, or experience. Specialty certification available through the Canadian Nurses Association is not a requirement for the CNS role, and only exists at a basic and not advanced level. The lack of regulation, title protection, and required credentials contributes to role confusion, poor stakeholder understanding of the role, and variability in the extent to which all CNS role domains and competencies can be fully implemented (Bryant-Lukosius et al. 2010; Kilpatrick et al. 2013).

6.8   Moving Forward: Challenges and Opportunities

In 2010, following completion of a national study of advanced practice nursing roles, a number of recommendations were made to improve the integration of CNSs within the health system: conduct research to examine workforce trends and factors influencing successful implementation and role impact, establish a common vision for the role in Canada, develop and establish national standards and competencies for CNS practice, and develop CNS-specific education (Bryant-Lukosius et al. 2010).

Since 2016, some progress has been made in implementing these recommendations (Bryant-Lukosius et al. 2018). Pan-Canadian strategies have raised the national profile and improved understanding of CNS practice. For example, two practice pattern studies were conducted to examine the CNS workforce and delineate the role (Jokiniemi et al. 2018; Kilpatrick et al. 2013). The results of both studies have or will be presented at national and provincial nursing forums. The Canadian Nurses Association developed a policy document (Canadian Nurses Association 2012b) and hosted a roundtable meeting (Canadian Nurses Association 2013) that led to the subsequent development of pan-Canadian CNS competencies. A national association of CNSs has been created to provide a voice for CNS practice and policy issues, and CNS education programs have been implemented in at least two provinces.

To maintain this momentum moving forward, CNSs and nursing leaders including regulators, educators, researchers, managers, and policy-makers will need to work collectively to agree on a common vision for the CNS role, establish a credentialing system, and articulate a clear business case, supported by national and international evidence, for how the role aligns to support policy priorities for improving the health of Canadians and creating sustainable healthcare services. Research is required to evaluate the impact and outcomes of CNS roles within the Canadian context. Priorities for research should parallel health system improvement priorities to demonstrate the value of CNSs for improving patient safety and quality of care, increasing access to care, providing chronic disease prevention and management, strengthening health systems integration, and addressing social determinants of health and health inequities (Canadian Nurses Association 2012a).

Lack of role clarity and poor stakeholder understanding of the CNS role are associated with underutilization and sub-optimal implementation of the role and poor CNS job satisfaction. These factors impact on CNS recruitment and retention and have contributed to a shrinking CNS workforce (Bryant-Lukosius et al. 2010; Kilpatrick et al. 2014b, 2016). Pan-Canadian efforts by national and provincial nursing associations and regulators will be necessary to stem the declining numbers of CNSs through policies to clarify the role; establish standardized role requirements and credentials; and educate the public, nurses, healthcare administrators, and government policy-makers about the role. Pan-Canadian approaches are needed to document master's prepared CNSs in each province in order to effectively monitor workforce trends and gaps in deployment.

A challenge for CNSs is that they are not well represented at decision-making and policy tables across all levels of the health system, and as a result CNS solutions for addressing healthcare needs are not considered (Bryant-Lukosius et al. 2010). CNSs tend to invest their energy to improve practice in their specialty area and not to advocate for the optimal development and utilization of the CNS role. If the role is to be sustained, CNSs must take a stronger leadership role, become more politically savvy, and be visible and influential at decision- and policy-making forums within healthcare organizations and professional nursing associations and in government.

In this time of economic restraint in health care, current funding models in which CNS salaries are paid through agency operating budgets are a major barrier to the introduction and sustainability of the role (Bryant-Lukosius et al. 2018). This has required courageous and creative nursing leaders to seek nontraditional sources of funding to recruit and develop novice CNSs in areas of high need for specialized expertise, such as mental health and addiction (Gehrs et al. 2016). Specific funding for priority healthcare needs has been useful for deploying CNSs where their expertise can be best utilized. For example, in 2005 Health Canada strategically recruited CNSs for 600 First Nations and Inuit communities to address population health needs and improve nursing practice in targeted areas including maternal/child health, mental health/addictions, chronic disease management, and diabetes (Veldorst n.d.). Healthcare leaders and CNSs should advocate for new funding envelopes and models to support CNS practice in areas of priority. Pay for performance models providing organizations with incentives to reach benchmarks for access and quality of care and bundled funding models for patients with complex chronic conditions are examples of potential funding approaches that may help to leverage CNS expertise.

6.9   Exemplar of CNS Practice in Oncology Palliative Care

This exemplar features a CNS working in palliative care in a cancer center offering highly specialized ambulatory cancer care services across large region in Southern Ontario, Canada. Patients (and their family members) diagnosed with cancer requiring complex symptom management and supportive care to address treatment side effects, manage the consequences of advanced disease, or receive comfort at end of life are the focus of the CNS role. This CNS demonstrates exemplary practice by fully operationalizing all four categories of Canadian CNS competencies (i.e., clinical practice, systems leadership, advancement of nursing practice, and evaluation and research) (Canadian Nurses Association 2014). These actions result in positive impacts at the patient, practice setting, and organizational/systems levels that are regional, provincial, national, and international in scope. This CNS has achieved exemplary practice through graduate and continuing education, national certification in both oncology and in palliative care, and 15+ years of CNS experience—she is an expert CNS (De Souza 2018).

Related to clinical care, the CNS has advanced in-depth knowledge and skills in cancer and palliative care. Working collaboratively within the interprofessional team, she conducts comprehensive patient and family assessments, triages patients to appropriate providers, navigates and refers the patient to community services, facilitates patient goal setting and care planning, provides patient education and self-management support, provides consultation to cancer center and community providers, and proactively assesses and manages patient symptoms and concerns through nurse-led clinics and telephone follow-up.

The CNS provides systems leadership to influence, implement, and manage change to improve care delivery within and across systems. In this regard she is politically strategic and goal and outcome oriented and effectively communicates and negotiates with the healthcare team and community stakeholders to innovate care. She improves access to and the quality of care by leading the implementation of evidence-based guidelines and policies and by assessing gaps in clinical care and designing new services to address these gaps. For example, she led the regional implementation of evidence-based strategies to improve cancer symptom screening and developed an interprofessional clinic to improve the management development of dyspnea for patients with advanced cancer. Within the cancer center, she develops palliative care expertise and services by mentoring students, nurses, and other providers.

Relevant to the advancement of nursing, this CNS leads initiatives to improve nursing practice as a board member for the national oncology nursing association, presents at conferences, and publishes her work. Nationally and internationally she improves nursing practice by developing and delivering palliative care education courses and programs. She fosters the development of CNS practice by articulating a clear vision of the CNS role to stakeholders (e.g., patients, team members, managers) and mentoring potential CNSs as a tutor in a graduate nursing education program. Provincially, she champions the development of CNS practice in cancer care by co-leading a community practice for advanced practice nurses.

In terms of evaluation and research, the CNS improves the quality of care at the cancer center by participating in interprofessional research, utilizing research evidence to design new policies, practices, and services; contributing to quality improvement initiatives; and leading the evaluation of new service delivery models, such as the dyspnea clinic described above.

References

Abela-Dimech F, Johnston K, Strudwick G (2017) Development and pilot implementation of a search protocol to improve patient safety on a psychiatric inpatient unit. Clin Nurs Spec 31(2):104–114

Asomaning N, Van Den Broek K (2011) Can Nurse 107(8):12

Bryant-Lukosius D, Carter N, Kilpatrick K, Martin-Misener R, Donald F, Kaasalainen S et al (2010) The clinical nurse specialist role in Canada. Can J Nurs Leadersh 23(Special Issue):140–166

Bryant-Lukosius D, Carter N, Reid K, Donald F, Martin-Misener R, Kilpatrick K et al (2015a) The clinical effectiveness and cost-effectiveness of clinical nurse specialist-led hospital to home transitional care: a systematic review. J Eval Clin Pract 21:763–781

Bryant-Lukosius D, Cosby R, Bakker D, Earle C, Burkoski V (2015b) Practice guideline on the effective use of advanced practice nurses in the delivery of adult cancer services in Ontario. Cancer Care Ontario, Toronto, ON. file:///C:/Users/Windows/Downloads/pebc16-4f_0.pdf. Accessed 16 May 2018

Bryant-Lukosius D, Martin-Misener R, Roussel J, Carter N, Kilpatrick K, Brousseau L (2018) Policy and the integration of advanced practice nursing roles in Canada: are we making progress? In: Goudreau KA, Smolenski M (eds) Health policy and advanced practice nursing, impact and implications, 2nd edn. Springer, New York, pp 357–374

Canadian Institute for Health Information (2017) Regulated nurses 2016. https://www.cihi.ca/sites/default/files/document/regulated-nurses-2016-report-en-web.pdf. Accessed 14 May 2018

Canadian Nurses Association (2006) 2005 workforce profile of registered nurses in Canada. Canadian Nurses Association, Ottawa, ON

Canadian Nurses Association (2012a) National expert commission. http://www.cna-aiic.ca/expert-commission/. Accessed 15 May 2018

Canadian Nurses Association (2012b) Strengthening the role of the CNS in Canada. Background paper. https://www.cna-aiic.ca/-/media/cna/files/en/strengthening_the_cns_role_background_paper_e.pdf?la=en&hash=E130029CE85AA0A8B3AD5FC96CF451E90415A4B3. Accessed 16 May 2018

Canadian Nurses Association (2013) Strengthening the role of the CNS in Canada. Pan-Canadian roundtable discussion summary report. https://www.cna-aiic.ca/-/media/cna/page-content/pdf-fr/clinical_nurse_specialist_role_roundtable_summary_e.pdf?la=en&hash=9994CE9E732B48FDA11FE6F51E4F0C4E3A4DCC08. Accessed 16 May 2018

Canadian Nurses Association (2014) Pan-Canadian core competencies for the clinical nurse specialist. https://www.cna-aiic.ca/-/media/cna/files/en/clinical_nurse_specialists_convention_handout_e.pdf?la=en&hash=E9DE6CADB7C0260D9CD969121DA79EB408B8466F. Accessed 13 May 2018

Canadian Nurses Association (2018) Clinical nurse specialists. https://www.cna-aiic.ca/en/nursing-practice/the-practice-of-nursing/advanced-nursing-practice/clinical-nurse-specialists. Accessed 13 May 2018

Canadian Nurses Association (n.d.) Advanced nursing practice. A national framework. https://www.cna-aiic.ca/~/media/cna/page-content/pdf-en/anp_national_framework_e.pdf. Accessed 16 May 2018

College and Association of Registered Nurses of Alberta (n.d.) Standard for the use of the title "Specialist" in registered nurse practice. http://nurses.ab.ca/content/dam/carna/pdfs/DocumentList/Standards/Standard-for-the-Use-of-the-Title-Specialist-in-RN-Practice.pdf. Accessed 16 May 2018

De Souza (2018) Cathy Kiteley. https://www.desouzainstitute.com/team_member/cathy-kiteley/

Desrochers F, Donivan E, Mehta A, Laizner AM (2016) A psychosocial oncology program: perceptions of the telephone-triage assessment. Support Care Cancer 24:2937–2944

Donald F, Martin-Misener R, Carter N, Donald EE, Kaasalainen S, Wickson-Griffiths A et al (2013) A systematic review of the effectiveness of advanced practices nurses in long-term care. J Adv Nurs 69(1):2148–2161

Easson-Bruno S (n.d.) Incoming President's address. Canadian Association of Advanced Practice Nurses Newsletter; 16: 1

Gehrs M, Ling S, Watson A, Cleverley K (2016) Capacity building through a professional development framework for clinical nurse specialist roles: addressing addiction population needs in the healthcare system. Can J Nurs Leadersh 29(3):23–36

Gordon J, Kenny E (2017) Bringing together a health region. Vascular Access 11(2):1–3

Jokiniemi K, Bryant-Lukosius D, Carr M, Kilpatrick K, Martin-Misener R, Rietkoetter S, et al Delineation of specialized and advanced practice nursing roles. Oral presentation accepted for the international nurse practitioner/advanced practice nurse network conference, Rotterdam, the Netherlands, 2018

Kaasalainen S, Ploeg J, Donald F, Coker E, Brazil K, Martin-Misener R, DiCenso A, Hadjistavropoulos T (2015) Positioning clinical nurse specialists and nurse practitioners as change champions to implement a pain protocol in long-term care. Pain Manag Nurs 16(2):78–88

Kilpatrick K, DiCenso A, Bryant-Lukosius D, Ritchie JA, Martin-Misener R, Carter N (2013) Practice patterns and perceived impact of clinical nurse specialist roles in Canada: results of a national survey. Int J Nurs Stud 50(11):1524–1536. https://doi.org/10.1016/j.ijnurstu.2013.03.005

Kilpatrick K, Kaasalainen S, Donald F, Reid K, Carter N, Bryant-Lukosius D et al (2014a) The effectiveness and cost effectiveness of clinical nurse specialists in outpatient roles: a systematic review. J Eval Clin Pract 20(6):1106–1123

Kilpatrick K, DiCenso A, Bryant-Lukosius D, Ritchie JA, Martin-Misener F, Carter N (2014b) Clinical nurse specialists in Canada: why are some not working in the role? Can J Nurs Leadersh 27(1):62–75

Kilpatrick K, Reid K, Carter N, Donald F, Bryant-Lukosius D, Martin-Misener R et al (2015) A systematic review of the cost effectiveness of clinical nurse specialists and nurse practitioners in inpatient roles. Can J Nurs Leadersh 28(3):56–76

Kilpatrick K, Tchouaket E, Carter N, Bryant-Lukosius D, DiCenso A (2016) Relationship between clinical nurse specialist role implementation, satisfaction, and intention to stay. Clinical nurse specialist. Int J Adv Nurs Pract 30(3):159–166

Marchand P (2010) The clinical nurse specialist as nurse navigator: ordinary role presents and extraordinary experience. Can Oncol Nurs J 20(3):80–83

Martin-Misener R, Bryant-Lukosius D, Harbman P, Donald F, Kaasalainen S, Carter N (2010) Education of advanced practice nurses in Canada. Can J Nurs Leadersh 23(Special Issue):61–84

McDonald D (2012) Who is the clinical nurse specialist. Can Nurse 108(6):22–25

National CNS Competency Task Force, National Association of Clinical Nurse Specialists (2010) Clinical nurse specialist core competencies. Executive summary 2006-2008. http://www.nacns. org/wp-content/uploads/2017/01/CNSCoreCompetenciesBroch.pdf. Accessed 13 May 2018

Ordre des infirmières et infirmiers du Québec (2011) A new specialty in infection prevention and control, A first in Canada. The Journal 5:1

Ordre des infirmières et infirmiers du Québec (2016) Pratique infirmière avancée. Réflexion sur le rôle de l'infirmière clinicienne spécialisée (Advanced practice nursing: Reflections on the role of the clinical nurse specialist). Publication no. 8456. http://www.anfiide-gic-repasi.com/wp-content/uploads/2014/07/8456-reflexion-role-ics.pdf. Accessed 16 May 2016

Smith Higuchi KA, Hagen B, Brown S, Zieber M (2006) A new role for advanced practice nurses in Canada. J Gerontol Nurs 32(7):49–55

Statistics Canada (2017a) Population size and growth in Canada: key results from the 2016 census. http://www.statcan.gc.ca/daily-quotidien/170208/dq170208a-eng.htm?HPA=1. Accessed 14 May 2018

Statistics Canada (2017b) Population trends by age and sex: 2016 census of population. https://www12.statcan.gc.ca/census-recensement/2016/rt-td/as-eng.cfm. Accessed 14 May 2018

Stilos K, Daines P (2013) Exploring the leadership role of the clinical nurse specialist on an inpatient palliative care consulting team. Nurs Res 26(1):70–78

Veldorst AJ (n.d.) Practice patterns of clinical nurse specialists working with first nations and Inuit communities. Master's thesis. McMaster University, Hamilton, ON

Wikipedia (2018) Geography of Canada. http://en.wikipedia.org/wiki/Geography_of_Canada. Accessed 14 May 2018

Part III

Europe

The Role and Practice of Clinical Nurse Specialists in the UK

7

Alison Leary

Abstract

Specialist practice in the UK has a long history, but the role of the clinical nurse specialist (CNS) remains unclear with no specific certification or regulatory framework.

This has resulted in a variety of levels of practice. In the UK the term CNS is not restricted to registered nurses or those in advanced practice, which could be seen as a risk.

This lack of regulatory framework has also meant that the development of practice has been unconstrained and innovative. Despite the variation in practice, the CNS role in the UK has largely evolved into an advanced practice role in order to meet patients' and family's needs.

In the UK there is a thriving specialist community across many areas of practice and patient populations which range from long-term conditions to more consultative expert roles.

There have been many studies that demonstrate the positive effect that specialist practice has on outcomes for patients, but the role is still poorly understood.

Keywords

Specialist · Advanced · Proactive case management · Innovation · Safety · Clinical nurse specialist · United Kingdom · Advanced practice nurse

---

This chapter has been written before the 2020 APN ICN guidelines were published and reflects the views of the authors.

A. Leary (✉)
London South Bank University, London, UK

© Springer Nature Switzerland AG 2021
J. S. Fulton, V. W. Holly (eds.), *Clinical Nurse Specialist Role and Practice*,
Advanced Practice in Nursing, https://doi.org/10.1007/978-3-319-97103-2_7

7.1   A Historical Perspective

The UK has a long history of specialist nursing practice. One of the first recorded specialist nurses was Dorothy Wyndlow Pattison (known more commonly as Sister Dora (1832–1878)) who practised in Walsall, England. Sister Dora became a specialist in the treatment of industrial injuries, particularly those related to working on the railway. Throughout the twentieth century, specialist nursing practice developed. In 1975 a cancer charity was founded by Douglas Macmillan, a civil servant, who established the first cancer and palliative care specialist nurse posts still known as Macmillan Nurses today.

The role of the clinical nurse specialist then began to establish itself outside of cancer in the late 1970s with pioneers such Elizabeth Anionwu who set up the first specialist service for people with sickle cell disease in Brent, London (Fig. 7.1).

Practice developed through the 1980s and 1990s in the UK. Various initiatives and policies promoted having a specialist nurse, and the charities that represented patient groups became powerful advocates of the role.

The Nurses, Midwives and Health Visitors Act 1979, which came into force on 1 July 1983, also created national boards. The English National Board (ENB) oversaw post-registration education in which specialist education was offered. This gave the clinical nurse specialist role its educational foundation as registered nurses were able to undertake specific courses in specialist areas such as urology, gynaecology or cancer care and then pursue work in those clinical areas. Towards the end of the twentieth century, undergraduate nurse education moved to being university based with a degree on qualification, and the ENB was phased out.

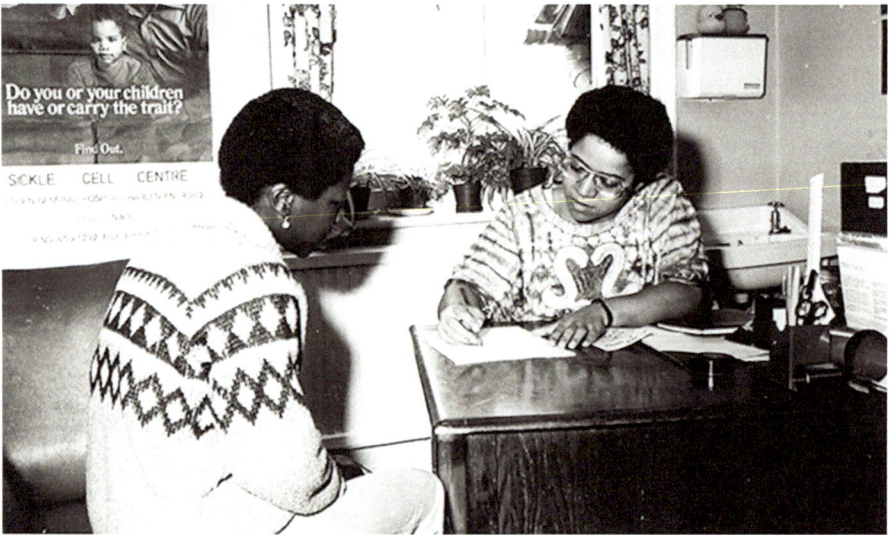

Fig. 7.1 Dame Professor Elizabeth Anionwu at work in Brent (right)

By the end of the 1990s, the CNS role was established, but there had been no strategic planning on how it was implemented—the roles and their deployment evolved over time meaning that their coverage was inequitable. In addition there was and still is no regulatory framework for specialist practice in the UK which meant that those performing the roles had a variety of practice levels and qualifications. By the start of the twenty-first century, their financial value to organisations facing austerity was doubted. This is in part because there is little common understanding of the roles which vary enormously by title and level of practice, or their contribution to patient care.

7.2   Defining Clinical Nurse Specialists in the UK

The definitions and scope of the CNS in the UK are confusing. As there is no regulatory framework, minimum qualification or little professional accreditation, the term CNS is not protected. This means the scope of practice and educational levels of those working in the role is very wide and the role is not solely associated with advanced practice. As there is no recognised regulatory or robust professional framework, the reality is that CNS work in the UK is essentially defined as an area of practice (e.g. a population or medical specialism) rather than a level of practice such as advanced.

In order to address this issue, the four UK countries have each adopted guidance on clinical nurse specialist practice.

Scotland was the first UK country to really formalise the role and the only UK country to explicitly state that clinical nurse specialists could be practising at an advanced level: "A clinical nurse specialist is a registered nursing professional who has acquired additional knowledge, skills and experience, together with a professionally and/or academically accredited post-registration qualification (if available) in a clinical specialty. They practise at an advanced level and may have sole responsibility for care episode or defined client/group" (ISD 2010). Although England has an advanced practice statement (DH 2010), it has tended to pay little policy attention to specialist practice. Wales took a multiprofessional approach and includes other health professions such as physiotherapists (physical therapists) but also refers to "specialist" as an area rather than level of practice (Welsh Government 2010). In Northern Ireland advanced practice has been defined (NIPEC 2014), but as with most of these documents, there is little mention of those in specialisms.

The primary employment model is still via an entity called the National Health Service (NHS). The NHS was founded in 1948, is centrally funded by taxation/national insurance and provides care free at point of use. There is a private healthcare sector in the UK, but employment of CNS in that sector has traditionally been limited. There is a growing market of other providers who are a mixture of different models such as community interest companies, non-profits, charities and private providers employing nurses, including CNSs, to run NHS services still within the universal healthcare model.

7.3   Models of CNS Practice

Generally, clinical nurse specialists in the UK provide complex services, many at advanced level in line with the International Council of Nurses' definition stating that an advanced practice nurse is a "registered nurse who has acquired the expert knowledge base, complex decision-making skills and clinical competencies for expanded practice, the characteristics of which are shaped by the context and/or country in which s/he is credentialed to practice. A master's degree is recommended for entry level" (ICN 2018).

The wide variety of levels of practice, services offered and education attained tends to be associated with different specialist groups and types of practice—despite this variation the term CNS has become ubiquitous, describing this entire population.

For example in the UK, CNSs, working in long-term conditions, tend to be proactive case managers. They manage a caseload of patients with a specific aetiology such rheumatology or neurology, often in collaboration with physician colleagues but taking the role as the primary provider of care. It's common to find CNS in these specialisms practising at an advanced level. They tend to be responsible for managing a caseload day to day including complex assessment, intervention (including psychosocial), prescribing medicines, brokering care and complex decision-making.

In areas such as cancer care where central government policy has supported the role or it has been enabled through the charitable sector, the workforce expansion was rapid meaning that there is more variation in levels of practice from development roles to advanced and consultant (attending) roles which lead entire services.

There has also been expansion in technical consulting specialist roles in the acute inpatient setting. These nurses rarely manage a caseload but act as a source of expertise. These roles are also often termed CNS and might specialise in areas such as pain, tissue viability or the management of inpatients with diabetes, for example. Acute hospitals have a high turnover of staff, and so these CNSs bring continuity of clinical standards, teach staff to manage the complexities of care and also review patients offering expert consultation services.

A summary of the types of specialist practice in the UK based on mining the authors' curated Cassandra dataset ($n = 18,000$ specialist nurses, approx. 70 million hours of work) is shown in Table 7.1.

7.4   CNS Practice Competencies

Although there are no agreed national competencies for CNS practice and little certification, many specialisms have developed their own competencies, for example, pain, diabetes and ophthalmology.

One of the most embedded is TREND which is for diabetes specialist practice (TREND 2015) and also includes a career framework. Some specialisms have

Table 7.1 The diversity of specialist nursing practice in the UK

Descriptor	Activity	Common areas of practice in UK
Proactive case manager	Day-to-day management of a caseload of patients—tends to be an advanced practice role, complex decision-making and clinical reasoning	Long-term conditions, acute and community
Reactive case manager	Day-to-day management of a caseload of patients—tends to be an advanced practice role but constrained by caseload numbers or complexity	Long-term conditions, acute and community
Consulting specialist	Expertise in a specific area of practice or patient population	Areas such as pain, tissue viability, infection control, inpatient diabetes care
Procedure-focussed specialist	Offers a holistic service including complex clinical decision-making	Areas such as colposcopy, endoscopy, central line insertion
Education-focussed roles	Provides clinical education often with specialist background	Supports education and practice development in specialist practice
Role substitution/ facilitation of others' work	Works to medical protocol may undertake activities such as physical examination/ prescribing but defers principal decision-making/works to protocol	Acute medical/surgical specialities, emergency care, ITU
Information and facilitation of others' work	Undertakes clinical administration, co-ordination of care, provision of information, largely protocolised care	Some long-term conditions or surgical pathways

competencies for services such as accreditation for endoscopy operators (JAG 2017); however these are not solely for specialist nurses. More recently in England, a framework for multiprofessional advanced clinical practice has been developed that may now add more uniformity to this level of practice across the different professions (Health Education England 2017).

7.5 Outcome Measures and Evaluation

The variability in levels of practice and services provided has made a common framework for the evaluation of these roles a challenge. Added to this lack of clarity are the current financial pressures that the employers of these post-holders find themselves, which means that the value of these roles is constantly questioned. This has led to repeated poor-quality local reviews based on time and motion type activity, which is of limited use in complex work (De Leon 1993, Raiborn 2004). Such activity analysis cannot handle relational work (Malloch 2015), and it generally results in underestimating nursing workload whilst also not considering outcomes at all.

Many of the evaluations have concentrated on quality aspects of services such as patient and family experience, which are generally very positive (Read 2015), and there is an increasing body of work which shows the benefit of CNSs in terms of efficiency and return on investment. These include reduction in the use of emergency care and acute inpatient care, more efficiently managed care, and better clinical outcomes for patients.

7.6   Credentialing, Regulatory and Legal Requirements

The term CNS is not a protected title in the UK and as such there is no regulatory or legal framework. A recent study by the author (Leary et al. 2017) discovered that job titles bore no association with levels of practice and that even individuals who were not registered nurses were conferred job titles such as "specialist nurse", "associate advanced nurse practitioner" or "clinical nurse specialist" by employers. This presents a challenge to the profession and a risk to the public who might assume they are dealing with a registered nurse.

Purposeful regulation of advanced practice has been tabled many times, but the last review by the council for healthcare and regulatory excellence (CHRE) stated in 2009 that "often what is termed advanced practice reflects career development within a profession and is appropriately governed by mechanisms other than additional statutory regulation" (CHRE 2009) and thus deemed regulation was unnecessary even though this assumption appears to be false.

The lack of regulatory framework does present a risk to patient safety—anyone in the UK, even those who are not registered nurses, can and does call themselves clinical nurse specialists or advanced practitioners (Jones-Berry 2018). The corollary is that there is little to impede the development of practice and many have found innovative ways to meet patient needs.

7.7   Moving Forward

Specialist nursing roles are at something of a crossroads in the UK. Policy in England is now prioritising a generalist "advanced clinical practitioner" role that can originate in any registered profession and can substitute for some medical roles. This has seen further scrutiny of CNS roles and their value rather than developing specialist practice.

Despite this there is tremendous support for these roles from charitable and other patient advocacy groups. Employers are also beginning to see the benefits of the CNS in contributing to better outcomes and more efficient services. There is an increasing amount of nurse-led work, for example, in areas such as gastroenterology where the majority of workload is managing day-to-day clinical care. This group of CNSs manages complex drug regimes, reviews patients in nurse clinics and provides case management functions whilst developing new ways of innovating service delivery (Leary and Punshon 2017). Such models are good exemplars of the further evolution of the CNS role in the UK.

7.8   Exemplars of Clinical Nurse Specialist Practice

7.8.1   Description of Specialty Area of Practice (Patient Population, Nature of Care, Etc.)

Yvonne Kana works as a specialist in ophthalmic care at a large specialist hospital in London. She sees a variety of patients with retinal problems and post-procedure dealing with any complications.

7.8.2   Describe a Case or Project that Is Exemplary of Practice in the Specialty

Yvonne offers a YAG laser service, a procedure which eliminates the cloudiness that occasionally interferes with a patient's vision after cataract/lens replacement surgery. She receives referrals from medical colleagues and assesses and treats patients.

7.8.3   Describe Practice Competencies Used in the Specialty Practice

Yvonne uses advanced assessment skills and her knowledge of specialist ophthalmic practice. There are competencies for ophthalmic nursing practice (RCN 2016) but no credentialing; however Yvonne has a master's degree in advanced practice.

7.8.4   Identify Typical Outcomes of Practice in the Specialty

Yvonne is able to manage the care and improve vision for many of her patients. Medical colleagues refer to her YAG laser service, and rates of satisfaction from patients are very high.

7.8.5   Description of Specialty Area of Practice (Patient Population, Nature of Care, Etc.)

Louisa Fluere works in a large central London acute hospital managing the care of men with advanced (metastatic) prostate cancer. She manages the care of around 100–140 patients per week across ambulatory care clinics.

7.8.6   Describe a Case or Project that Is Exemplary of Practice in the Specialty

Healthy hormones—introduction of seminar-based education to help men on androgen deprivation therapy.

Long-term androgen deprivation therapy (ADT) for advanced prostate cancer can result in significant and distressing side effects and longer-term adverse metabolic effects. A seminar-based service improvement initiative was developed to provide information and strategies to understand ADT, to manage side effects and to provide lifestyle advice regarding cardiovascular and bone issues. The seminars were evaluated with patient questionnaires and were positively received. This approach has proven to be a valuable tool in the care of this patient group and has been presented worldwide.

7.8.7 Describe Practice Competencies Used in the Specialty Practice

To run this service, Louisa utilises advanced assessment skills, prescribing of medicines (ADT, side effect management, supportive medication for symptom control, systemic anticancer therapies and chemotherapies). She is responsible for management of side effects using pharmacological, lifestyle and psychological approaches. Her role includes treatment initiation and monitoring, psychosocial care and education of patients, families and staff.

7.8.8 Identify Typical Outcomes of Practice in the Specialty

This is a high-volume, largely ambulatory service which manages the majority of the service workload with input as required from physicians and other members of the team. Louisa's service ensures timely, person-centred care that is cost-effective and valued by patients.

7.8.9 Description of Specialty Area of Practice (Patient Population, Nature of Care, Etc.)

Tony Kemp works as a specialist in prehospital care. He qualified as a registered nurse in 1983 and went on to work in a range of acute care settings including anaesthetics and intensive care. Alongside this he trained and worked within aeromedical care. Tony practises at an advanced level of practice specialising in prehospital immediate care in the British Association of Immediate Care Scheme (BASICS); he is also a teacher and researcher.

7.8.10 Describe a Case or Project that Is Exemplary of Practice in the Specialty

Nursing is not often utilised in prehospital immediate care due to the emerging dominance of helicopter (HEMS) doctors and the emergence of paramedic critical care pathways. Tony emphasises that a major part of his advanced practice specialist role extends beyond the immediate needs of the patient.

Recognising and preparing for the potential problems and the need to provide care that reduces onward negative physiological insult as part of the extended emergency care team is very much a significant part of his role. This is well evidenced in the care of an entrapped and seriously injured driver whose survival to the arrival of the emergency services was largely due to the intra-abdominal compression from the vehicle intrusion. Whilst recognising the devastating lower limb injuries, freeing the driver would lead to their rapid demise due to the lack of access to their legs and the presumed serious crush injuries present. Under Tony's advice the extrication was managed by the fire and rescue commander as a staged event with medical care being provided with a view to optimising the patient throughout prior to final release. The patient went on to make a full recovery, albeit following bilateral amputation, and was neurologically intact.

7.8.11 Identify Typical Outcomes of Practice in the Specialty

Tony's outcomes are not only in the clinical effectiveness of bringing a high level of complex care to patients out of hospitals but also a leadership role within a multidisciplinary team. This includes the application of a research base and also teaching other professionals in high-risk, high-pressure situations.

References

CHRE (2009) Advanced practice: report to the four UK health departments. https://www.professionalstandards.org.uk/docs/default-source/publications/advice-to-ministers/advanced-practice-2009.pdf?sfvrsn=6. Accessed April 2018

De Leon E (1993) Industrial psychology. Rex Publishing, London

Department of Health (2010) Advanced level practice—a position statement. https://www.gov.uk/government/publications/advanced-level-nursing-a-position-statement

Health Education England (2017) Advanced practice framework. https://hee.nhs.uk/our-work/advanced-clinical-practice. Accessed May 2018

ICN (2018) Nurse practitioner and advanced practice roles definition and characteristics of the role. International Council of Nurses, Geneva. https://international.aanp.org/Practice/APNRoles

ISD (2010) The advanced practice framework for Scotland. ISD Scottish Government. http://www.advancedpractice.scot.nhs.uk/definitions/aligning-frameworks.aspx. Accessed April 2018

JAG (2017) Guide to the JAG accreditation scheme. Royal College of Physicians. https://www.thejag.org.uk/Downloads/Accreditation/170131%20-%20guidance%20-%20guide%20to%20the%20JAG%20accreditation%20scheme%20v3.0.pdf. Accessed May 2018

Jones-Berry S (2018) The false job titles that are undermining trust in nurses. Nurs Stand. https://rcni.com/nursing-standard/newsroom/analysis/exclusive-false-job-titles-are-undermining-trust-nurses-128971. Accessed May 2018

Leary A, Punshon G (2017) Optimum caseload calculations for gastroenterology specialist nurses. Cohn's & Colitis UK, St Albans

Leary A, Maclaine K, Trevatt P, Radford M, Punshon G (2017) Variation in job titles within the nursing workforce. J Clin Nurs 26:4945–4950

Malloch K (2015) Measurement of nursing's complex health care work: Evolution of the science for determining the required staffing for safe and effective patient care. Nurs Econ 33(1):20–25

NIPEC (2014) Advanced nursing practice framework. https://www.health-ni.gov.uk/sites/default/files/publications/dhssps/advanced-nursing-practice-framework.pdf. Accessed May 2018

Raiborn CA (2004) Managerial accounting. Nelson Thomson Learning, Melbourne

RCN (2016) The nature, scope and value of ophthalmic nursing. Royal College of Nursing, London

Read C (2015) Time for some advanced thinking? Health Service J Suppl. https://www.hsj.co.uk/download?ac=1298457. Accessed May 2018

TREND (2015) An integrated career and competency framework for diabetes nursing. TREND, UK. http://trend-uk.org/wp-content/uploads/2017/02/TREND_4th-edn-V10.pdf. Accessed May 2018

Welsh Government (2010) Framework for advanced nursing, midwifery and allied health professional practice in Wales. http://www.wales.nhs.uk/sitesplus/documents/829/NLIAH%20Advanced%20Practice%20Framework.pdf

CNS Role and Practice in Ireland

8

Owen Doody

Abstract

CNS posts have a short history in Ireland, but none the less they have developed across all practice areas and disciplines of nursing (mental health, children, adult/general, intellectual disability) and midwifery. CNSs practise within the core concepts of the role (patient/client care, patient/client advocacy, education and training, audit and research, consultancy) and exhibit a range of competencies related to their knowledge, communication, organization, liaison, management, leadership, care/service provision, teamwork and decision-making. However, given the different pathways to CNS post, there is a need for those CNSs who did not hold the education level to engage in continuing education, and this education should be a postgraduate diploma (level 9) to master's level. In addition, there is a need for regulatory support to guide the development of national standards for CNS posts through key performance indicators to facilitate benchmarking and standardization of CNS roles. While the expectation to fulfil many roles can lead to role overload, there is also a need to ensure CNS fulfil each component of their role including research and audit in order to demonstrate their value and make their contribution visible. Thereby administration support may be a necessary consideration for services/organizations in order to support CNSs to fulfil their role and reach their full potential and grow advanced nurse practitioners (ANPs).

This chapter has been written before the 2020 APN ICN guidelines were published and reflects the views of the authors.

O. Doody (✉)
Department of Nursing and Midwifery, University of Limerick, Limerick, Ireland
e-mail: owen.doody@ul.ie

© Springer Nature Switzerland AG 2021
J. S. Fulton, V. W. Holly (eds.), *Clinical Nurse Specialist Role and Practice*,
Advanced Practice in Nursing, https://doi.org/10.1007/978-3-319-97103-2_8

Keywords

Ireland · Clinical nurse specialist · Intellectual disability · Decision-making
Autonomy · Multiple sclerosis

8.1 Brief History of CNS Role and Practice

The origins of Irish CNSs stem back to the Working Party on General Nursing
Report (Department of Health—DoH 1980). However, the role of CNS was not
recognized until the late 1990s when after a period of industrial unrest, the nursing
board and health service employers produced a collaborative report. The resulting
Report of the Commission on Nursing (Government of Ireland—GoI 1998) recommended the establishment of the National Council for the Professional Development
of Nursing and Midwifery (NCPDNM) and recognized the need to endorse nursing
as a career. The NCPDNM was established in 1999; however, in the absence of a
framework for CNS development, it resulted in a diverse group of individuals practising with minimal support (Doody and Bailey 2011). To address this issue, the
NCPDNM published a framework for CNS which identified three independent
pathways (immediate, intermediate and future) through which nurses working in a
specialty could attain acknowledgement of their experience and learning (NCPDNM
2001, 2004a, 2007, 2008). The introduction of a formal pathway, definition and core
functions of CNS in 2001 permitted the development of CNS posts in Ireland to
begin. The introduction of CNS posts in Ireland supported a key function of the
NCPDNM which was to develop a clinical career pathway for nurses working in a
specialist area of practice in order to progress from staff nurse to CNS (NCPDNM
2002) and supported national policy (Department of Health and Children—DoHC
2001). CNS posts are one of two clinical career posts available to staff in Ireland
with the NCPDNM developing advanced nurse practitioner (ANP) posts in tandem
with CNS.

8.2 Definition of CNS

In Ireland a CNS is defined as a nurse specialist in clinical practice who has
undertaken formal recognized post-registration education relevant to his/her area
of specialist practice at level 8 or above on the National Qualification Authority of
Ireland (NQAI) framework. Such formal education is underpinned by extensive
experience and clinical expertise in the relevant specialist area. The level of practice of a CNS is higher than that expected of a staff nurse (NCPDNM 2008). In
conjunction with defining CNS, the NCPDNM (2007, 2008) defined an area of
specialty as an area of nursing practice that requires application of specially
focused knowledge and skills, which are both in demand and required to improve
the quality of client/patient care.

8.3   Conceptualizations/Model(s) of CNS Practice

In Ireland CNS practice is conceptualized within what the NCPDNM described as the five core concepts of the CNS role. These core concepts were adapted from Hamric's (1989) role components (expert practitioner, educator, consultant and researcher) and broadened to include advocacy (Doody and Bailey 2011). Each core concept needs to be embraced within CNS practice, and to support CNSs the NCPDNM identified broad descriptors attributed to each core concept (Table 8.1).

8.4   CNS Practice Competencies

Within Ireland competence of a CNS encompasses those of a nurse and those for specialist practice, which are based on the core concepts of the role (NCPDNM 2008) and specific employer/specialist job descriptions (Table 8.2). The core competencies of the CNS are shared by all who practise at specialist level based on the core concepts of the role. Specific competencies are those identified as specific to the practice role and setting, and the responsibility for detailing specific competencies lies with service providers and should be outlined in the job description.

8.5   Outcome Measures and Evaluation

Irish research studies indicate that CNSs contribute positively to patient/client and healthcare outcomes. However, such studies are descriptive and small-scale and do not involve comparisons. Nationally two evaluations (NCPDNM 2004b and Begley

Table 8.1 Core concepts for the CNS specialist role (NCPDNM 2004a, 2007, 2008)

Core concept	Description
Client focus	Work must have a strong patient focus whereby the specialty defines itself as nursing and subscribes to the overall purpose, functions and ethical standards of nursing. The clinical practice role may be divided into direct and indirect care
Patient/client advocate	Role involves communication, negotiation and representation of the patient/client values and decisions in collaboration with other healthcare workers and community resource providers
Education and training	Remit for education and training consists of structured and impromptu educational opportunities to facilitate staff development and patient/client education. Each CNS is responsible for his/her continuing professional development, thereby ensuring sustained clinical credibility among nursing, medical and paramedical colleagues
Audit and research	Audit of current nursing practice and evaluation of improvements in the quality of patient/client care. Knowledge of relevant current research to ensure evidence-based practice and research utilization. Contribute to nursing research relevant to his/her particular area of practice. Any outcomes of audit and/or research should contribute to the next service plan
Consultancy	Interdisciplinary and intra-disciplinary consultations, across sites and services. This consultative role also contributes to improved patient/client management

Table 8.2 Area and associated competencies as per core concepts (NCPDNM) and employer job description

Core concept	Associated competencies	Domain	Associated competencies
Client focused	Articulates and demonstrates the concept of nursing specialist practice within the framework of relevant legislation, the *Scope of Nursing and Midwifery Practice Framework* (An Bord Altranais 2000a), *The Code of Professional Conduct and Ethics* (An Bord Altranais 2000c) and *Guidelines for Midwives* (An Bord Altranais 2001)	Professional knowledge	Practice in accordance with relevant legislation and with regard to the Scope of Nursing and Midwifery Practice Framework (Nursing and Midwifery Board of Ireland 2015) and the Code of Professional Conduct and Ethics for Registered Nurses and Registered Midwives (Nursing and Midwifery Board of Ireland 2014)
	Possesses specially focused knowledge and skills in a defined area of nursing practice at a higher level than that of a staff nurse		Maintain a high standard of professional behaviour and be professionally accountable for actions/omissions. Take measures to develop and maintain the competences required for professional practice
	Performs a nursing assessment, plans and initiates care and treatment modalities within agreed interdisciplinary protocols to achieve patient-/client-centred outcomes and evaluates their effectiveness		Adhere to the nursing and midwifery values of care, compassion and commitment (DoH 2016)
	Identifies health promotion priorities in the area of specialist practice		Adhere to national, regional and local HSE pathways and policies, procedures, protocols and guidelines
	Implements health promotion strategies for patient/client groups in accordance with public health agenda		Adhere to relevant legislation and regulation
			Adhere to appropriate lines of authority within the nurse/midwife management structure In-depth knowledge of the pathophysiology

Table 8.2 (continued)

Core concept	Associated competencies	Domain	Associated competencies
			The ability to undertake a comprehensive assessment of the patient, including taking an accurate history of their condition and presenting problem
			The ability to employ appropriate diagnostic interventions to support clinical decision-making and the patients' self-management planning
			The ability to formulate a plan of care based on findings and evidence-based standards of care and practice guidelines
			The ability to follow up and evaluate a plan of care
			Knowledge of health promotion principles/coaching/self-management strategies that will enable people to take greater control over decisions and actions that affect their health and wellbeing
			An understanding of the principles of clinical governance and risk management as they apply directly to their role and the wider health service
			Evidence of teaching in the clinical area
			A working knowledge of audit and research processes
			Evidence of computer skills including use of Microsoft Word, Excel, e-mail, PowerPoint
Patient/client advocacy	Enables patients/clients, families and communities to participate in decisions about their health needs	Communication and interpersonal skills	Effective communication skills
	Articulates and represents patient/client interests in collaboration with the interdisciplinary team		Ability to build and maintain relationships particularly in the context of MDT working

(continued)

Table 8.2 (continued)

Core concept	Associated competencies	Domain	Associated competencies
	Implements changes in healthcare service in response to patient/client need and service demand		Ability to present information in a clear and concise manner
			Ability to manage groups through the learning process
			Ability to provide constructive feedback to encourage future learning
			Effective presentation skills
Education and training	Provides mentorship, preceptorship, teaching, facilitation and professional supervisory skills for nurses training and other healthcare workers	Organization and management skills	Evidence of effective organizational skills including awareness of appropriate resource management
	Educates patients/clients, families and communities in relation to their healthcare needs in the specialist area of practice		Ability to attain designated targets, manage deadlines and multiple tasks
	Identifies own continuing professional development (CPD) needs and engages accordingly		Ability to be self-directed, work on own initiative
			A willingness to be flexible in response to changing local/organizational requirements
Audit and research	Identifies, critically analyses, disseminates and integrates nursing and other evidence into the area of specialist practice	Building and maintaining relationships including team and leadership skills	Leadership, change management and team management skills including the ability to work with MDT colleagues
	Initiates, participates in and evaluates audit		
	Uses the outcomes of audit to improve service provision		
	Contributes to service planning and budgetary processes through use of audit data and specialist knowledge		
Consultancy	Provides leadership in clinical practice and acts as a resource and role model for specialist practice	Commitment to providing a quality service	Awareness and respect for the patient's views in relation to their care
	Generates and contributes to the development of clinical standards and guidelines		Evidence of providing quality improvement programmes

Table 8.2 (continued)

Core concept	Associated competencies	Domain	Associated competencies
	Uses specialist knowledge to support and enhance generalist nursing practice		Evidence of conducting audit
			Evidence of motivation by ongoing professional development
		Analysing and decision-making	Effective analytical, problem-solving and decision-making skills

et al. 2010) have been conducted in Ireland. Within the NCPDNM (2004b), evaluation outcomes related to patient/client care were evident (numbers seen, effectiveness of interventions, referrals received/made, telephone consultations, waiting times, patient/client satisfaction, quality of life indicators and a reduction in hospital general practitioner/emergency department admissions/attendance/visits). Of note within the evaluation was the recognition that some CNS roles lend themselves to performance measurement more readily than others, that many CNSs were executing outcome measurement but were using different terminology to describe the task and that, when measurements become more complex, the number of CNSs measuring those decreases (NCPDNM 2004b). Building on the 2004 evaluation, Begley et al's. (2010) evaluation identified patient/client, staff and service/healthcare outcomes. Patient/client outcomes identified include patient satisfaction, reduction of morbidity and promotion of self-management. Staff-related outcomes include increased knowledge, empowerment, retention and work satisfaction. Service/healthcare (delivery/development, quality) outcomes include waiting times, continuity, research, leadership and collaboration (Begley et al. 2010). Broader research identifies Irish CNS's contribution to the management of cystic fibrosis (Savage 2007), views of nurse prescribing (Lockwood and Fealy 2008), use of dependency and prioritization tools in palliative care (Bracken et al. 2011), activities in an acute hospital (Wickham 2011), community palliative care CNSs (Quinn and Bailey 2011), lesser recognized roles (Wickham 2015), perceived outcomes of research and audit activities (Begley et al. 2015), examining the contribution of intellectual disability CNSs (Doody et al. 2017a), activities of intellectual disability CNSs (Doody et al. 2017b), families' perception of intellectual disability CNSs (Doody et al. 2018) and multidisciplinary team members' perspectives on intellectual disability CNSs contribution (Doody et al. 2019).

8.6   CNS Education

The expectation for CNS is a recognized post-registration education programme relevant to his/her area of specialist practice at level 8 or above on the National Qualification Authority of Ireland (NQAI) framework. However, in the establishment of CNS post in Ireland, three pathways were in operation. First is the immediate pathway, for registered nurses already performing in the role of CNS at the time of implementation of the framework where the nurse held an appropriate post-registration qualification and/or a minimum of 5 years' experience in the area of specialty. This route was available up to 30 April 2001. The second pathway was the intermediate pathway for newly appointed CNSs (1 May 2001–31 August 2010) where a newly appointed CNS must achieve the academic qualifications and professional experience within a specified timeframe of appointment (agreed locally). Finally, the future pathway which identifies the academic qualifications and professional experience which a newly appointed CNS must hold prior to appointment (minimum of 5 years' post-registration experience, 2 years of practice in a specialist area and a post-registration diploma minimum level 8 of the National Qualifications Authority of Ireland related to the area of specialist practice). This pathway took effect on 1 September 2010. These pathways have given rise to a diverse group of CNSs who may or may not have an advanced level of education.

8.7   Credentialing: Regulatory, Legal and Certification Requirements

To become a CNS, one should fulfil the requirements determined by the NCPDNM (2008) in their framework for the establishment of CNS posts. After the Nurse Act (2011), the NCPDNM was subsumed under the Nursing and Midwifery Board of Ireland (NMBI), and the responsibility for CNS approval lies with the Health Service Executive (HSE) Office of the Nursing and Midwifery Services Director (ONMSD) for applications from HSE-funded organizations on an interim basis under the delegated authority of the DoH, while the Nursing and Midwifery Planning and Development Units (NMPDUs) and the ONMSD will approve applications for statutory and voluntary organizations on an interim basis under the delegated authority of the DoH.

The CNS is guided by their Scope of Nursing and Midwifery Practice Framework which considers:

- Competence
- Responsibility, accountability and autonomy
- Continuing professional development
- Support for professional nursing and midwifery practice
- Delegation and supervision
- Practice setting
- Collaborative practice
- Expanded practice and emergency situations

In addition as a specialist, the CNS also has an expanded scope of practice that incorporates the interpretation and application of advanced nursing theory and research, higher-level decision-making and autonomy in practice, which are consistent with their education level and clinical experience.

All registered nurses in Ireland are bound by the Code of Professional Conduct and Ethics for Registered Nurses and Registered Midwives (Nursing and Midwifery Board of Ireland 2014) which guides nurses in their day-to-day practice and helps them to understand their professional responsibilities in caring for patients in a safe, ethical and effective way. The code is guided by five principles:

- Principle 1: Respect for the dignity of the person
- Principle 2: Professional responsibility and accountability
- Principle 3: Quality of practice
- Principle 4: Trust and confidentiality
- Principle 5: Collaboration with others

8.8 Moving Forward: Challenges and Opportunities

CNSs play an important role in providing specialist knowledge and skills; but they need ongoing support from their managers and medical colleagues, and they require real opportunities to participate in continuing professional development for the CNS to operate at a higher level of practice, making decisions at specialist practice level, and where appropriate to develop nurse-led services. CNSs must claim ownership of their own practice; highlight their contribution to quality, safe and cost-effective care; and make their role visible. In addition there is a need for CNSs who entered on the immediate or intermediate pathway to advance their educational level to that of their international colleagues if they have not done so to date.

Given the different pathways individuals may have taken to their CNS post, there is a need for those CNSs who did not hold the education level to engage in continuing education, and this education should be a postgraduate diploma (level 9) to master's level in order to support them in their role particularly audit and research. With the diverse roles and practice areas that CNSs are employed, there is a need for regulatory support and guidance and to development national standards for CNS posts highlighting key performance indicators that would facilitate benchmarking and standardization of CNS roles. CNSs fulfil many roles which can lead to role overload, and this has to be considered in light of the fact that CNSs also need to ensure they fulfil each component of their role including research and audit in order to demonstrate their value and make their contribution visible. Thereby administration support may be a necessary consideration for services/organizations in order to support CNSs to fulfil their role and reach their full potential and grow advanced nurse practitioners (ANPs).

8.9 Exemplar of Clinical Nurse Specialist Practice: The MS CNS

(a) Description of specialty area of practice (patient population, nature of care, etc.).
    Multiple sclerosis (MS) is a chronic, progressive neurological disease affecting the central nervous system (Harrison 2014) that tends to manifest early in

life, usually between the ages of 20 and 40 years (Bjorgvinsdottir and Halldorsdottir 2014). It is an autoimmune disease which causes neuroinflammation, demyelination and axonal degeneration, resulting in lesion formation throughout the central nervous system which alters function (Kalb and Reitman 2014). It is estimated that 2.5 million people worldwide are affected by the disease, and there is evidence that the incidence and prevalence of MS is increasing globally (Multiple Sclerosis International Federation—MSIF 2016; Lonergan et al. 2011; O'Connell et al. 2017). Disease-modifying therapies (DMTs) in MS have hugely expanded in recent years, as has the high cost of drug treatment. Furthermore, recommendations from MS experts advise that DMTs should be initiated early in the disease course in order to prevent demyelination and brain atrophy, as damage to the brain and nervous system starts long before the first clinical symptom (Giovannoni et al. 2017).

(b) Describe a case or project that is exemplary of CNS practice in the specialty.

CNS roles are a comparatively new specialism in the care of MS patients internationally, and there can be huge variation in the actual role of the CNS in terms of levels of clinical autonomy, education and clinical setting (Matthews 2015). Many CNSs are not just involved with MS but also 'general neurology' responsible for caring for patients with a wide range of neurological diseases, i.e. epilepsy, motor neurone disease and Parkinson's disease, while some CNS roles purely focus on MS patients. The CNS also has varying titles as well as roles, such as specialist nurse, MS nurse specialist, CNS MS, MS nurse and neurology nurse specialist.

In working with patients with MS, a key aspect of care provision is the education and support to both patients, families and carers throughout their journey. Adjustment to the diagnosis of MS for patients and families is difficult due to the complex unpredictable nature of the disease. The chronic nature of the disease means patients are never discharged from care, and MS is a disease that impacts on the whole family unit. Therefore, long-term relationships can develop between the MS patients, their families and carers and the CNS. The purpose of CNS's roles includes improving the quality of clinical care, providing leadership, auditing and research activity in the nursing profession. The role has expanded recently and is more involved with diagnosis, management and support of MS patients. CNSs also play a significant role in the overall management of DMTs and particularly in promoting adherence to therapy (Burke et al. 2011). The huge expansion in pharmacological MS therapies has impacted significantly on the workload of the CNS, the role has moved more towards a 'high-tech' monitoring role, and this may have implications on the workload and ability of the CNS to provide care to patients. MS CNSs need to be highly educated and skilled to monitor patients on drug therapies, as some of the potential side effects are fatal (Abel and Embrey 2018). Also MS CNSs play an important role in averting accident and emergency admissions and unnecessary hospital admissions (Mynors et al. 2015). However, the role of the CNS is changing rapidly with the explosion of pharmacological treatments, and this may impact on patient care.

Management of MS endeavours to shorten and prevent relapses, and reduce severity of relapses, preventing the accumulation of disability. There are currently 14 approved drug therapies, and huge advancements have been made in the treatment of MS which has radically altered how drug therapies are initiated (Comi et al. 2017). This has resulted in an individualized, tailored approach to DMT, which requires the CNS MS to have an in-depth knowledge of drug mechanisms and side effects to monitor the patient safely. However, there are limited treatments for those with advanced MS, and many patients with advanced MS feel abandoned and that resources and are concentrated on pharmacological treatments for relapsing-remitting multiple sclerosis (RRMS) patients (Abel and Embrey 2018).

(c) Describe practice competencies used in the specialty practice.

Within the role of MS CNS, competencies relate to professional knowledge, condition/specialist knowledge, communication and interpersonal skills, organization, liaison and management skills, building and maintaining relationships (individual, family and team), leadership skills, providing a quality care/service, analysing and decision-making are utilized and demonstrated across the core concepts of the role: client/patient focused, patient/client advocacy, education and training, audit and research and consultancy. CNS competencies are supported and guided in practice by the HSE and NCPDNM (2008) resource pack.

(d) Identify typical outcomes of CNS practice in the specialty.

Warner et al. (2005) demonstrate how specialist nursing services can initiate change in service delivery that ultimately improves outcomes in patient care identifying a threefold increase in treatment and at least 85% of patients are treated within 10 days of reporting symptoms to a CNS as compared to the previous 12% rate of treatment within 10 days, demonstrating that CNSs work at an advanced-level, developed specialist practice which can effectively manage patients experiencing a relapse through enabling prompt access to services and treatment. Smithson et al. (2006) highlight that CNSs are identified as being the most knowledgeable of all healthcare professionals by patients who also expressed a desire for seeing the CNS rather than any other professional and regarded the CNS as an alternative to the neurologist. In addition, patients saw the CNS as a link between primary and secondary care and in the best position to provide individualized co-ordinated care as they knew the patient and understand their unique needs (Aspinal et al. 2012; Smithson et al. 2006).

Having a CNS involved in care impacts positively and helps sustain improvements in the choice, quality and the delivery of MS care (Forbes et al. 2006), and CNSs are seen as the appropriate professionals to provide specialist care (While et al. 2009). The MS CNS addresses many broad care needs, including information regarding MS and general health, bowel and bladder problems, sexual dysfunction, financial advice, weight loss, relapse management, advice regarding family planning and pain (While et al. 2009). The MS CNS is a versatile role where the CNS contributes to all elements of continuity of care for people with long-term neurological conditions (Aspinal et al. 2012) as the MS

CNS has specialist knowledge, knowledge of local services and a co-ordinating role and are flexible, holistic and collaborative in their approach to practice, all of which are key attributes in the promotion of continuity of care (Methley et al. 2017; Aspinal et al. 2012). Key within the care process is 'person-centred care', where the MS CNS has developed a relationship based on trust and continuity and this provides psychosocial support and reduced anxiety levels for patients (Methley et al. 2017). Being person-centred and involving patients in their care enabled patients to feel listened to, and as a result they reported feeling more satisfied with their treatment choices and overall experiences of healthcare services (Methley et al. 2017; Tintoré et al. 2017). However, Mynors et al. (2015) findings from the 'Generating Evidence in Multiple Sclerosis Services (GEMSS) MS specialist nurse evaluation project' highlighted that CNSs lack the skills, time, tools and motivation to collect data about their service. This raises the question of their visibility and contribution which would help define their value and demonstrate the service they provide is effective.

References

Abel N, Embrey N (2018) Multiple sclerosis: dealing with complex treatment decisions. Br J Nurs 27(3):132–136

Aspinal F, Gridley K, Bernard S, Parker G (2012) Promoting continuity of care for people with long-term neurological conditions: the role of the neurology nurse specialist. J Adv Nurs 68(10):2309–2319

Begley C, Murphy K, Higgins A et al (2010) Evaluation of clinical nurse and midwife specialist and advanced nurse and midwife practitioner roles in Ireland (SCAPE) final report. National Council for the Professional Development of Nursing and Midwifery, Dublin

Begley C, Elliott N, Lalor JG, Higgins A (2015) Perceived outcomes of research and audit activities of clinical specialists in Ireland. Clin Nurs Spec 29(2):100–111

Bjorgvinsdottir K, Halldorsdottir S (2014) Silent, invisible and unacknowledged: experiences of young caregivers of single parents diagnosed with multiple sclerosis. Scand J Caring Sci 28(1):38–48

Bracken M, McLoughlin K, McGilloway S, McMahon E (2011) Use of dependency and prioritization tools by clinical nurse specialists in palliative care: an exploratory study. Int J Palliat Nurs 17(12):599–606

Burke T, Dishon S, McEwan L, Smrtka J (2011) The evolving role of the multiple sclerosis nurse: an international perspective. Int J MS Care 13(3):105–112

Comi G, Radaelli M, Sørensen PS (2017) Evolving concepts in the treatment of relapsing multiple sclerosis. Lancet 389(10076):1347–1356

Department of Health (1980) The working party on general nursing report, Tierney report. Department of Health, Dublin

Department of Health (2016) Values for nurses and midwives in Ireland. Stationery Office, Department of Health and Children, Dublin

Department of Health and Children (2001) Quality and fairness: a health system for you. Stationery Office, Department of Health and Children, Dublin

Doody O, Bailey ME (2011) The development of clinical nurse specialist roles in Ireland. Br J Nurs 20(14):868–872

Doody O, Slevin E, Taggart L (2017a) Focus group interviews examining the contribution of intellectual disability clinical nurse specialists in Ireland. J Clin Nurs 26(19–20):2964–2975

Doody O, Slevin E, Taggart L (2017b) Activities of intellectual disability clinical nurse specialists in Ireland. Clin Nurs Spec 31(2):89–96

Doody O, Slevin E, Taggart L (2018) Families' perceptions of the contribution of intellectual disability clinical nurse specialists in Ireland. J Clin Nurs 27(1–2):e80–e90

Doody O, Slevin E, Taggart L (2019) A survey of nursing and multidisciplinary team members' perspectives on the perceived contribution of intellectual disability clinical nurse specialists. J Clin Nurs Spec 28(21–22):3879–3889

Forbes A, While A, Mathes L, Griffiths P (2006) Evaluation of a MS specialist nurse programme. Int J Nurs Stud 43(8):985–1000

Giovannoni G, Butzkueven H, Dhib-Jalbut S, Hobart J, Kobelt G, Pepper G, Sormani MP, Thalheim C, Traboulsee A, Vollmer T (2017) Brain health—time matters in multiple sclerosis. Oxford Pharma Genesis Ltd, Oxford

Government of Ireland (1998) Report of the commission on nursing: a blueprint for the future. Stationery Office, Government of Ireland, Dublin, p 1998

Hamric AB (1989) History and overview of the CNS role. In: Hamric AB, Spross JA (eds) The clinical nurse specialist in theory and practice, 2nd edn. WB Saunders, Philadelphia

Harrison K (2014) Fingolimod for multiple sclerosis: a review for the specialist nurse. Br J Nurs 23(11):582–589

Health Service Executive and National Council for the Professional Development of Nursing and Midwifery (2008) Clinical nurse/midwife specialist role resource pack. National Council for the Professional Development of Nursing and Midwifery and Nursing and Midwifery Planning and Development Unit HSE–South, Dublin

Kalb R, Reitman N (2014) Multiple sclerosis: a model of psychosocial support, 5th edn. National MS Society, New York

Lockwood EB, Fealy GM (2008) Nurse prescribing as an aspect of future role expansion: the views of Irish clinical nurse specialists. J Nurs Manag 16(7):813–820

Lonergan R, Kinsella K, Fitzpatrick P, Brady J, Murray B, Dunne C, Hagan R, Duggan M, Jordan S, Mckenna M, Hutchinson M (2011) Multiple sclerosis prevalence in Ireland: relationship to vitamin D status and HLA genotype. J Neurol Neurosurg Psychiatry 82(3):317–322

Matthews V (2015) Delivering expert care to people with multiple sclerosis across Europe: an update. Br J Neurosci Nurs 11(5):235–237

Methley A, Campbell S, Cheraghi-Sohi S, Chew-Graham C (2017) Meeting the mental health needs of people with multiple sclerosis: a qualitative study of patients and professionals. Disabil Rehabil 39(11):1097–1105

Multiple Sclerosis International Federation—MSIF (2016) What is MS. https://www.msif.org/about-ms/what-is-ms/. Accessed 2 Apr 2018

Mynors G, Suppiah J, Bowen A (2015) Evidence for MS specialist services: findings from the GEMSS MS specialist nurse evaluation project. Hertfordshire, MS Trust

National Council for the Professional Development of Nursing and Midwifery (2001) Approval process for clinical nurse/midwife specialists (CNS/CMS). National Council for the Professional Development of Nursing and Midwifery, Dublin

National Council for the Professional Development of Nursing and Midwifery (2002) Guidelines on the development of courses preparing nurses and midwives as clinical nurse/midwife specialists and advanced nurse/midwife practitioners. National Council for the Professional Development of Nursing and Midwifery, Dublin

National Council for the Professional Development of Nursing and Midwifery (2004a) Framework for the establishment of clinical nurse/midwife specialist posts, 2nd edn. National Council for the Professional Development of Nursing and Midwifery, Dublin

National Council for the Professional Development of Nursing and Midwifery (2004b) An evaluation of the effectiveness of the role of the clinical nurse/midwife specialist. National Council for the Professional Development of Nursing and Midwifery, Dublin

National Council for the Professional Development of Nursing and Midwifery (2007) Framework for the establishment of clinical nurse/midwife specialist posts, 3rd edn. National Council for the Professional Development of Nursing and Midwifery, Dublin

National Council for the Professional Development of Nursing and Midwifery (2008) Framework for the establishment of clinical nurse/midwife specialist posts, 4th edn. National Council for the Professional Development of Nursing and Midwifery, Dublin

Nursing and Midwifery Board of Ireland (2014) Code of professional conduct and ethics for registered nurses and registered midwives, Nursing and Midwifery Board of Ireland, Dublin

O'Connell K, Tubridy N, Hutchinson M, McGuigan C (2017) Incidence of multiple sclerosis in the Republic of Ireland: a prospective population-based study. Mult Scler Relat Dis 13:75–80

Quinn C, Bailey ME (2011) Caring for children and families in the community: experiences of Irish palliative care clinical nurse specialists. Int J Palliat Nurs 17(11):561–567

Savage E (2007) The contribution of specialist nurses to the management of cystic fibrosis in Ireland. J Child Young People Nurs 1(4):180–185

Smithson WH, Hukins D, Jones L (2006) How general practice can help improve care of people with neurological conditions: a qualitative study. Prim Health Care Res 7(3):201–210

Tintoré M, Alexander M, Costello K, Duddy M, Jones DE, Law N, O'Neill G, Uccelli A, Weissert R, Wray S (2017) The state of multiple sclerosis: current insight into the patient/health care provider relationship, treatment challenges, and satisfaction. Patient Prefer Adher 11:33–45

Warner R, Thomas D, Martin R (2005) Improving service delivery for relapse management in multiple sclerosis. Br J Nurs 14(14):746–753

While A, Forbes A, Ullman R, Mathes L (2009) The role of specialist and general nurses working with people with multiple sclerosis. J Clin Nurs 18(18):2635–2648

Wickham S (2011) The clinical nurse specialist in an Irish hospital. Clin Nurs Spec 25(2):57–62

Wickham S (2015) Lesser recognised important roles of the clinical nurse specialist. J Nurs Care 4(3):251–253

Clinical Nurse Specialist Role and Practice in Finland

9

Krista Jokiniemi, Riitta Meretoja, and Jaana Kotila

Abstract

In Finland, the advanced practice nursing roles emerged in the early 2000s in university hospital settings. By 2018, there are around 80 clinical nurse specialists, and the numbers continue to rise. Currently the clinical nurse specialist roles are not regulated in Finland, and there is no title protection for these roles. Healthcare organizations control the use of titles and job descriptions; however, the need to push forward the regulation and licensure has been recognized as an important national goal concerning the development of these roles. The first national frameworks to guide the role development and implementation have commenced only recently. Although the national advanced practice nursing frameworks have taken time to evolve, the development of the clinical nurse specialist competencies is well on its way giving guidance to the role and practice development and implementation. Several central stakeholders, such

---

This chapter has been written before the 2020 APN ICN guidelines were published and reflects the views of the authors.

K. Jokiniemi (✉)
Faculty of Health Sciences, Department of Nursing Science, University of Eastern Finland, Kuopio, Finland
e-mail: krista.jokiniemi@uef.fi

R. Meretoja
Hospital District of Helsinki and Uusimaa, Helsinki, Finland

J. Kotila
Neuro Center, Hospital District of Helsinki and Uusimaa, Helsinki, Finland
e-mail: jaana.kotila@hus.fi

© Springer Nature Switzerland AG 2021
J. S. Fulton, V. W. Holly (eds.), *Clinical Nurse Specialist Role and Practice*,
Advanced Practice in Nursing, https://doi.org/10.1007/978-3-319-97103-2_9

as the Finnish Nurses Association, ministries, administrators, educators, and researchers, are working in close collaboration to support the clinical nurse specialist role and practice development.

Keywords
Finland · Clinical nurse specialist · Advanced practice nurse · Competence · Role Education

9.1 Brief History of CNS Role and Practice

In Finland, the advanced practice nursing (APN) roles emerged in the early 2000s to respond to the increasing complexity and needs of the healthcare environment, such as requirements of rapid access to high-quality care, managing changing environments, and developing evidence-based practices (EBP) (Fagerström 2009; Jokiniemi 2014). The first implementation of the APN role, the clinical nurse specialist (CNS), was carried out in 2001 at the Helsinki University Hospital (Meretoja and Vuorinen 2000; Meretoja et al. 2002). During the past 5 years, the numbers of CNS positions have tripled, with around 80 CNSs working around the country in 2018. The numbers of CNS positions continue to rise as the healthcare organizations are increasingly investing to these roles. By the year of 2025, the CNS positions are expected to double.

The CNS role and practice was initially developed and implemented in university hospital settings, and majority of the CNSs today practice in in-hospital practice settings. The CNS's central focus of practice is advanced clinical nursing. The primary practice goal is to ensure and improve the quality of clinical care, support staff and multidisciplinary teams in clinical care provision, endorse organizations' clinical performance, and foster the advancement of clinical nursing through scholarship activities (Jokiniemi 2014). In a country with 5.5 million people, Finland has around 80,000 registered nurses (RN), which account for 14.7 per 1000 population which is 4 times higher than the number of physicians (3.2 per 1000 population) (OECD. Stat 2018). As the numbers of CNSs are still low, representing less than 0.5% of the nursing population, a challenge is whether the CNSs are able to work in close proximity from the direct patient care. In several organizations, in this early phase of role development, placing the very few first CNSs has been strategic aiming to benefit and support healthcare organizations in increasing the quality of patient care and EBP by scholarship activities. Only in few instances, the CNS practice involves 50% of time allocated to advanced clinical nursing domain. More resources are needed to revenue the scope of practice into advanced clinical direct patient care.

9.2 Definition of CNS

The role and practice of the CNS is evolving in Finland. There is a national consensus definition of the role and scope of practice and recommendations for future development (Kotila et al. 2016; Jokiniemi et al. 2020). Based on the national research (Jokiniemi

2014; Jokiniemi et al. 2015a, 2018) and role and practice development (Kotila et al. 2016, 2018; Jokiniemi 2018, 2020), the CNS role may be defined as follows:

> *Clinical nurse specialist is an experienced master's or doctoral prepared registered nurse whose central focus of practice is advanced clinical nursing. The aim of the role is to support healthcare organizations to achieve their strategic goals, to assure and increase the quality and effectiveness of patient care, and to improve the merging of evidence-based practice and scholarship activities. Clinical nurse specialist role domains are advanced clinical practice and practice development, consultation and staff education, transformational leadership, and scholarship activities. The role actualizes through direct and indirect evidence-based patient care influencing positively to the patient care, nursing profession, organization, scholarship, and the community at large.*

9.3   Conceptualizations/Model(s) of CNS Practice

CNS is an APN role. In Finland, the APN roles currently include the roles of the CNS and nurse practitioner (NP). The CNS role development in Finland, while following closely to the international role development and visions, has been impacted by the healthcare needs and the current reform of the social and healthcare services. The initial CNS role conceptualization took place in the national doctoral dissertation study in 2014 (Jokiniemi 2014), where the CNS role conceptualization, implementation, and evaluation framework was developed. In this framework, the central concepts of the CNS roles and practice as well as continuous phases of analyzing the CNS role need, designing and implementing the role, and evaluating the role, were described. Following this initial research, the Finnish Nursing Association's expert group has taken an active role in modeling nurses' career from registered nurse to APN. The nurses' clinical career model includes three competency levels: registered nurse, specialized nurse, and advanced practice nurse, which includes the roles of CNS and NP (Fig. 9.1). Furthermore, advanced practice nurses have an opportunity to get limited prescription rights, by completing a separate postgraduate training worth 45 European Credit Transfer and Accumulation System (ECTS) credits. Nurse prescribers are licensed by the National Supervisory Authority for Welfare and Health (Kotila et al. 2016).

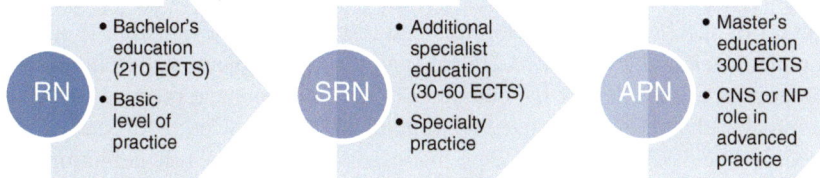

Fig. 9.1 Nurses' clinical career (Modified from Jokiniemi et al. 2018). *RN* registered nurse, *SRN* specialized registered nurse, *APN* advanced practice nurse, *CNS* clinical nurse specialist, *NP* nurse practitioner, *ECTS* European Credit Transfer and Accumulation System

9.4   CNS Practice Competencies

To achieve the role expectations, CNSs need clinical knowledge and skills beyond the level of frontline nursing. Uppermost of importance in developing the advanced competencies needed are prior nursing experience and an education at master's or doctoral level (ICN 2014; Sheer and Wong 2008). Furthermore, within the dynamic healthcare environment, the characteristics of capability, such as knowledge on learning, creativity, self-efficacy, and working with others, are utilized to support better role achievement (Hase and Davis 1999; Gardner et al. 2008).

The development of the CNS practice competency descriptions is ongoing in Finland. The initial competency descriptions were scientifically validated and first published in 2014 (Jokiniemi 2014). Hence in 2014, these competency descriptions have been further validated in a national study through rigorous mixed-method research project. The development of a competency scale for CNSs involved examination and comparison of the Finnish competencies against the US and Canadian competency sets (Baldwin et al. 2007; CNA 2014), as well as expert and practicing CNS evaluations of the competency scale. This scale has demonstrated strong content validity within the national context (Jokiniemi et al. 2018). It has been tested in terms of content and construct validity within the Scandinavian context (Jokiniemi et al. 2020).

The Finnish CNS competencies cover the spheres of patient, nursing, organization, and scholarship. The *patient sphere* encompasses evidence-based clinical practice, management of complex patient populations, and promotion of ethical patient-centered care. The *nursing sphere* involves CNS activities to ensure the quality of the nursing practice and support of staff knowledge as well as facilitation of healthy work environment. *Organizational sphere* competencies, in turn, involve integration and promotion of EBP, support of practice development and innovation, and transformational leadership. Lastly, the *scholarship sphere* competencies contain leadership and assessment of quality improvement projects/EBP as well as promotion of research and knowledge translation activities within the organization. The advanced-level competencies of the CNSs overlap with each other and are utilized in direct and indirect patient care to achieve the role expectations (Jokiniemi 2014; Jokiniemi et al. 2018, 2020).

9.5   Outcome Measures and Evaluation

Definition of specific outcome measures and research-based evaluation is still the most underdeveloped area of the CNS role and practice implementation in Finland. The importance of evaluating the outcomes of the CNS role and practice as well as economical evaluation is recognized (Jokiniemi 2018). However, in this early phase of the CNS role development, there are inconsistencies with the role definitions and the scope of practice within various healthcare organizations. Therefore, defining and measuring the CNS-sensitive outcomes in the role domains of advanced clinical practice and practice development, consultation and staff education, as well as transformational leadership and scholarship activities is challenging.

Individual PhD researchers and master's students have conducted outcome assessments of the CNS roles, which have centered on the first experiences of the role implementation and perceptions of the roles (Viholainen 2018; Jokiniemi et al. 2015b). Evaluation research projects are greatly needed to show evidence of the CNS role impact on various aspects of direct and indirect patient care and EBP. Besides the outcomes in clinical nursing, the CNS role is influencing positively to the nursing profession, scholarship, and the community at large. In the future, it is imperative to collect evaluation data, conduct larger-scale national studies, and take part in international outcome studies, in order to evaluate the CNS practice structures, processes, and outcomes (Donabedian 2005; Kilpatrick et al. 2016) from the perspectives of patient, nursing, organization, and the community at large.

9.6   CNS Education

Finland has a dual system of higher education, with both universities and universities of applied sciences (UAS) offering master's-level education in nursing. The entry requirement to both education systems is a bachelor's degree in nursing (Ministry of Education and Culture 2014*). It takes 3.5 years to complete bachelor-level degree (210 European Credit Transfer and Accumulation System [ECTS] credits) and between 1½ and 3 years to get the master's degree in nursing (300 ECTS credits). The content of master's-level education that prepares nurses for advanced clinical nursing roles and practice, both in UAS (90 ECTS credits) and universities (300 ECTS credits), is currently under evaluation and further development. Universities have provided master's-level education for nurses since 1979 with advanced clinical nursing programs in place since 1991 (Suominen and Leino-Kilpi 1995). The UAS, in turn, piloted degree program in advanced nursing practice the first time in 2006 (Fagerström and Glasberg 2011), which was formalized by the Ministry of Education and Culture in 2010. Typically, the CNSs have attained their education from the university.

Despite the rather long history of specialist-level practice and existing master's-level educational programs, there is no nationally congruent curriculum for advanced practitioners or no uniform national education programs in place for these roles (Jokiniemi 2014; Hukkanen and Vallimes-Patomäki 2005). There are only singular governing national documents on the concept of advanced practitioners and their responsibilities or education. To better answer to the requirements of the advanced practitioner education, several stakeholders and institutions are presently examining the curriculums.

It is generally accepted that the minimum requirement for the CNS role is the master's-level education. However, currently several CNSs in Finland held a doctoral degree or are pursuing one in nursing science. The doctoral degree in nursing science is a thesis based, and therefore is not clinically weighed, but prepares the CNSs to better achieve the scholarship aspects of the CNS role. Based on the initial national recommendations for nurse training, it may be concluded that the registered nurse has a possibility to advance in clinical nursing through three steps: (1) specializing in nursing (30 to 60 ECTS credits), (2) master's-level advanced practice nurse education (210 + 90/300 ECTS credits), and (3) doctorate-level education (Jokiniemi 2014, 2020; MSAH 2012).

9.7   Credentialing: Regulatory, Legal, and Certification Requirements

National legislation closely regulates the professional practice of healthcare personnel. The National Supervisory Authority for Welfare and Health (Valvira) grants upon application the right to practice as a licensed or authorized professional and authorizes the use of the occupational title of healthcare professional. Currently there are no legislative and regulatory mechanisms or protected titles in place for advanced practitioners. The CNS roles are regulated by the legislation on registered nurses and guided by individual organizational policies (Kotila et al. 2016; Jokiniemi et al. 2014).

Although the need for credentialing the CNS roles was recognized within a national policy Delphi study, the probability of taking forward the individual aspects of credentialing such as title protection, national registration, and regulation was perceived as low (Jokiniemi et al. 2015a). Although regulatory issues may take a long time to actualize (Arslanian-Engoren et al. 2011; Bryant-Lukosius et al. 2010), and despite the challenges, developing the prospects of the role regulation and credentialing is the ambition of the central CNS role developers/pioneers. The Finnish Nurses Association's APN expert group, set up in 2013, continues to strive for the clarification and integration of the advanced nursing roles and practice. Following the conceptualization of the advanced practice roles completed in 2016 (Kotila et al. 2016; Jokiniemi et al. 2020), the next step is to press for the development of the education and credentialing of these roles. The FNA's expert group involves members from several facets such as education, healthcare organizations, researchers, as well as collaborators from the Ministries of Social Affairs and Health and Education and Culture, thus involving valuable expertise and leveraging on role development.

9.8   Moving Forward: Challenges and Opportunities

Some of the role and practice *challenges* for APN in Finland include further development of the scope of practice for CNSs as well as for NPs. The educational preparation/curriculum for these new advanced clinical roles needs to answer to the challenges in patient population and the society. Educational preparation for advanced clinical nursing requires high educator competencies in clinical nursing and clinical nursing science. It also requires strong educational collaboration with the medical faculty members and clinicians. Moreover, there is a need to develop continuous training possibilities for practicing CNSs to maintain and update their knowledge.

Despite recent progress on the CNS role and practice development in Finland, we still have many challenges ahead. In the future, we need to focus more closely to the clinical aspects of the advanced direct patient care and to further develop the implementation of full scope of APN and autonomous role to better answer to the needs of patient population and the society. Furthermore, we need to push for credentialing of these roles to foster the role and practice recognition and sustainability of these roles.

The role and practice *opportunities* of the CNSs are vast yet underutilized in Finland. There is great interest to develop and create these roles with the ongoing social and healthcare reform; thus the advanced nursing roles have a significant position in the production of future healthcare services. Significant factors for success are the influential national APN expert network engaged in advancing the APN role development and visibility. This work is supported by the involvement and close collaboration of Ministry of Social Affairs and Health and Ministry of Education and Culture in the development of the APN roles.

Furthermore, the research in the area of CNS role development and implementation is expanding rapidly. There is a growing body of national research on the CNS role and practice from master's to postdoctoral study. Funding is available for strong proposals on the CNS/APN research. Furthermore, the development and research of these roles is supported by the national legislation regulating the healthcare and healthcare professionals (Healthcare Professionals Act 1994, Health Care Act 2010) supporting the continuous efforts of CNS practice and role development.

9.9   Exemplar of Clinical Nurse Specialist Practice

9.9.1   Description of Neuroscience Specialty Practice

In specialist medical healthcare, the CNSs work usually within specialty patient population; however, CNS practice varies across different organizations. In some organizations, it has been specified that the CNS should spent 50% of time in clinical practice and 50% in other activities, but it is not the case in all of the organizations. Our example of specialty practice area comes from neuroscience nursing. The Neuro Center (NC) consists of 5 hospitals, with neurology or neurosurgery polyclinics and 14 wards. Surgery, emergency, and power control operations are mainly concentrated in main Helsinki University Hospital area. NC has 670 staff, of which 127 are doctors and 442 are nurses. The NC has almost 17,000 transcripts every year; it manages approximately 9500 emergency patients and makes approximately 3500 operations. The NC also has national responsibility for the leadership of the neuroscience specialty. One CNS works at the NC, where her practice focuses on facilitating EBP within the specialty, supporting the multidisciplinary team, and working at a system level to foster change. To enact these priorities, the CNS serves as an expert educator, consultant, transformational leader, a mentor, and a facilitator of research.

9.9.2   Exemplary CNS Project in the Specialty of Neuroscience

One exemplary CNS-led project relates to prevention of ventilator-associated pneumonia (VAP). The goal was to focus on VAP prevention by utilizing endotracheal tubes with subglottic secretion drainage ports for patients expected to require greater than 48 or 72 hours of mechanical ventilation. During the project, the CNS-led team developed a VAP prevention protocol (VAP-PP) and education program for NC. The CNS implemented the staff education, carefully explaining each VAP-PP step to the nursing staff to build up their skill and confidence level. During the initial implementation of the VAP-PP, it was important for the CNS, nurse manager, and the critical care physician to provide support for staff and lead by example to demonstrate the skills necessary to facilitate the desired change.

Another CNS-led project was the creation of the Nurses' Neuroscience Handbook (NNH) (2021). The idea was drawn from nursing students' quality improvement project. The goal of the NNH was to provide nurses an easy access guide related to neuroscience nursing, its policies, procedures, and outcomes. The NNH encompasses both research evidence and the silent knowledge gathered from the organization. The creation of the NNH actualized through series of steps and decisions. Today NNH works as an evidence-based road map for nurses on how to operate within neuroscience nursing. Standardized practice protocols, such as the NNH, incorporate evidence into the nursing practice and assist nurses to improve their performance.

9.9.3   Practice Competencies Used in the Projects

In the described projects, the CNS had a vital role in applying research evidence into nursing practice, educating and consulting staff, and leading the transformation of nursing practice. Moreover, several competencies were required to accomplish the projects' goals. The CNS utilized competencies within all of the spheres of patient, nursing, organization, and scholarship working in close collaboration with the multidisciplinary team within the NC.

9.9.4   Outcomes of CNS Practice Within the Projects

The VAP-PP was developed, implemented, and reinforced by the CNS-led team. The CNS leadership of the project was time-consuming and required extensive preparation for meetings, assisting nurses with their work, providing feedback to the units, and facilitating the multidisciplinary involvement in the project. Implementation of evidence-informed VAP prevention protocol reduced significantly the incidence of VAP.

Challenges in the implementation of the NNH existed at each stage of the process due to general opposition from multiple areas to practice change, as well as the diversity of specialties (such as neurosurgery and neurology) which had their own customs of practice. Despite the challenges, it is imperative to CNS practice to focus on providing the best possible care for patients. Implementing the NNH created an opportunity to engage staff nurses in EBP and to improve the care of patients by harmonizing and integrating the nursing practices within the NC. Nowadays, the NNH is widely used in other university hospitals in Finland. Next step is to develop digital NNH as a part of digital Health Village.

References

Arslanian-Engoren C, Struble L, Sullivan B (2011) An innovative approach to revising a clinical nurse specialist curriculum to meet core competencies in 3 specialty tracks (adult health, gerontology, and psychiatric-mental health). 2011 National Association of clinical nurse specialists National Conference Abstracts, Baltimore, Maryland, March 10 to 12. Clin Nurse Spec 25:77–77

Baldwin KM, Lyon BL, Clark AP, Fulton J, Davidson S, Dayhoff N (2007) Developing clinical nurse specialist practice competencies. Clin Nurse Spec 21:297–303

Bryant-Lukosius D, Carter N, Kilpatrick K, Martin-Misener R, Donald F, Kaasalainen S et al (2010) The clinical nurse specialist role in Canada. Nurs Leadersh 23:140–166

CNA (2014) Pan-Canadian core competencies for the clinical nurse specialist. https://www.cna-aiic.ca/~/media/cna/files/en/clinical_nurse_specialists_convention_handout_e.pdf?la=en. Accessed 15 May 2018

Donabedian A (2005) Evaluating the quality of medical care. Milbank Q 83:691–729

Fagerström L (2009) Developing the scope of practice and education for advanced practice nurses in Finland. Int Nurs Rev 56:269–272

Fagerström L, Glasberg A (2011) The first evaluation of the advanced practice nurse role in Finland—the perspective of nurse leaders. J Nurs Manag 19:925–932

Gardner A, Hase S, Gardner G, Dunn SV, Carryer J (2008) From competence to capability: a study of nurse practitioners in clinical practice. J Clin Nurs 17:250–258

Hase S, Davis L From competence to capability: the implications for human resource development and management. Paper presented to Millennial challenges in management, education, cybertechnology, and leadership: Association of International Management, 17th Annual Conference, San Diego, 6–8 August 1999. https://epubs.scu.edu.au/cgi/viewcontent.cgi?referer=https://scholar.google.ca/&httpsredir=1&article=1126&context=gcm_pubs. Accessed 15 May 2018

Healthcare Professionals Act. No. 559/1994. [English]. http://www.finlex.fi/en/laki/kaannokset/1994/en19940559.pdf. Accessed 15 May 2018

Health Care Act. No. 1326/2010. [English]. https://www.finlex.fi/fi/laki/kaannokset/2010/en20101326_20131293.pdf. Accessed 22 April 2021

Hukkanen E, Vallimes-Patomäki M Co-operation and Division of Labour in securing access to care. A survey of the pilot projects on Labour Division carried out within the National Health Care Project. Reports of the Ministry of Social Affairs and Health: 21, Finland. 2005

ICN. International Council of Nurses (2014) Definition of nurse practitioner/advance practice nurse. Definition and characteristics of the role. http://international.aanp.org/Practice/APNRoles. Accessed 15 May 2018

Jokiniemi K (2014) Clinical nurse specialist role in Finnish Health Care. Doctoral dissertation, University of Eastern Finland. http://epublications.uef.fi/pub/urn_isbn_978-952-61-1579-5/urn_isbn_978-952-61-1579-5.pdf. Accessed 15 May 2018

Jokiniemi K (2018) Advanced practice nursing roles—towards optimal role utilization. Pro Terveys. [Finnish]

Jokiniemi K, Haatainen K, Pietilä A (2014) Advanced practice nursing roles: the phases of the successful role implementation process. Int J Caring Sci 7:946

Jokiniemi K, Haatainen K, Meretoja R, Pietilä A (2015a) The future of the clinical nurse specialist role in Finland. J Nurs Scholarsh 47:78–86

Jokiniemi K, Haatainen K, Pietilä A (2015b) From challenges to advanced practice registered nursing role development: qualitative interview study. Int J Nurs Pract 21:896–903

Jokiniemi K, Pietilä A, Meretoja R (2018) Constructing content validity of clinical nurse specialist core competencies. Scand J Caring Sci 32(4):1428–1436

Jokiniemi K, Suutarla A, Meretoja R, Kotila J, Axelin A, Flinkman M, Fagerström L (2020) Evidence-informed policymaking: modelling nurses' career pathway from registered nurse to advanced practice nurse. Int J Nurs Pract 26(1):e12777. https://doi.org/10.1111/ijn.12777

Jokiniemi K, Pietilä AM, Mikkonen S (2020) Construct validity of clinical nurse specialist core competency scale: an exploratory factor analysis. J Clin Nurs https://doi.org/10.1111/jocn.15587

Kilpatrick K, Tchouaket E, Carter N, Bryant-Lukosius D, DiCenso A (2016) Structural and process factors that influence clinical nurse specialist role implementation. Clin Nurse Spec 30:89–100

Kotila J, Axelin A, Fagerström L, Flinkman M, Heikkinen K, Jokiniemi K et al (2016) New roles for nurses—quality to future social welfare and health care services. Publication of the Finnish Nurses Association, Helsinki

Kotila J, Salonen A, Meretoja R (2018) Competence framework clarifies work roles. Pro Terveys. [Finnish]

Meretoja R, Vuorinen R (2000) Clinical nurse specialist in clinical practice. Sairaanhoitaja 73:24–25. [Finnish]

Meretoja R, Kaira A, Puualainen A, Santala I, Vuorinen R (2002) Asiantuntijasairaanhoitaja muutoksen tekijä kliinisessä hoitotyössä. Clinical nurse specialist: a change-maker in clinical nursing. Sairaanhoitaja 75:8–9. [Finnish]

Ministry of Social Affairs and Health, Finland Healthcare Professionals Act. No. 559/1994. [English]. http://www.finlex.fi/en/laki/kaannokset/1994/en19940559.pdf. Accessed 15 May 2018

Ministry of Social Affairs and Health, Finland. Health Care Act. No. 1326/2010. [English]. http://www.finlex.fi/en/laki/kaannokset/2010/en20101326.pdf. Accessed 15 May 2018

MSAH (2012) Koulutuksella osaamista asiakaskeskeisiin ja moniammatillisiin palveluihin. Ehdotukset hoitotyön toimintaohjelman pohjalta. Publications of the Ministry of Social Affairs and Health vol 7, pp 1–29. [Finnish] https://julkaisut.valtioneuvosto.fi/bitstream/handle/10024/71627/URN%3ANBN%3Afi-fe201504224497.pdf?sequence=1. Accessed 15 May 2018

Nurses' Neuroscience Handbook. Publications of The Neuro Center. Helsinki University Hospital, Helsinki 2021

OECD.Stat (2018). http://stats.oecd.org/index.aspx?DataSetCode=HEALTH_STAT. Accessed 15 May 2018

Sheer B, Wong F (2008) The development of advanced nursing practice globally. J Nurs Scholarsh 40:204–211

Suominen T, Leino-Kilpi H (1995) More expertise to nursing. Sairaanhoitaja 68:35–36. [Finnish]

Viholainen K (2018) Nurses' expertise in advanced practice nursing in specialised medical care. Master's thesis, University of Eastern Finland. [Finnish]

From the Nurse Specialist in Clinical Nursing to the Advanced Practice Nurse with Prescribing Rights: The French Case

10

Christophe Debout

Abstract

Advanced practice nursing was officially recognized in France in 2018. This legislative development marks the culmination of a process that originated in the late 1980s in a project led by the nursing profession to promote the development of clinical nursing expertise. However, this recognition was only possible after lengthy negotiations whose main objective was to adopt a strategy to guarantee the population access to care in a context of increased demand and medical shortages. Now that this legislative step has been taken, the goal is to introduce the first advanced practice nurses in practice environments, to sustain this type of practice and to allow it to develop in order to effectively meet the needs of the population while maintaining this new function in the nursing realm.

Keywords

French nursing · Clinical nurse specialist · Certified nurse clinician · French advanced practice nurse

---

This chapter has been written before the 2020 APN ICN guidelines were published and reflects the views of the authors.

C. Debout (✉)
IFITS, Paris, France

Sciences Po Paris, Paris, France

© Springer Nature Switzerland AG 2021
J. S. Fulton, V. W. Holly (eds.), *Clinical Nurse Specialist Role and Practice*,
Advanced Practice in Nursing, https://doi.org/10.1007/978-3-319-97103-2_10

10.1   Introduction

France is often better known abroad for the universal health coverage offered to its population than for the nature of the specific contribution nurses make to the health system (World Health Organization 2000).

The profile of the modern nurse, introduced in France in 1878, has been described by Poisson as the "French republican model" (Poisson 1998). Its characteristics were shaped by the political, demographic, social and medical context of the France of the Third Republic, which was marked in particular by a fundamentally anticlerical government (Poisson 1998).

This model breaks with the organization of French healthcare institutions which, until that period, was entrusted to religious congregations such as the Daughters of Charity of Saint Vincent de Paul or the Augustinian Sisters of the Hôtel Dieu in Paris (Leroux-Hugon 1992).

Initially very dependent on the medical profession which had been at the origin of its creation, the nursing group followed a slow process of professionalization. This process began at the end of the First World War under the impetus of an emblematic figure in the French nursing pantheon: Léonie Chaptal (Debout and Magnon 2014).

The apogee of this movement of emancipation and affirmation of the nursing profession in the field of health will be observed especially during the last quarter of the twentieth century.

It will manifest itself in different fields: organization of nursing care, nursing leadership in hospital management, reform of education but also development of clinical nursing. The development of the clinical nursing practice observed in France since the beginning of the 1990s can be considered as one of the factors for asserting the specificity of the nursing perspective and positioning this function in the multi-professional team (Debout 2014). This initiative will be one of the major factors that will foster the emergence of the concept of advanced nursing practice in France. Nurses involved in the development of clinical nursing will strive to ensure that advanced practice is not only understood as a palliative to the medical shortage in a substitution logic but also as an innovative nursing role constituting a new link in the patient care chain.

It will take more than 16 years of discussions, consultations and experimentations before the legislator finally decides to introduce advanced nursing practice in France at a time when the supply of care, particularly in the medical field, has continued to deteriorate. The profile of advanced practice nurses introduced in France in 2018 focuses on a specific area of intervention, currently there are four, but this number will probably change in the years to come in order to adapt to the needs of the population and the inadequacies of the healthcare supply. Compared with the international reference frameworks defined by the International Council of Nurses (ICN) Advanced Practice Nurse Network (Schober 2016), the advanced practice nurse as defined in France is very similar to the profile of clinical nurse specialist. In France, the advanced practice nurse certainly has autonomy and the authority to prescribe, or more precisely to renew or adapt a prescription, but his/her autonomy is still very much supervised by the physician who refers the patient to her and is not positioned as a first-line healthcare provider (Debout 2018).

After clarifying a few elements relating to the context of health in France and the characteristics of the nursing profession in this country, the factors that will lead to the introduction into French legislation of advanced practice for nurses during the summer of 2018 will be specified, in particular the development of clinical nursing. The many challenges that remain to be met in the introduction phase of advanced practice nurses will finally be identified, in particular the evaluation of the service provided.

10.2   Health in France

Before outlining the contribution made by the nursing profession to the supply of care in France and identifying the characteristics of advanced practice nursing, it is appropriate to present the main characteristics of the French health context, focusing on identifying the needs and expectations of the population in this field, but also the organization of the supply of care and the structure of the health professions.

The state of health of the population living in France is generally good. Life expectancy in 2015 was 85 years for women and 78.9 years for men. These figures are constantly rising. Cancers and cardiovascular diseases are the most frequent causes of death (27.6 and 25.1%) in France (Directorate of Research 2017).

However, high-risk health behaviours can be observed in the population, particularly in terms of nutrition and tobacco consumption. Similarly, heavy alcohol consumption among young people is a cause for concern (Research Directorate 2017).

France's economic situation influences the health status of its population. Significant differences are noted between the well-off social classes and those in a more precarious financial situation; the latter have a combination of risk factors (Direction de la recherche 2017).

In addition, disparities are observed in health between French regions, which impact on the life span of individuals.

10.2.1 Organization of the Health System and Healthcare Provision in France

The French health system and social security have provided the population with universal health coverage since the end of the Second World War (Tabuteau 2013). The approach adopted for many years favoured curative rather than preventive care (OECD 2017). Highly hospital-centred, the health system has long given primacy to university hospitals. Its governance is now guided by the principles of New Public Management applied to the health sector (Simonet 2014). The provision of care in the community is largely based on the private practice of physicians, nurses and other health professionals. The notion of the healthcare team in the community is therefore fragmented.

Changes in the demographic and epidemiological characteristics of the French population have necessitated a profound reorientation of the healthcare system in recent years. An ambulatory shift has been initiated in order to better meet the health needs of an aging population increasingly affected by non-communicable diseases but also to reduce health expenditures (Debout 2016).

This reform has profoundly transformed healthcare institutions; a hyper-concentration of supply is underway in hospital superstructures (Vigneron 2018). The search for productivity gains is very significant in these hospitals, making environments less and less favourable to the practice of professionals (Brami et al. 2012). The result is high turnover in teams and an increase in the incidence of burn-out phenomena (Desailly-Chanson et al. 2016).

10.2.2 Structure of the Health Professions

The model that structures the health professions in France can be described as old-fashioned. It gives primacy to the physician, who is always placed as first-line provider in the health system.

The other health professions are subject to medical authority and are referred to as "medical auxiliaries" in the Public Health Code. Although some professions, such as nurses or physiotherapists, have an autonomous role since 1978, they are still considered auxiliary professions.

The contribution made by nurses to the system is significant: there are more than 600,000 nurses in France working in a wide variety of environments (DREES 2018). However, there are only three nursing specialties recognized in the Public Health Code (childcare nurse, nurse anaesthetist and operating room nurse). This very small number of nursing specialties is surprising given that hospital care environments are increasingly specialized (Mossé 2018); the notion of versatility is favoured for nurses in order to facilitate human resource management. A large majority of nurses are employed in the public sector (DREES 2018). Most home care nursing care is provided by nurses who practise independently (Bourgueil et al. 2005). The nursing profession obtained a self-regulating body in 2006, the National Nursing Order.

On the other hand, the academization of nursing education started very late. It was not until 2009 that a bachelor's degree was required to enter the nursing profession. This delay impeded the development of nursing research capacity.

France does not currently have a nursing shortage. However, a prospective study points out that the system will have to increase its nursing workforce by more than 50% by 2040 in order to cope with increasing healthcare needs (DREES 2018).

The current and future challenges that the healthcare system will have to face in order to meet the growing needs of the population will be a major challenge.

10.3   The Development of Clinical Nursing: The Roots of Advanced Nursing Practice

To fully use the autonomy given to nurse by legislation, it was necessary to offer them additional education enabling them to reflect on their practice and to use theoretical frameworks developed by the nursing discipline. It was the prerequisite to redefine their professional contribution within the multi-professional team and to use their autonomous therapeutic role for the benefit of patients and their relatives. It was also necessary to promote the development of clinical nursing expertise in practice environments.

10.3.1 The Origins of a Project

The development of the clinical nursing began in the 1980s in response to the changing needs and expectations of the population in terms of health and nursing care but also to the aspirations of nurses.

This project was launched jointly between French-speaking Switzerland and France under the impetus of Rosette Poletti, a Swiss nurse (Debout 2014).

10.3.2 Shaping a Profile

The targeted profile was influenced by the clinical nurse specialist function that has been established for many years in North America. It directs the activity of this type of nurse, certainly towards patients and their families but also towards healthcare professionals and organizations. The aim is for these nurses to be change agent and to make a significant contribution to continuous quality improvement and risk management. This clinical curriculum represents a new type of career pathway for nurses outside of management or education.

When it was created, the clinical career pathway was conceived as gradual including three levels spread over several years:

- Level 1: Certified Clinical Nurse
- Level 2: Clinical nurse specialist (in French the term was translated as "infirmière spécialiste clinique" in France which means "nurse specialist in clinical nursing") the transformative power of this function is emphasized within nursing teams in order to change the organization of care and the practice of nurses.
- Level 3: Nurse consultant
  A rather generalist approach was preferred even if some more specialised training courses have also been proposed, notably in the field of cancerology.

10.3.3 Characteristics of the Curriculum

The modular curriculum, spread over several years, is implemented on a part-time basis; allowing the nursing to reain on her job, which favours the integration of the contents.

The programme is mainly offered by private school working outside the academic environment. Numerous attempts to establish partnerships with French and foreign universities have not yielded positive results.

Nurses who benefit from this programme develop the skills enabling them to fully invest the autonomy granted to their profession with the aim of improving the care provided to patients and achieving positive care results in a global approach to their health. One of the major objectives of this type of programme is to increase the level of expertise of clinical reasoning and to promote the use of nursing taxonomies, particularly nursing diagnoses, in order to clarify nurses' clinical judgements. The autonomous therapeutic role of the nurse is strongly developed in the programme.

This programme is characterized by a strong porosity to the knowledge produced by the nursing discipline that provides nurses with theoretical frameworks for their clinical practice. The contribution of physicians in this programme is almost non-existent.

In addition to these purely clinical contents, the programme also encourages nurses to acquire a systemic understanding of organizations. It develops in the trainees the skills required to support the professional development of healthcare teams and to exercise effective clinical leadership that facilitates the introduction of innovation and support for change in healthcare sectors.

The final certification is organized before a jury of peers, which was initially international in nature.

10.3.4 A Formal Recognition of the Role That Was Narrowly Missed

In 1995, as part of the reform of the education programme of nurse managers, consideration was given to giving statutory and financial recognition to nurses who became certified in clinical nursing. Unfortunately, this project could not become a reality. A French society of clinical nurses having registered the title of clinical nurse, the reaction of schools wishing to continue offering these programmes was not long in coming, opening up legal proceedings for many years before a decision was handed down in their favour.

In this context of internal tension within the profession, the Ministry of Health decided to refrain from recognizing this role. 1995 therefore remains the year of missed opportunity for clinical nurse specialists.

10.3.5 Difficult Census of Certified Clinical Nurse Specialists

It is difficult to identify certified professionals at the various levels of the clinical career pathway; it should be remembered that the law establishing a National Order of Nurses dates only from 2006 (Hamel 2008). However, it can be estimated that many nurses have been certified at level 1, much fewer at level 2 and a very small number at level 3 (ANFIIDE 2016).

The majority of these nurses have reinvested the knowledge and skills gained from this programme in their clinical practice, whether they are employed or working in private practice.

10.3.6 Reinvestment of Clinical Competencies in Healthcare Environments

This type of programme has been attractive to nurses. While nurses initially enrol in these courses on an individual basis, the positive results obtained by certified nurses led hospitals to set up in-service training programmes in order to certify many nurses in the hospital.

There was no shortage of opportunities for reinvestment, as many changes were introduced in the healthcare sector during this period requiring clinical nursing expertise.

Examples include public health plans focusing on pain management, AIDS, the development of palliative care or cancer care. The increase in the prevalence and incidence of patients living with a chronic disease has also created new needs that clinical nurse specialists could meet, particularly in the area of therapeutic education.

In addition, the introduction of hospital accreditation in the late 1990s made it necessary to rely on this type of nurse prepared to implement the continuous quality improvement process.

Despite the added value generated by clinical nurse specialists, they did not obtain legislation change and financial recognition commensurate with their investment. The great majority of them did not agree to remain on the status quo of 1995.

A specific common interest group was created at the beginning of 2000 within the national nursing association (ANFIIDE); it quickly took the name of Advanced Practice Nursing Network (RéPASI). The work of this group is mainly based on the publications of the Advanced Practice Nurse Network of the International Council of Nurses.

10.4 From Clinical Nursing to Advanced Practice in Nursing

In a context marked by a search for a better match between the supply and demand for care, two dynamics have converged since the early 2000s to lead to the introduction of advanced practice in French legislation and regulations, which was achieved in July 2018. These two trends take a different view of the concept of advanced practice.

The first initiative emanates from nursing professionals who aspire to develop their clinical expertise. This desire results from the evolution of patients' needs (complex situations, end-of-life support, support for people living with a chronic disease, etc.) and the process of professionalization of the nursing group. This movement has its origins in the development of the clinical career pathway and in the positions taken by the professional organizations of clinical nurse and clinical nurse specialists, in particular the RéPASI. Advanced practice is approached by the nursing profession as a strategy that could bring a nursing contribution to the problem of access to care while encouraging the development of nursing expertise for the benefit of patients. Frames of reference developed by ICN nurse practitioner/advanced practice nursing network and lessons learned from foreign experiences in this field were integrated into this vision of advanced practice carried by the nursing profession.

The second initiative, which emerged in the early 2000s, approaches advanced practice as an effective strategy to address the problem of medical shortages. This shortage is the consequence of the application of a very strict *numerus clausus* at the end of the first year of medical studies coupled with the complete freedom left to young physicians to choose where they wish to practise in France, even though their university training is largely subsidized by the state within public universities. The main aim of this strategy is to save medical time by transferring to other professionals activities that were previously the exclusive medical prerogative of the state. This vision of advanced practice is influenced by the concept of task shifting introduced by the WHO (World Health Organization 2007). These recommendations were formulated in a report written in 2003 by Professor Berland, Dean of the Faculty of Medicine of Marseille (Berland 2003).

The bibliographical search carried out in the context of the preparation of this report highlighted the benefits of advanced nursing practice in the countries that have implemented it. However, the proponents of this trend retain only certain characteristics of the concept. The approach remains strongly centred on the patient's health problem addressed primarily from the biophysical perspective and often omits the added value of the holistic nursing approach centred on the patient's experience that characterizes advanced practice.

It can therefore be observed that a plural vision of advanced practice animates the stakeholders involved in the reflection aimed at evaluating the relevance of its introduction in the French context. However, political decision-makers seem much more influenced by the second current in their understanding of the concept.

10.5   Experimentations and Lengthy Negotiations

Changing the structure of the health professions and transferring to "medical auxiliaries" activities previously exclusively implemented by physicians is always a sensitive subject in France. For some physicians and for many medical professional organizations, in particular the private practice physicians' unions, it gives rise to a feeling of loss of monopoly in the field of health and, for some, potential financial loss as well. Didier Tabuteau points out that this fear might be linked to the history of the medical profession, which lost its monopoly during the French Revolution with the creation of health officers (Tabuteau 2012); it took a century to the medical profession to recover it at the end of the nineteenth century, and now they want to keep it.

This highly political subject has, in fact, undergone many changes in line with the orientations of successive governments during the 15 years of discussions surrounding this project.

Reports and experiments have multiplied, generating a significant latency in decision-making. In 2011 in particular, the Hénart-Berland-Cadet report nevertheless stressed the urgency of reaching decisions in this field in view of the constant increase in the population's health needs and the growing difficulties of access to care (Hénart et al. 2011). This latency has had harmful consequences in clinical environments, forcing professionals to find solutions to the difficulties encountered, even if it means going beyond their scope of practice, as highlighted by the public survey conducted by the HAS in 2007 (Haute Autorité de Santé 2007).

In 2009, as part of the adoption of a broader public health law, an article introduced the concept of cooperation between health professionals based on protocols (Ministry of Health 2009). These protocols, drafted by the professionals concerned at local level (hospital, health centre, etc.), must be validated by the Regional Health Agency (ARS) and the High Authority for Health (HAS). The aim of this article was to legalize the transfer of activities by describing them in an explicit protocol. This mechanism is directly inspired by the concept of task shifting introduced in 2007 by the WHO (World Health Organization 2007). However, the methodology imposed to draft a protocol is very cumbersome to implement by teams wishing to engage in a project of this nature. Moreover, the nominative nature of these protocols sometimes creates difficulties for professionals and institutions in terms of continuity of care provision. Indeed, if the delegator (the physician) or the delegate (e.g. the nurse) is absent, the activity can no longer be implemented. Similarly, a nurse forced to move to another hospital for personal reasons does not retain the benefit of the skills developed in the position he/she just left. There was no economic model attached to this type of practice until 2019: a nurse who develops these complementary skills and implements these derogatory activities does not receive additional remuneration. Finally, the additional education required to develop the skills needed to implement the activity delegated by the physician is very focused on the intervention and does not necessarily include the development of nursing expertise, which would be essential for the effective implementation of a protocol of this nature in a patient-centred approach. These shortcomings were identified in the evaluations of the methodology carried out by the HAS (Haute Autorité de Santé 2015). However, and despite these shortcomings, this system will be maintained; the methodology will simply be simplified (Ministry of Solidarity and Health 2018a). These cooperation protocols have been criticized by many professional organizations, including the National Nursing Order. Implemented in conjunction with the discussions on the introduction of advanced nursing practice, this project has created a lot of confusion, creating the false impression that any nurse included in a cooperation protocol could be considered an advanced practice nurse.

As the publication of legislation introducing advanced practice in nursing was repeatedly announced as imminent by successive ministers of health but was repeatedly postponed until later, some universities wanted to take the lead in anticipating the education of future advanced practice nurses. Two master's programmes dedicated to advanced practice have thus been proposed by two French universities. In the absence of legislation defining the function of advanced practice nurse in France and in order to avoid encouraging nurses for the illegal practice of medicine, the expected profile of these programmes was that of clinical nurse specialist, but the commonly used name was advanced practice nurse. From 2012, the political changes that have taken place lead the ministers of health and higher education to veto the development of other programmes of this type in the absence of legislation governing advanced practice in France.

In 2016, a study performed by ANFIIDE identified approximately 103 nurses graduated from these programmes (ANFIIDE 2016). The introduction of these professionals in often unprepared practice environments has made it difficult for them to reinvest the gains they have made from their master's and has led many of them to feel frustrated. In addition, some of these advanced practice nurses have integrated a cooperation protocol in order to benefit from a legal framework for their practice.

These phenomena have increased the confusion between advanced practice and cooperation protocol in the French context.

Finally, the Ile-de-France Regional Health Agency (ARS) launched an initiative in 2014, the PREFICS project, with the aim of encouraging hospitals and health centres in this region to create advanced practice nursing positions. Some master's degree programmes were identified within the framework of this project in order to prepare the future nurses included in this initiative, but great heterogeneity can be observed in these programmes (Agence Régionale de Santé-Ile-de-France 2016).

It should be noted that all of these professionals coming from different educational pathways considered themselves to be in advanced practice.

10.6   A Lengthy Process of Developing Legislation and Regulations for Advanced Nursing Practice

Article 119 of the law on the modernization of the health system voted in 2016 (Safon 2016) was obtained after long negotiations; in the future it will allow all professions qualified as "medical auxiliaries" to get access to advanced practice. Many professional organizations have worked to achieve this outcome, targeting not only decision-makers but also the nursing profession in all its diversity.

After this law was passed, the aim was to maintain lobbying activities on the subject in order to obtain text to implement this article of the law.

It took almost a year for the Ministry of Health to begin the process of drafting these texts.

A first step towards this goal has been taken from December 2016 to April 2017. The Ministry of Health has set up a large group of experts in a process that was announced as "participatory". Hearings of professionals and managers from clinical environments have been organized in order to better identify needs but also to identify innovations in this field. Many graduates from the two clinical master's programmes were thus able to present their approach to care to this group of experts. The experiences gathered were diverse, hospital, ambulatory and occupational health sectors, and addressed somatic as well as psychiatric health problems. However, the Ministry of Health did not wish to involve the three existing nursing specialties in the reflection on the introduction of advanced practice creating a profound resentment.

Following these hearings, a final meeting was held in April 2017 during which a draft text was presented by the representatives of the Ministry of Health to the experts of the working group. The latter considered that the proposals made did not reflect the work of the group stressing that the Ministry of Health opted for a very restrictive vision of advanced practice imposing a strong dependency of advanced practice nurses to the medical authority. This proposal was rejected by the nursing representatives.

French political events then interrupted this work for several months. After the election of a new President and a new National Assembly as well as the appointment of a new government in the first half of 2017, the debate only resumed in the autumn of 2017 part of a national plan to improve access to healthcare (Ministry of Solidarity and Health 2017).

However, the methodology adopted by the new ministers in charge of the project was different from the previous one. Three very tight groups were set up and a very tight schedule was imposed on them. The number of nurses around the negotiating table was small.

The first group, led by the Ministry of Health, was tasked with drafting the texts governing the practice of advanced practice nurses. Areas of tension were quickly identified during the negotiation process within this group, particularly about the lack of positioning first-line healthcare provider, the autonomy granted to advanced practice nurses, etc. The areas of certification selected were also the subject of controversy. The initial project planned to propose four areas of certification: chronic disease, oncology/hemato-oncology, chronic kidney disease/dialysis/renal transplantation and psychiatry/mental health. However, despite the major needs identified in the area of psychiatry and mental healthcare provision in France, representatives of psychiatrists refused to introduce advanced practice nurses in this field. In order not to delay the publication of the texts, the Ministry of Health decided to create three areas in 2018 and to continue negotiations for an additional year for the psychiatry and mental health area.

The second group was led by the Ministry of Higher Education and Research. The aim was to define the curriculum in order to be alabl to admit first students in autumn 2018. A list of activities and a competency framework (Fig. 10.1) were

1. Assess the health status of patients as a relay for medical consultations for identified pathologies.

2. Define and implement the patient's care plan based on the overall assessment of the patient's state of health.

3. Design and implement prevention and therapeutic education actions.

4. Organising patient care and health pathways in collaboration with all the actors concerned.

5. Implement and conduct actions to evaluate and improve professional practices by exercising clinical leadership.

6. Research, analyse and produce professional and scientific data

Fig. 10.1 French advanced practice nurse competency framework

developed as well as a national curriculum which sets out the broad outlines of the educational pathway advanced practice nursing students must follow. The criteria for university accreditation have also been defined.

Finally, the third group's mission was to propose an economic model that would enable this type of exercise to be paid.

It should be noted that all of these texts were prepared quickly in order to meet the ambitious timetable set by the government. The first two groups began their work at the same time, while the third group was postponed.

Moreover, in the context of the final validation of these draft texts, the High Council of Paramedical Professions (HCPP), which brings together representatives of the professions qualified as "medical auxiliaries", did not give its approval, considering them insufficiently ambitious.

Despite this lack of validation by this consultative body, the implementing texts were published in July 2018. They were then amended in August 2019 in order to introduce the field of psychiatry-mental health certification finally accepted by psychiatrists after an additional year of negotiations.

10.7 Summary of the Texts Published in July 2018 and August 2019 Defining the Advanced Practice Nursing Practice

The implementation texts, published in July 2018 and amended in August 2019, are based on the elements already set by Article 119 of the law on the modernization of our health system voted in 2016 (Ministère des Affaires Sociales et de la Santé 2016).

The advanced practice nurse in France is therefore governed by one law (Ministère des Affaires Sociales et de la Santé 2016), two decrees (Ministère de l'enseignement supérieur, de la recherche et de l'innovation 2018; Ministère des solidarités et de la santé 2018b) and three acts (Ministère des solidarités et de la santé 2018c, d; Ministère des solidarités et de la santé-Ministère de l'enseignement supérieur, de la recherche et de l'innovation 2018). They establish a specific protected title for this role.

An analysis of these texts reveals the salient aspects of the advanced practice nurse profile in France.

- The advanced practice nurse must necessarily be part of a team, and his/her activity is therefore interdependent with that of the other members of the team he/she works with in a hospital or in the community.
- Advanced practice nurse can be employed in the public (civilian sector as well as in the military health service) or private sector; he/she can as well work in private practice.
- The advanced practice nurse's scope of practice is broader than that of other nurses; they have prescribing authority. However, the autonomy granted to this category of nurses is supervised by the physician who decides to refer patients with stabilized chronic disease to an advanced practice nurse. Patients may refuse this proposition. The physician identifies beforehand patient's diagnosis and prescribes the treatment. The advanced practice nurse organizes the patient's care pathway.

An organization protocol written and signed by the physician and the advanced practice nurse determines their methods of intervention and collaboration. Within this collaborative practice with the physician, the advanced practice nurse is responsible for its decisions and actions.

An advanced practice nurse is certified in one of the four areas of intervention currently defined by the texts:

- Stabilized chronic disease, prevention and common polypathologies in primary care
- Oncology and hemato-oncology
- Chronic kidney disease, dialysis, kidney transplantation
- Psychiatry-mental health

Any patient with a pathology included in one of these fields can benefit from the intervention of an advanced practice nurse regardless of age if his/her condition is deemed stable by his physician.

More specifically, advanced practice nurse's activities fall into two categories: clinical and focused on team/organisation.

10.7.1 Clinical Activities

Advanced practice nurse's area of certification determines the nature of the clinical activities that the nurse can implement in the follow-up of patients living with a chronic disease considered to be stabilized who are referred to it by a physician. The nurse mobilizes his/her skills with the aim of working with the patient to maintain this state of stability by implementing a wide range of activities:

- Preventive activities, in particular therapeutic education of the patient
- Renewal or adaptation of the treatment plan initially prescribed by the physician

- Prescription of diagnostic tests (lab test, X-ray, etc.) in order to support the nurse's clinical reasoning or that of the physician (the list of tests that an advanced practice nurse is authorized to prescribe is set by an act)
- Performance of specific technical procedures
- Prescription of nursing care provided by home care nurses
- Referral of patients to the appropriate health professional to meet their needs

In addition, advanced practice nurse implements activities relating to the clinic within the framework of the missions assigned to it.

10.7.2 Activities Focused on Team/Organisation

They are essentially team-centred and aim to improve the quality and safety of care as well as individual/team performance.

The range of activities that the advanced practice nurse can implement to achieve this objective is varied: knowledge transfer to staff, promotion of evidence-based nursing, implementation of continuous quality improvement and risk management process, introduction of clinical innovations, continuous professional development of nurse, contribution to research, etc.

In hospitals, these activities are implemented in the context of a collaborative practice established with nurse managers.

10.8 Curriculum

Section 119 of the law passed in 2016 insisted on the need to validate qualifying programme to obtain the title of advanced practice nurse. This programme must be provided in a university setting. Universities (schools of medicine) wishing to offer this type of programme must be accredited by the Ministry of Higher Education, Research and Innovation (MESRI).

A decree and an act set the outline of the national curriculum. The curriculum is based on a competency-based approach.

The curriculum published in 2018 includes innovative elements in the nursing education scheme. In order to respect the autonomy of universities, flexibility has thus been left to the faculties in the implementation of the national curriculum, and the pedagogical choices are validated by the university internal authorities. The final certification is issued by the university.

Flexibility can be introduced in particular in:

- The design of the pedagogical project based on the curriculum
- The modalities of implementation of the programme (face-to-face, distance learning or mixed model)
- The student selection process
- The summative evaluation framework

For the first time in France, a curriculum dedicated for nurses will be fully implemented by the university (faculties of medicine), while preregistration nursing education (baccalaureate level) and graduate programme for nurse anaesthetists are implemented within the framework of a partnership between the school of nursing and the university. Physicians and nurses will contribute their respective skills to the programme in both its theoretical and clinical components.

At the end of the programme, the student receives a state diploma that allows him/her to practise in advanced practice (protected title), and the level of study that he/she has attained is recognized at the master's degree level, but the national master's degree is not awarded.

The implementation of this programme is evaluated by the High Council for the Evaluation of Research and Higher Education (HCERES) as part of the periodic evaluation of all the missions and activities of the university concerned.

10.8.1 Selection of Students

The methods of selection of students differ from those previously used in nursing education. No annual admission quota is set at either national or regional level. Each university determines its students intake capacity according to the educational resources it is able to mobilize.

The selection process is determined by each university in accordance with the criteria and procedures determined by the university itself. Only one condition is imposed at national level: the candidate must have a nursing diploma or an equivalent title giving him/her authorization to practise in France.

Another particularity of the selection process is the possibility to enter in the programme directly after the preregistration course. However, in this situation, the newly graduated will only be able to practise as an advanced practice nurse after obtaining a diploma if he/she attests to a minimum of 3 years of experience as a nurse.

A validation of prior learning is possible allowing direct entry into semester 3. Nurses with a master's degree in clinical nursing can, if they wish, apply to take advantage of this pathway. However, no specific collective measures (grandfathering) have been planned for this candidate profile, so they must undertake an individual approach, the results of which are linked to their career path but also to their ability to make the most of it in the resumé they write.

10.8.2 Programme Structure

The programme is Y-shaped and is spread over four semesters. Clinically oriented teaching units are predominant in this programme, given the centrality of this type of activity to the work of advanced practice nurse.

It is implemented by a teaching team made up of physician/nurse pairs.

Semesters 1 and 2 constitute the common core of the programme. A 2 months of clinical internship is scheduled during the second semester.

At the end of the second semester, the student selects the domain in which he/she wishes to be certified at the end of the programme.

Semesters 3 and 4 are specific to each domain.

During semester 3, clinical teaching remains central. Students can deepen their knowledge and apply their skills in their chosen field of practice, thus reinforcing fundamental knowledge and developing mastery of clinical reasoning as well as skills to efficiently coordinate a pathway of patients.

Semester 4 has a different format; students need to perform a 4-month internship and must write a master's thesis allowing students to implement the research process while benefiting from supervision.

10.8.3 Clinical Internships

The two internships allow students to benefit from the integration of theory and practice. The student also benefits from tutoring during the internship period implemented by a pair of physician and nurse.

The first clinical placement, of a minimum duration of 2 months, must be validated during semester 2. It allows the student to understand the activities and the scope of the role he or she aspires to exercise. This internship also allows him/her to develop skills in clinical reasoning, in particular the performance of clinical examinations.

The second internship, carried out during semester 4, lasts a minimum of 4 months. This internship should enable the student to reinvest the clinical knowledge acquired during the previous semesters in a specific clinical domain. In addition, it enables the student to implement all the missions assigned to advanced practice nurse, particularly activities dedicated for healthcare teams, by exercising effective clinical leadership.

10.8.4 The Master's Thesis

An important part of semester 4 is devoted to activities related to the thesis to be completed by the student under the supervision of a nurse or an advanced practice nurse.

The curriculum offers four modalities for the realization of this master's thesis:

- A literature review
- An analysis of professional practices
- A critical analysis, based on clinical experience, inspired by a specific theoretical framework
- A research study

At the end of their programme, students are awarded a state diploma as well as a master's degree attesting to the academic level reached by the university where they studied. In this system, the structure that prepares the student is the same as that which certifies the advanced practice nurse.

Equipped with this professional title, the newly graduated advanced practice nurse can then register his or her new qualification with the Nursing Order and practise his or her role.

10.9   Stakeholder Reactions After the Publication of the Texts

The publication of the texts governing the practice and education of advanced practice nurse has generated a great deal of reactions.

Curiously, patient associations have expressed little opinion on this subject.

On the other hand, there was no lack of reactions from medical professional organizations. The unions of private practice physician in particular expressed their positions more strongly, stating that physicians did not need advanced practice nurses but rather administrative assistants who would allow them to have more clinical time. The fear of a loss of remuneration in the private practice sector was also perceptible. Some medical professional organizations adopted a protective discourse towards patients and population, insisting on the supervision that physicians will perform on the clinical activity of advanced practice nurses, thus creating a potentially negative image of the competency and skills developed by this new category of nurses.

Nursing organizations did not fail to react to the profile of advanced practice nurse created by the legislation, especially since the draft texts had been disapproved by the HCPP. While ANFIIDE welcomed the introduction of this role in the health system, the lack of ambition in the texts was deplored. Many professional nursing organizations regretted the medical suzerainty imposed on this new role, which reduced advanced practice nurse's autonomy; the level of competency and skills attained by students at the end of their education seems to be underestimated. They are also surprised by the low porosity of French texts with international evidence, despite the large amount of international data available on the subject. The lack of positioning of advanced practice nurse as first-line health provider is also deplored in view of the insufficient supply of primary care in many French regions. Finally, they underline the semantic choices made in the texts that reserve certain terms such as diagnosis, consultation, etc. for the physician.

These positions taken by professional organizations have been relayed by the media and social networks.

Graduates from Master of Clinical Nursing also expressed bitterness and dissatisfaction in the summer of 2018. The legislator did not wish to introduce a grandfathering process or a bridge dedicated to this group of nurses. The files of those who wish to benefit from a validation are therefore examined individually by the programme managers of the universities in which they are applying, which may lead to variable validations.

10.10 Perspectives

The introduction of advanced practice nurses in the French health system suggests that, in the long term, benefits similar to those evaluated in other national environments will be observable:

– Improved access to healthcare for the population, particularly for people living with chronic diseases
– Highlighting the added value for patients benefiting from advanced practice nurses' interventions
– Creation of practice environments more favourable to nursing practice in synergy with nursing management
– Production of evidence showing the benefits for patients of a comprehensive nursing approach
– Evolution of social representations of nurses

However, many challenges remain to be met in order to introduce this new nursing function into the health system and to ensure its sustainability.

10.10.1 Effective Implementation of the National Curriculum

While educational programmes are most often implemented by medical faculties, it is essential for this programme to be anchored in the nursing discipline and that nursing leadership can be exercised throughout it. Although the national curriculum provides for the establishment of nurse/physician pairs to ensure the coordination of units, the academic status of the nurse is not specified, unlike that of the physician; this observation may seem paradoxical when at the same time a body of nursing faculty was created in France in 2019.

In view of the innovative nature of this role, it is necessary to adequately prepare tutors. The first students will indeed be tutored by expert nurses and physicians, and then, as advanced practice nurses' staff grows, this tutoring can be carried out by their peers.

The pioneering spirit often motivates the first students who take up this new role. This pioneering position also prevents them from benefiting from the modelling process that is nevertheless essential to the development of professional identity or more precisely to its adaptation to the specificities of advanced practice nursing.

During the first years, students will have to work hard to make known this new role for which they are destined, all the more so as many misconceptions still surround advanced practice in France.

It will also be necessary to observe the career paths of students who have undertaken this programme immediately after registration. There is a significant risk of loss of skills and competency if the newly graduated advanced practice nurse cannot carry out its role during this 3-year period.

Finally, the autonomy left to the universities in the implementation of the programme combined with the role of certifier that has been assigned to them exposes them to the risk of heterogeneity of advanced practice nurse profiles.

10.10.2 Successful Deployment of Advanced Practice Nurses in Clinical Environments

The phases of introduction of the advanced practice nurse and deployment of the first qualified professionals are always singular moments within a health system. It is therefore necessary to anticipate their deployment in clinical environments and to provide them with a favourable practice environment in order to create attractiveness for this type of position.

Indeed, it is not enough to succumb to the fashion effect by simply creating one or more advanced practice nurse positions in the hope that they will find their place in the multi-professional team. Initiating a project of this nature implies rethinking the organization of care within a team in order to integrate this new player (Schober 2017). Models of care organization should be developed both in hospitals and in the community, taking into account the available evidence in this field.

The advanced practice nurse will have to establish a collaborative practice with physicians.

They will also have to gain the legitimacy and credibility necessary to exercise effective clinical leadership within the nursing team. It is essential that the first advanced practice nurses continue to identify themselves with the nursing profession.

It will also be important for those who will be working in a hospital to create synergy with the nursing management in order to avoid any impression of competition between the two roles.

10.10.3 Assessing the Added Value of Advanced Practice Nurse

French Members of Parliament have asked the Ministry of Health to carry out an initial assessment of the impact of the introduction of advanced practice nurses in the health system by the end of 2021. The results of this evaluation will be decisive for the future of this role. However, the Ministry of Health has not yet communicated on the method that will be used. It is crucial that the choice of indicators as well as the methods of evaluation be adapted; it is absolutely necessary to avoid an evaluation of the activity that is too focused on the medical time saved and does not take into account the added value of the global approach adopted by the advanced practice nurse.

10.10.4 Propose an Economic Model That Is Commensurate with the Contribution Made

The economic model designed to remunerate the activity of the advanced practice nurses working in the public or private sector as well as in independent practice is not yet fully known. The first decisions made in this area concern the advanced practice nurse who will be working in private practice, and they fall far short of the expectations of advanced practice nurse students. Moreover, the first projections concerning remuneration in the public sector have also led to disappointment for future advanced practice nurses.

The economic model chosen will reflect the social recognition attributed to this role and will also be a factor of attractiveness towards this clinical career.

10.10.5 Changing Profile and Creating New Areas of Intervention

Healthcare is being restructured in France. In this dynamic context, it will be necessary in the future to influence the ministerial positions regarding advanced practice nurse as first-line health provider. It would improve access to primary healthcare and relieve congestion in the emergency services.

New areas of intervention could be created to better meet the health needs of the population. For example, a consultation was launched in November 2019 to examine the potential contribution of advanced practice nurse in emergency departments. Other sectors have also expressed a desire to benefit from advanced practice nurse, such as the army health service as well as occupational health teams.

However, it will be necessary to avoid too great a fragmentation of the areas of certification, which would expose to the risk of overlapping fields of intervention of advanced practice nurses.

10.11 Conclusion

At the end of this description of the French situation, it appears that the profile of advanced practice nurse that has been introduced into the health system is certainly an evolution for the healthcare supply and for the nursing profession, but not a real revolution. Following the example of foreign experiences in this field, it is likely that this first legislative decision opens the way for further developments, particularly in terms of the autonomy granted to advanced practice nurse.

The process of introducing advanced nursing practice in France began with initiatives in the field of education combined with changes in the practice of nurses who had benefited from these skill developments before obtaining an appropriate legislative framework. A significant latency has been deplored coupled with highly fluctuating political orientations on this topic. Three profiles of advanced practice nurses have thus followed one another, resulting from three educational systems: nonacademic, master's degree, and university education recognized at master's level. This sequence can be frustrating for professionals who, due to the lack of a legislative framework and a suitable practice environment, have had difficulty putting into practice the skills developed during their course of study.

The long negotiation process that preceded the publication of the legislative texts and the content of these texts are also indicative of the sociology of the health professions in France and the way nursing professional leadership is exercised in France. The current context of healthcare in France is marked by an erosion of leadership exercised by nurses and nurse managers to the benefit of the medical profession, which, at clinical level, in management and in education, seems to wish to occupy a predominant position. The choices made related to the scope of practice of advanced practice nurse fail to take into account certain population needs, ignoring the recommendations published in this field (Bryant-Lukosius and DiCenso 2004) with the aim of maintaining the initial structure of the health professions between the medical profession on the one hand and "medical auxiliaries" on the other. The semantic analysis of the terms used in the legislation and regulations is indicative of the frame of reference used by those who wrote them, as are the terms that seem to have been deliberately avoided because they are considered to be exclusively reserved for physicians. However, it is interesting to highlight the essential role of the national nursing association in this project but also to note that even before the first advanced practice nurse graduated, a dedicated trade union was created to defend their interests and their future working conditions as well as their remuneration. This is a rather singular phenomenon in the nursing profession.

A new phase in the history of nurses in France is therefore underway. In the future, advanced practice nurses will undoubtedly contribute to preserving universal health coverage and, consequently, the health of the population living in France.

This topic will also offer many objects to explore through research.

References

Agence Régionale de Santé-Ile-de-France (2016) Projet "Préfiguration d'Infirmiers Cliniciens Spécialisés". Rapport final—Synthèse

ANFIIDE (2016) L'infirmière de pratique avancée, bilan d'étape, état des lieux en France

Berland Y (2003) Mission "Coopération des professions de sante: le transfert de tâches et de compétences". Rapport d'étape

Bourgueil Y, Marek A, Mousquès J (2005) La participation des infirmières aux soins primaires dans six pays européens et au Canada

Brami L, Damart S, Kletz F (2012) Réformes de l'hôpital, crise à l'hôpital: une étude des liens entre réformes hospitalières et absentéisme des personnels soignants. Politiques et management public 29:541–561

Bryant-Lukosius D, DiCenso A (2004) A framework for the introduction and evaluation of advanced practice nursing roles. J Adv Nurs 48:530–540

Debout C (2014) [The clinical nursing practice some elements of clarification in the French context]. Soins; la revue de reference infirmiere 26–31

Debout C (2016) Vieillissement, chronicité et virage ambulatoire: impact sur les soins à domicile. Journal de droit de la santé et de l'assurance maladie 25–29

Debout C (2018) Infirmière de pratique avancée en France: première esquisse. Soins 63:59–65

Debout C, Magnon R (2014) Léonie Chaptal, un leader visionnaire. Les Tribunes de la santé 73–83

Desailly-Chanson MA, Siahmed H, Elshoud S (2016) Etablissements de santé Risques psychosociaux des personnels médicaux: recommandations pour une meilleure prise en charge Mise en responsabilité médicale: recommandations pour une amélioration des pratiques. Rapport Inspection Générale des Affaires Sociales [Report of the Inspector General of Social Affairs]

Direction de la recherche, des études, de l'évaluation et des statistiques (2017) L'état de santé de la population en France: rapport 2017

DREES (2018) 53% d'infirmiers en plus entre 2014 et 2040, une forte hausse qui répond à la demande de soins. Etudes et rapports

Hamel F (2008) Mouvements infirmiers, représentation professionnelle et conflits sociaux. Rech Soins Infirm 44–48

Haute Autorité de Santé (2007) Les pratiques actuelles de coopération: analyse des témoignages des professionnels de santé

Haute Autorité de Santé (2015) Les protocoles de coopération art 51

Hénart L, Berland Y, Cadet D (2011) Rapport relatif aux métiers en santé de niveau intermédiaire

Leroux-Hugon V (1992) Des saintes laïques. Les infirmières à l'aube de la IIIe République, Paris. Sciences en situation

Ministère de l'enseignement supérieur, de la recherche et de l'innovation (2018) Décret no 2018-633 du 18 juillet 2018 relatif au diplôme d'Etat d'infirmier en pratique avancée

Ministère de la Santé (2009) Loi Hôpital, patients, santé et territoires (HPST)

Ministère des Affaires Sociales et de la Santé (2016) LOI n° 2016-41 du 26 janvier 2016 de modernisation de notre système de santé

Ministère des solidarités et de la santé (2017) Renforcer l'accès territorial aux soins

Ministère des solidarités et de la santé (2018a) Ma santé 2022: un engagement collectif

Ministère des solidarités et de la santé (2018b) Décret no 2018-629 du 18 juillet 2018 relatif à l'exercice infirmier en pratique avancée

Ministère des solidarités et de la santé (2018c) Arrêté du 18 juillet 2018 fixant la liste des pathologies chroniques stabilisées prévue à l'article R. 4301-2 du code de santé publique

Ministère des solidarités et de la santé (2018d) Arrêté du 18 juillet 2018 fixant les listes permettant l'exercice infirmier en pratique avancée en application de l'article R. 4301-3 du code de santé publique

Ministère des solidarités et de la santé-Ministère de l'enseignement supérieur, de la recherche et de l'innovation (2018) Arrêté du 18 juillet 2018 relatif au régime des études en vue du diplôme d'Etat d'infirmier en pratique avancée. JORF

Mossé P (2018) Une économie politique de l'hôpital-contre Procuste

OECD (2017) How much do OECD countries spend on prevention? (OECD health working papers no. 101). https://doi.org/10.1787/f19e803c-en

Poisson M (1998) Origines républicaines d'un modèle infirmier, (1870-1900): histoire de la profession infirmière en France. Editions hospitalières, Vincennes

Safon M-O (2016) Loi de modernisation de notre système de santé. IRDES, Paris

Schober M (2016) Introduction to advanced nursing practice: an international focus. Springer

Schober M (2017) Strategic planning for advanced nursing practice. In: Strategic planning for advanced nursing practice. Springer, pp 9–33

Simonet D (2014) Assessment of new public management in health care: the French case. Health Res Policy Syst 12:57

Tabuteau D (2012) Santé et politique en France. Rech Soins Infirm 6–15

Tabuteau D (2013) Les pouvoirs de la santé: la complexité d'un système en quête de régulation. Les tribunes de la santé

Vigneron E (2018) Histoire et Préhistoire de la coopération hospitalière et des groupements hospitaliers de territoire (GHT). Bull Acad Natl Med 202:1967–1979

World Health Organization (2000) The world health report 2000: health systems: improving performance. World Health Organization

World Health Organization (2007) Task shifting: rational redistribution of tasks among health workforce teams: global recommendations and guidelines

CNS Role and Practice in Germany

11

Elke Keinath

Abstract

This chapter presents an overview about advanced nursing practice in Germany, which is an emerging concept in the healthcare service. Currently the spheres of work of the majority of advanced practice nurses are comparable to clinical nurse specialists. They provide direct clinical care to patients, support and empower nurses and/or other healthcare staff as well as strive towards changes within the organisation. Widely used are Hamric's Integrative Model of Advanced Practice Nursing and the PEPPA framework to provide guidance regarding the competencies and implementation of ANP. Missing regulation within nursing poses a big hinderance in this process. As an example of ANP practice in Germany serves the implementation of delirium management. Also described are education and professional developments with regard to ANP. An outlook finishes this chapter.

Keywords

Clinical nurse specialist · Advanced practice nurse · Delirium management
Emerging ANP practice · Germany · Hamric's Integrative Model of Advanced
Practice Nursing

This chapter has been written before the 2020 APN ICN guidelines were published and reflects the views of the authors.

E. Keinath (✉)
Pflegeexpertin APN, Klinikum Darmstadt, Darmstadt, Germany
e-mail: elke.keinath@mail.klinikum-darmstadt.de

This chapter describes the role and practices of advanced practice nurses (APNs) in Germany. It outlines common notions regarding advanced nursing practice (ANP), looks at issues such as evaluation and education, provides an example of ANP practice and presents professional issues regarding ANP as well as an outlook.

The vast majority of APNs currently practising in Germany are comparable to clinical nurse specialists (CNS) (Mendel and Feuchtinger 2009; Feuchtinger 2016) as they are covering the three spheres of CNS practice: direct patient care, nursing and nursing staff and the organisation (Chan and Cartwright 2014: 359).

As described in previous monographs of this series (Schober 2016, 2017), ANP in Germany is still at an early stage (Maier et al. 2017). The first publications regarding ANP appeared in the 2000s (Sachs 2007; Advisory Council on the Assessment of Developments in the Health Care System (SVR) 2007; Mendel and Feuchtinger 2009). A decade later, one still finds phrases like "cultural lag" (Schaeffer 2017: 27) or words like exotic (Teigeler 2014: 12). In the mid-1990s the university hospital in Freiburg employed the first academically qualified nurse in a clinical setting (Feuchtinger 2016). In the new millennium, increasingly more and more APN roles were implemented, particularly within hospital settings (Teigeler 2014; Boeckler and Dorgerloh 2014; Weskamm 2017; Feuchtinger 2016). As role models, they open clinical settings as a possible career pathway for academically qualified nurses, next to management, education or science. However, clinical careers remain rare.

For many within the German nursing community, the term "expert" is firmly connected to Benner's "From Novice to Expert" (Benner 2001). An in-depth discussion about commonalities and differences, and consequently a clear distinction between basic, expert and advanced level (Spross 2014: 29), is still pending. However, in conjunction with international notions, there are common understandings regarding APN roles:

- That advanced practice is synonymous with clinical expertise (Dowling et al. 2013: 132).
- That they need to have a clinical focus, working with patients and/or their families. Direct patient care is understood to be there where the patient is (Spirig and DeGeest 2004: 233).
- That ANP should be an extension and expansion of the original nursing field of action (Gaidys 2011: 17; DBfK 2017: 1).
- That these roles require further training and education beyond the basic nursing training and that these roles possess additional competencies and responsibilities (Spross 2014).
- That nursing development across wards or departments remains an important feature of APN roles (Kaden et al. 2012; Schmitte et al. 2014; Hock et al. 2017).
- That successful implementation needs managerial support and a regular exchange between the APN and the nursing management. To ensure that APNs are implemented in accordance with the strategic development and objectives of the organisation, it is pivotal that the director of nursing is part of the board (Sniatecki et al. 2017: 280).

The position paper of the three German-speaking professional organisations (Germany, Austria and Switzerland) in 2013 was an important milestone as it provided a definition of an APN as well as with "Pflegeexperte APN" (translated: nursing expert APN) a possible title for these roles (DBfK et al. 2013: 2). While this title is not protected by law, the addition of the letters "APN" distinguishes it from other, not academically qualified, nursing experts and connects it to the international concept of advanced practice. However, this title does not differ between APN roles such as nurse practitioner (NP)[1] or CNS.

11.1   Utilised ANP Models in Germany

Fitting with the general developmental stage of ANP in Germany, the discussion regarding differing ANP models and concepts is much in their infancy. The most widely known and utilised models are Hamric's "Integrative Model of Advanced Practice Nursing" (Hamric et al. 2014), which is relevant for the discussion regarding competencies (DBfK et al. 2013: 1), and the PEPPA framework[2] of Bryant-Lukosius and DiCenso (2004), which guides the implementation of APN roles in Germany (Feuchtinger 2016).

Most APNs describe their tasks and competencies along Hamric's model (Teigeler 2014; Drexler and Weidlich 2016; Naegele et al. 2016; Schmitte 2016; Weskamm 2017). While all emphasise the importance of working in a clinical setting with patients and/or their families, the other competencies from Hamric's model[3] are present to varying degrees according to the setting and job description of the individual APN. It is apparent; some of these roles have a more general and some a more specialist focus in their daily routines. In the latter the emphasis lies on supporting the patient, while in the former the emphasis lies on supporting nurses and other staff caring for a specialised group of patients (Drexler et al. 2017: 266).

APNs are either assigned to a department and work, due to interdepartmental tasks, in a matrix organisation (Boeckler and Dorgerloh 2014: 14) or form a leadership team, in which they take the clinical lead, while another person occupies the managerial lead (Drube et al. 2016: 94).

11.2   Evaluation of ANP in Germany

Evaluation of ANP practice is not optional (Kleinpell 2013: 27). At this early stage of APN roles in Germany, evaluation is pertinent to identify needs of patients, families, teams or healthcare services and to promote role clarity by ensuring a good

---

[1] Nurse practitioners (NPs) are understood to work foremost in primary care and frequently carry out task traditionally performed by doctors. In Germany NPs are discussed as a possible solution for the lack of medical staff in rural areas (Feuchtinger 2016: 49; Maier 2017: 62).

[2] Participatory, evidence-based, patient-focused process, for guiding the development, implementation and evaluation of advanced practice nursing (PEPPA) (Bryant-Lukosius and DiCenso 2004).

[3] Guidance and coaching, consultation, evidence-based practice, leadership, collaboration, ethical decision-making (Spross 2014: 44).

match between the identified needs and the APN, her role, competencies and scope of practice (Bryant-Lukosius et al. 2016: 37). Expanding on the PEPPA framework (Bryant-Lukosius and DiCenso 2004), PEPPA-Plus guides the development of stage-specific questions for APN-role evaluation (Bryant-Lukosius et al. 2016). It is conceivable that PEPPA-Plus is suitable for and applicable to the German context, but more applications are needed to confirm this.

Evaluation is a complex process as APNs cannot be seen in isolation due to the multifactorial impact of their roles (Schaeffer 2017: 28). A suitable approach to evaluate complex interventions includes qualitative and quantitative methods and builds on formative and summative steps (Höhmann and Bartholomeyczik 2013). Currently the majority of evaluations are formative and encompass descriptive statistical data such as number of training sessions and number of participants (Höhmann and Bartholomeyczik 2013: 308). Lack of regulation and licensing of APN further complicates evaluation of these roles.

11.3   Education of APNs in Germany

There is no doubt that an established nursing science plus academically qualified nurses in clinical settings are essential factors for the successful development and implementation of ANP. However, in Germany academic structures in nursing have been established with great delay. The first academic nursing courses were not established until the 1990s (Robert Bosch Stiftung 1992); initially offered courses were aimed at experienced nurses, who were interested to move into management or teaching. As late as 2004, the first bachelor's degree in nursing, which combined academic training with a nursing exam, was commenced (Friesacher 2014: 35). This late implementation of nursing science and lack of research funding contributes to the difficult data situation in nursing and ANP (Schaeffer 2017: 29).

Presently ANP curricula in Germany are not standardised, the courses on offer vary, and their contents are heterogeneous (Maier 2017: 62). A nationwide curriculum for ANP courses is missing. In 2013 Ullmann and Lehwaldt postulated a demand for more clinically focused and patient-orientated ANP-course content that furthers autonomous (nursing) practice plus the necessary decision-making skills. Pulcini (2014: 142) recommends that faculty members remain embedded in APN practice. In Germany, this is a challenging notion due to little overlap between the differing sectors of education and clinical practice. Course leaders may not possess own personal work experience as an APN.

11.4   An Example of APNs in the Hospital Setting

Exemplary for APN roles in the hospital setting are APNs working with patients with delirium, either in a general hospital setting (Bürger and Kugler 2016) or within the setting of an intensive care unit (ICU) (Krotsetis and Nydahl 2014;

Sniatecki 2016, 2017). APNs are well educated and placed to successfully implement and conduct a structured and interprofessional management of these patients.

The occurrence of a delirium results in significant consequences for the patient with regard to the healing process and treatment outcomes (Arbeitsgemeinschaft der Wissenschaftlichen Medizinischen Fachgesellschaften e.V. (AWMF) 2015: 6).

With published incidence rates from 30% to over 80%, delirium belongs to the most commonly observed syndromes in critical care patients (AWMF 2015: 6). Its signs are an impaired cognitive function or perception and a disturbed consciousness, and it presents with an acute onset and fluctuating course. It is usually reversible (AWMF 2015: 24).

A delirium can present itself in various subforms: hyperactive, hypoactive or as a mixed form. The hyperactive form is more easily recognised as the patients can be restless or agitated; patients with a hypoactive delirium can be sleepy, quiet and withdrawn. As a consequence, it is estimated that two-thirds of patients with delirium syndromes are not recognised during a routine clinical assessment (AWMF 2015: 26). Guidelines therefore recommend a structured screening with a suitable delirium assessment tool on at least 8 hourly basis (AWMF 2015: 13), to ensure that patients with a hypoactive or a mixed delirium are identified. An early delirium management can positively influence the outcome (AWMF 2015: 3). Preventative measures play a particularly pivotal role, especially as non-pharmacological options such as reorientation strategies (e.g. intensive communication or ensuring the use of glasses or hearing aids) take here centre stage (AWMF 2015: 8–9), one of the many opportunities for nurses to directly impact on the patients' wellbeing.

Working in direct clinical practice with delirious patients revealed the need for a structured management for these patients regarding assessment, prevention, monitoring, therapy and evaluation (Sniatecki 2016: 278). Having identified the need, the aim was to improve the quality of delivered care and health services. For this, the issue was raised within the management structures within the unit and the hospital, ultimately leading to changes in service provision of the organisation (Sniatecki et al. 2017: 286–287). After the implementation of a structured assessment tool in form of the confusion assessment method for the intensive care unit (CAM-ICU) (Ely et al. 2001), a formative evaluation revealed that the numbers of patients with delirium were higher than prior to the implementation. This confirmed the assumption that particularly patients with hypoactive or mixed form of delirium were not identified earlier and did not receive any support or treatment because of this (Sniatecki et al. 2017: 287).

Spending time in direct clinical practice supports the development of a deepened relationship between patient and the APN that allows for early detection of (mood) changes and empowering staff to act in a timely manner (personal communication with S. Sniatecki 27/04/2018).

While preventative and non-pharmacological treatment options are mainly influenced by nurses (Bürger and Kugler 2016), another pivotal strategy to reduce the risk for developing a delirium is avoiding sedation and its medication (AWMF

2015: 8). Therefore, an interprofessional approach and close collaboration with medical staff is a prerequisite for success (Sniatecki 2016). Consultation with the families of patients with delirium can contribute numerous information about patients' usual behaviour or likes and dislikes; notwithstanding families also need guidance in dealing with the situation (Krotsetis and Nydahl 2014).

APNs provide clinical leadership through utilisation of their advanced skills in the direct patient contact but also by empowering nurses and other staff through mentoring or teaching, in either formal or informal teaching sessions, either in groups or one to one (Sniatecki 2016), or facilitating evidence-based practice through the development of an easy-to-use evidence-based pocket card (Bürger and Kugler 2016). This corresponds with their perception as "change agents" and as an intermediary between nursing science and practice (Mendel and Feuchtinger 2009: 208).

Leadership is also displayed by contributing to the nursing and ANP community through articles or conference presentations, which allowed others to benefit from their strategies and their findings (Krotsetis and Nydahl 2014; Sniatecki 2016; Bürger and Kugler 2016; Sniatecki et al. 2017; Bürger 2017; Nydahl 2018).

11.5   Professional Issues Regarding ANP

Like many countries, the healthcare service in Germany is facing multiple challenges due to the demographic and epidemiological changes. The need for change in the provision of health care has been recognised by politicians as well as professional organisations, such as Deutscher Pflegerat (DPR) and Deutscher Berufsverband für Pflegeberufe (DBfK), who support the development of APN roles (DBfK 2013). However, just transferring tasks between professions will fail; instead processes need to be changed (Wolke 2017: 37).

Specific challenges to the implementation of ANP are due to a lack of registration and self-government in nursing and, as a consequence, not regulated APN roles. This is a major hinderance to push the notion of ANP, as regulation means role clarity (Maier et al. 2017: 34) and contributes to the sustainability of ANP (Schober 2016: 124). Currently, APN roles are implemented in Germany without being clearly defined. There is a lack of funding for education and research into ANP (Schaeffer 2017: 29). Clinical salary structures are just beginning to consider academic qualifications (DBfK 2016: 2).

The central professions within the healthcare services in Germany are, by law, physicians. New professional groups such as physician assistants (PAs) have been discussed and implemented in recent years. In 2017 the Federal Medical Council agreed to support the implementation of delegatory practice of PAs (Bundesärztekammer 2017: 113), not autonomous practice like APN. While it is possible that PA may pose a suitable career move for some nurses, the nursing association Deutscher Berufsverband für Pflegeberufe (DBfK) emphasises that this is not an extension and expansion of nursing, but rather stands in competition to developments such as ANP (DBfK 2017: 1).

11.6 Outlook

While ANP is getting more known within nursing, it is still not general knowledge in politics or society. Plenty of APNs are professionally and politically engaged to further ANP. By presenting and discussing their roles as well as demonstrating positive patients' experiences to the public, either locally or through liaison with the media, they create an awareness within society regarding APN-supported healthcare services. National and international networking and exchange supports that German APNs benefit from experiences with the implementation of ANP in other countries.

It can be assumed that with an increasing number of academically qualified nurses as well as more role models in clinical practice, the interest in a clinical career will grow and in the midterm/long term enhance the numbers of APNs in Germany.

Future plans for nursing take ANP already into account, as seen in case studies presented on a website regarding the skill mix. There it is shown how APNs contribute to the provision of health care by enhancing the nursing team (Robert Bosch Stiftung 2018).

In the coming years, ANP and APNs will continue to develop into an important building block for the delivery of a patient-focused health care, particularly for patients with complex needs in and across all settings and areas. However, this requires structured implementation, regulation and evaluation of APN roles as well as an education, which is internationally compatible.

References

Advisory Council on the Assessment of Developments in the Health Care System/Sachverständigenrat zur Begutachtung der Entwicklung im Gesundheitswesen (SVR) (2007) Kooperation und Verantwortung: Voraussetzungen einer zielorientierten Gesundheitsversorgung. http://www.svr-gesundheit.de/fileadmin/user_upload/Gutachten/2007/Kurzfassung_2007.pdf. Accesssed 14 May 2018

Arbeitsgemeinschaft der Wissenschaftlichen Medizinischen Fachgesellschaften e.V. (AWMF) (2015) S3-Leitlinie Analgesie, Sedierung und Delirmanagement in der Intensivmedizin: AWMF-Registernummer: 001/012

Benner PE (2001) From novice to expert: excellence and power in clinical nursing practice. Prentice Hall, Upper Saddle River, NJ

Boeckler U, Dorgerloh S (2014) Advanced nursing practice: Eine Option für deutsche Kliniken. CNE Pflegemanagement 2:14–15

Bryant-Lukosius D, DiCenso A (2004) A framework for the introduction and evaluation of advanced practice nursing roles. J Adv Nurs 48(5):530–540. https://doi.org/10.1111/j.1365-2648.2004.03235.x

Bryant-Lukosius D, Callens B, DeGeest S, Degen Kellerhals S, Fliedner M, Grossmann F, et al (2016) Advanced nursing practice roles in Switzerland: a proposed framework for evaluation. Basel. http://www.swiss-anp.ch/fileadmin/2_ANP-Wissen_Forschung/PEPPA_Plus_final_Version.pdf. Accessed 8 Apr 2018

Bundesärztekammer (2017) Beschlussprotokoll des 120. Deutschen Ärztetages vom 23. bis 26.05.2017 in Freiburg. http://www.bundesaerztekammer.de/fileadmin/user_upload/downloads/pdf-Ordner/120.DAET/Beschlussprotokoll_120_DAET.pdf. Accessed 25 May 2018

Bürger F (2017) Development of an evidence-based pocket card for non-pharmacological Delir Prevention Entwicklung einer evidenz-basierten Pocket Card für die nicht-pharmakologische Delirprävention. Vortrag auf dem Acute Care Symposium. https://www.uniklinik-freiburg.de/acute-care-symposium/programm.html. Accessed 14 May 2018

Bürger F, Kugler C (2016) Die Entwicklung einer evidenzbasierten Pocketcard non-pharmakologischer Interventionen für die Pflege von Menschen mit Delir im Akutkrankenhaus. Pflegewissenschaft 18(3/4):140–150. https://doi.org/10.3936/1335

Chan GK, Cartwright CC (2014) The clinical nurse specialist. In: Hamric AB, Hanson CM, Tracy MF, O'Grady ET (eds) Advanced practice nursing: an integrative approach, 5th edn. Elsevier, St. Louis, pp 359–395

Deutscher Berufsverband für Pflegeberufe (DBfK) (2013) Advanced nursing practice: Pflegerische Expertise für eine leistungsfähige Gesundheitsversorgung

Deutscher Berufsverband für Pflegeberufe (DBfK) e.V (2016) Infoblatt Entgeltordnung TVöD 2017. https://www.dbfk.de/media/docs/download/Allgemein/Infoblatt-Entgeltordnung-TVoeD-2017.pdf. Accessed 25 May 2018

Deutscher Berufsverband für Pflegeberufe (DBfK), Österreichischer Gesundheits- und Krankenpflegeverband (ÖGKV), Schweizer Berufsverband der Pflegefachfrauen und Pflegefachmänner (SBK-ASI) (2013) Advanced nursing practice in Deutschland, Österreich und der Schweiz. www.dbfk.de/de/veroeffentlichungen/Positionspapiere.php. Accessed 13 May 2018

Deutscher Berufsverband für Pflegeberufe e.V (2017) Position des Deutschen Berufsverbandes für Pflegeberufe zu, Physician Assistants'. https://www.dbfk.de/media/docs/download/DBfK-Positionen/Position-DBfK-zu-Physician-Assistants-2017.pdf. Accessed 13 May 2018

Dowling M, Beauchesne M, Farrelly F, Murphy K (2013) Advanced practice nursing: a concept analysis. Int J Nurs Pract 19(2):131–140. https://doi.org/10.1111/ijn.12050

Drexler S, Weidlich S (2016) Patientensetting im Blick. Heilberufe 68(9):54–55. https://doi.org/10.1007/s00058-016-2346-6

Drexler S, Garbe K, Feuchtinger J, Kaiser S, Köberich S, Mielke J et al (2017) Pflegeentwicklung am Universitätsklinikum Freiburg und dem Universität-Herzzentrum Freiburg Bad Krozingen. In: Stemmer R, Remmel-Faßbender R, Schmid M, Wolke R, Anderl-Doliwa B (eds) Aufgabenverteilung und Versorgungsmanagement im Krankenhaus gestalten: Von erfolgreicher Praxis lernen. Medhochzwei, Heidelberg, pp 253–271

Drube I, Wegner Y, Steinhauer M, Pavelcsik S, Bruch A (2016) Pflege im Gesundheitszentrum Glantal- auf dem Weg zur evidenzbasierten Pflegepraxis. In: Deutsches Netzwerk APN & ANP g.e.V (ed) Advanced Practice Nurses Magazin. Deutsches Netzwerk APN & ANP g.e.V, Goch, pp 92–99

Ely EW, Inouye SK, Bernard GR, Gordon S, Francis J, May L et al (2001) Delirium in mechanically ventilated patients: validity and reliability of the confusion assessment method for the intensive care unit (CAM-ICU). JAMA 286(21):2703–2710. https://doi.org/10.1001/jama.286.21.2703

Feuchtinger J (2016) ANP—Studiert und doch nah an der Praxis. Heilberufe 68(6):48–49

Friesacher H (2014) Studienmöglichkeiten in der Pflege. Im OP 20(01):34–44. https://doi.org/10.1055/s-0033-1363927

Gaidys U (2011) Qualität braucht Kompetenz und Verantwortung—Herausforderungen und Perspektiven einer Advanced Nursing Practice für die Gesundheitsversorgung aus pflegewissenschaftlicher Sicht. Pflege 24(1):15–20. https://doi.org/10.1024/1012-5302/a000087

Hamric AB, Hanson CM, Tracy MF, O'Grady ET (eds) (2014) Advanced practice nursing: an integrative approach, 5th edn. Elsevier, St. Louis

Hock S, Lang J, Meissner K, Schmitt A, Werner J (2017) Praxisentwicklung durch APN in der Kinderintensivpflege intensiv 25(6):314–22. https://doi.org/10.1055/s-0043-119091

Höhmann U, Bartholomeyczik S (2013) Komplexe Wirkungszusammenhänge in der Pflege erforschen: Konzepte statt Rezepte. Pflege & Gesellschaft 18(4):293–312

Kaden A, Keinath E, Knisch A, Marquard S, Müller A, Schmitte H (2012) Pflegeentscheidungen treffen—am Fall lernen. PADUA 7(3):122–126. https://doi.org/10.1024/1861-6186/a000058

Kleinpell RM (2013) Measuring outcomes in advanced practice nursing. In: Kleinpell RM (ed) Outcome assessment in advanced practice nursing, 3rd edn. Springer, New York, NY, pp 1–43

Krotsetis S, Nydahl P (2014) Delir und Angehörige auf ITS—ein ganzheitlicher Ansatz intensiv 22(4):198–201. https://doi.org/10.1055/s-0034-1383876

Maier CB (2017) Advanced practice nurses (APN) in der Primärversorgung. Die Schwester Der Pfleger. 56(11):60–63

Maier CB, Aiken LH, Busse R (2017) Nurses in advanced roles in primary care: Policy levers for implementation. OECD health working papers, no. 98. Paris. https://doi.org/10.1787/a8756593-en

Mendel S, Feuchtinger J (2009) Aufgabengebiete klinisch tätiger Pflegeexperten in Deutschland und deren Verortung in der internationalen Advanced Nursing Practice. Pflege 22(3):208–216. https://doi.org/10.1024/1012-5302.22.3.208

Naegele M, Rebafka A, Leppla L, Mößner U, Engelhardt M, Haseman M (2016) Onkologische Pflege zwischen Forschung und Praxis. Heilberufe 68(7–8):56–58. https://doi.org/10.1007/s00058-016-2288-z

Nydahl P (2018) Wenn auf den Schlaganfall ein Delir folgt. Die Schwester Der Pfleger. 57(1):86–90

Pulcini J (2014) International development of advanced practice nursing. In: Hamric AB, Hanson CM, Tracy MF, O'Grady ET (eds) Advanced practice nursing: an integrative approach, 5th edn. Elsevier, St. Louis, pp 133–145

Robert Bosch Stiftung (1992) Pflege braucht Eliten: Denkschrift der Kommission der Robert-Bosch-Stiftung zur Hochschulausbildung für Lehr- und Leitungskräfte in der Pflege; mit systematischer Begründung und Materialien. Bleicher, Gerlingen

Robert Bosch Stiftung (2018) 360° Pflege. https://www.qualifikationsmix-pflege.de/qualifikationsmix/fallbeispiele/. Accessed 3 May 2018

Sachs M (2007) "Advanced Nursing Practice"-Trends: Implikationen für die deutsche Pflege: Ein Literaturüberblick mit Beispielen aus den USA, Großbritannien und den Niederlanden. Pflege & Gesellschaft 12(2):101–117

Schaeffer D (2017) Advanced Nursing Practice Erweiterte Rollen und Aufgaben der Pflege in der Primärversorgung in Ontario/Kanada. Pflege & Gesellschaft. 22(1):18–35

Schmitte H (2016) Grenzen überwinden in der psychiatrischen Versorgung. Heilberufe 68(11):58–60. https://doi.org/10.1007/s00058-016-2464-1

Schmitte H, Kaden A, Keinath E, Knisch A, Meißner K, Müller A (2014) Die Pflege voranbringen. Die Schwester Der Pfleger. 53(1):18–23

Schober M (2016) Introduction to advanced nursing practice: an international focus. Springer International Publishing, Cham

Schober M (2017) Strategic planning for advanced nursing practice. Springer International Publishing, Cham

Sniatecki S (2016) Keine Party auf Station? intensiv 24(5):276–80. https://doi.org/10.1055/s-0042-111708

Sniatecki S, Keinath E, Knisch A, Herrmann V, Meißner K, Werner J (2017) ANP konkret: Entwicklung einer advanced nursing practice (ANP) im Florence-nightingale-Krankenhaus. In: Stemmer R, Remmel-Faßbender R, Schmid M, Wolke R, Anderl-Doliwa B (eds) Aufgabenverteilung und Versorgungsmanagement im Krankenhaus gestalten: Von erfolgreicher Praxis lernen. Medhochzwei, Heidelberg, pp 273–289

Spirig R, DeGeest S (2004) Editorial: "advanced nursing practice" lohnt sich! Pflege 17(4):233–236. https://doi.org/10.1024/1012-5302.17.4.233

Spross J (2014) Conceptualizations of advanced practice nursing. In: Hamric AB, Hanson CM, Tracy MF, O'Grady ET (eds) Advanced practice nursing: an integrative approach, 5th edn. Elsevier, St. Louis, pp 27–66

Teigeler B (2014) Mit master am Patientenbett: advanced nursing practice. Die Schwester Der Pfleger 53(01):12–15

Ullmann P, Lehwaldt D (2013) Hochschulische Masterprogramme im Kontext der modernen Pflegebildung: die nationale Perspektive. In: Darmann-Finck I, Hülsken-Giesler M, eds.

bwp@ Spezial 6–17. Hochschultage Berufliche Bildung 2013, Fachtagung 14: FT14-Pflege Pflegebildung im Zeichen des demographischen Wandels, pp 1–14. https://www.bwpat.de/ausgabe/ht2013/fachtagungen/fachtagung-14. Accessed 1 May 2018

Weskamm A (2017) "Das Bestmögliche für den Patienten herausholen": Pflegeexperten APN in der Praxis. Die Schwester Der Pfleger. 56(3):40–44

Wolke R (2017) Ökonomische Aspekt von Aufgabenneuverteilung und Einsatz akademisch qualifizierter Pflegender im Krankenhaus. In: Stemmer R, Remmel-Faßbender R, Schmid M, Wolke R, Anderl-Doliwa B (eds) Aufgabenverteilung und Versorgungsmanagement im Krankenhaus gestalten: Von erfolgreicher Praxis lernen. Medhochzwei, Heidelberg, pp 21–51

Part IV
Asia

CNS Role and Practice in Japan

12

Pamela A. Minarik, Garrett K. Chan, and Shiori Usami

Abstract

The aim of this chapter is to describe the Certified Nurse Specialist (CNS) role and practice in Japan from the history of the role's development to current challenges and opportunities. The CNS was the first post-RN role in Japan, a developed country with a high proportion of elderly people and a high healthy life expectancy. Included in the chapter is a brief history of modern Japanese nursing since 1874 noting the first CNS practice in hospitals began in the early 1990s. In Japan, laws governing health professional scope of practice are national. National law stipulates the qualifications for licensure of Japanese health care professionals. In the chapter, definition of CNS role and practice is described. A case exemplar described the practice of an expert Japanese CNS. The U.S. CNS was the

---

This chapter has been written before the 2020 APN ICN guidelines were published and reflects the views of the authors.

P. A. Minarik
College of Nursing, Samuel Merritt University, Oakland, CA, USA

Aomori University of Health and Welfare, Aomori, Japan
e-mail: pminarik@samuelmerritt.edu

G. K. Chan (✉)
School of Nursing, University of California, San Francisco, CA, USA

S. Usami
Department of Nursing, Shitennoji University, Advanced Practice Nursing Institution, Habikino City, Osaka, Japan

Kumamoto University, Kumamoto, Japan
e-mail: susami@shitennoji.ac.jp

© Springer Nature Switzerland AG 2021
J. S. Fulton, V. W. Holly (eds.), *Clinical Nurse Specialist Role and Practice*,
Advanced Practice in Nursing, https://doi.org/10.1007/978-3-319-97103-2_12

model for the Japanese CNS. Initially the role focused on inpatient hospital care with both direct and indirect care activities. In Japan, practice competencies for CNSs are jointly endorsed among three organizations: the Japanese Nurses Association (JNA), the Japanese Association of Nursing Programs in University (JANPU) and professional nursing specialty organizations. JNA certifies individual CNSs. The JANPU accredits CNS educational programs.

Discussion of research on CNS outcomes includes recommendations for additional research. Psychiatric CNS outcomes research has demonstrated the effectiveness of psychiatric liaison CNSs, influencing health policy. Current issues in advanced practice nursing development are reviewed in relation to challenges and opportunities for the future.

Keywords
Certified nurse specialist (CNS) role · History Japanese CNS · Research on CNS effectiveness · Advanced practice nurse (APN) in Japan · CNS credentialing system · CNS practice competencies · Licensure · Case exemplar

12.1 Introduction

In this chapter, we will describe the certified nurse specialist (CNS) role and practice in Japan from the history of the role's development to current challenges and opportunities. We will also provide a case exemplar to describe the practice of an expert Japanese CNS.

Japan is a developed country that is undergoing many social changes. The proportion of elderly people in the population is increasing, and there is a decline in people under the age of 15. Health-related indicators have constantly improved, and healthy life expectancy is high (Japanese Nursing Association (JNA) 2016). Japan has a universal healthcare insurance system in which all citizens benefit (JNA 2016). Certified nurse specialists are an integral part of the healthcare system to provide expert specialist nursing practice to advance the health of Japanese people.

12.2 Brief History of the CNS Role

Modern Japanese nursing developed with a change from traditional Chinese medicine to western medicine in 1874 after the Meiji Restoration (1868) (JNA 2016). In 1987, the Ministry of Health, Labor, and Welfare published a report about the need for nurse specialists (Komatsu 2010). This was the first reference to the CNS role (Dr. Keiko Okaya, personal communication, 6/11/18). Prior to the 1987 report, nurses were trained and educated as generalist nurses without any specialization. Because of increasing challenges with the introduction of more technologies, the growing number of patients with complex health conditions, increasing complexity of nursing care, and the challenges of infection rates and multidrug-resistant organisms within the hospitals at that time, the government realized the need for the CNS in Japan.

JNA founded a Credentials Committee that worked for 7 years to develop a CNS system, influenced by the CNS role in the USA (Dr. Keiko Okaya, personal communication, 6/11/18; Komatsu 2010). In 1994, the CNS system was established by JNA and the rules and bylaws completed in 1995. In 1996, JNA contracted with the Japanese Association of Nursing Programs in Universities (JANPU) about the roles of each organization in relation to the CNS. The role of JNA is to certify the individual CNS; the role of JANPU is to accredit education programs preparing CNS students. From 1996, JNA began certifying CNSs in three specialties: cancer nursing, psychiatric and mental health nursing, and community nursing. In 1998, JANPU began accrediting CNS education programs at the master's level (Dr. Keiko Okaya, personal communication, 6/11/18). As of December 2017, there were 2104 certified specialists in Japan who were working in hospitals, outpatient clinics, and community settings in 13 specialties. The specialties are cancer, psychiatric mental health, community health, gerontology, child health, women's health, chronic care, critical care, infection control, family health, home care, genetic, and disaster nursing. The top three specialties by number were cancer, psychiatric mental health, and critical care nursing (JNA, n.d.).

In 2007, the Japanese Association of Certified Nurse Specialists (JACNS) (http:// jpncns.org/) was formed with goals of improving nursing care quality, being involved in quality assurance, and making policy recommendations to promote people's health (Komatsu 2010). Inclusive of all specialties, the JACNS has held conferences since 2014. Of all CNSs, 70% belong to the JACNS. The JACNS promotes research to show the effectiveness of CNSs and makes policy recommendations to the government (Usami 2015a, b).

The CNS was the first advanced practice nurse (APN) role in Japan; they encountered problems with intraprofessional collaboration. Many CNSs experienced problems with effective utilization in healthcare due to misunderstanding by administrators about how to best use CNSs to improve patient care, possibly because of the social importance of age-based seniority and a perceived difficulty of individual CNSs fitting into organizations where the social culture involves belonging to a group. Early visionary nurse administrators and those who later worked with CNSs provided strong support. Over time, however, hospitals began to receive funding from the central government healthcare financing system for CNS services in selected specialties such as oncology and palliative care and the psychiatric liaison consultation team. Currently, the JACNS is advocating for reimbursement for dementia teams.

There are far fewer numbers of CNSs than RNs in Japan. CNSs have been practicing in Japanese hospitals since the early 1990s but often work in staff nurse roles with one day per week to work as a CNS. Many CNSs are faculty in graduate schools of nursing. Some CNSs practice as a CNS and teach part-time in a school of nursing. Prefectures farther away from Tokyo and rural prefectures are less likely to have CNS roles in healthcare institutions. Appropriate utilization of CNSs will increase their visibility and show their effectiveness.

12.3 Definition and Practice of the Certified Nurse Specialist

The CNS credentialing system of JNA contributes to the development of health-care and welfare as well as improves nursing science by credentialing CNSs with specific advanced specialty nursing knowledge and skills. The CNS provides efficient, high-level nursing care to individuals, families, and groups that have complex nursing problems (JNA 2016). CNS roles and activities include providing excellent nursing practice to patients, families, and communities, consultation with nurses and other healthcare providers, coordination, ethical coordination to protect the rights of individuals and others, education of nurses, and research activities (JNA 2016).

12.4 Conceptualizations/Models of CNS Practice

The US CNS was the model for the Japanese CNS. Initially, the model focused on inpatient hospital care with both direct and indirect care activities. The emphasis is on excellent direct patient care, but indirect activities are also important. One of the original motivations for developing the psychiatric liaison CNS role in the late 1980s to early 1990s was to provide nurse support in hospitals (an indirect care activity) (Minarik and Sato 2016). Now, approximately 30% of CNSs practice in community settings such as home visiting centers and outpatient clinics (Dr. Mieko Tanaka, personal communication, 6/11/18).

12.5 CNS Practice Competencies

Competencies are commonly defined as the knowledge, skill, and behavior/attitude/ aptitude to deliver high-quality and safe patient care. In Japan, practice competencies for CNSs are jointly endorsed among three organizations: the JNA, the JANPU, and professional nursing specialty organizations (JANPU 2015; Komatsu 2010). CNS competencies build upon registered nurse competencies (Komatsu 2010). These competencies are attained during the educational program through courses and supervised clinical experiences. Komatsu (2010) urged the Japanese Society of Cancer Nursing to develop core competencies along with curriculum and job descriptions for certification examinations. The JACNS has developed a CNS clinical ladder, based on Benner (Usami 2014). However, there is no standard list of core CNS competencies applying to all CNSs in all specialties.

12.6 Outcome Measures and Evaluation

Japanese nursing needs CNS outcomes data to show the effectiveness of CNS interventions and the impact of CNSs on quality of care. According to Komatsu (2010), cancer CNS outcomes data is limited to descriptive data in 14 years of published case reports. Komatsu (2010) called for well-designed trials to measure the outcomes of cancer CNS interventions with complex patients. Currently, there are no published studies on CNS outcomes except by psychiatric CNSs (Dr. Atsuko Uchinuno, personal communication, 8/6/18).

Psychiatric CNS outcomes research has demonstrated the effectiveness of psychiatric liaison CNSs and has influenced health policy. Usami (2015) and Nozue et al. (2016) showed that psychiatric mental health CNS intervention improved depression scores in hospitalized physically ill patients. Research by Usami et al. (2009) demonstrated the effectiveness of the psychiatric liaison consultation team in the general hospital. Teams were comprised of CNS, psychiatrist, clinical psychologist, a nurse, and a social worker, usually led by the CNS. Usami and her colleagues submitted the 2009 paper to the government, and that resulted in a change in policy to fund hospitals for psychiatric liaison consultation teams. This reimbursement of liaison psychiatric CNS was the first time among psychiatric CNSs.

12.7 Education of CNSs

The Japanese Association of Nursing Programs in Universities (JANPU) accredits CNS programs. For CNS programs, there is a 26-unit, a 38-unit, or a 46-unit option. All CNS curricula must include the following common subjects (Common Subjects A): Nursing Education, Nursing Management, Nursing Theory, Nursing Research, Consultation, Nursing Ethics, and Nursing Politics (JANPU 2015). The 38- and 46-unit CNS curriculum must include Physical Assessment, Pathophysiology, and Clinical Pharmacology (Common Subjects B) in addition to the Common Subjects A. Additionally, all three CNS curricula must include a specialty educational curriculum as determined by the JANPU. An example of the specialty content for the education of a psychiatric mental health CNS is described in "An introduction to psychiatric liaison nursing in Japan" (Minarik and Sato 2016). Komatsu (2010) described the history, education, and practice of the oncology certified nurse specialist, including specialty educational content.

Although the goal of the CNS master's education is to produce an expert in clinical practice, Japanese curricula may not require enough supervised hours with a practicing CNS, constraining graduates' readiness for expert practice (Minarik and Chan 2014). In addition, practicing CNSs may not be geographically close, requiring CNS students to travel for supervised clinical experiences.

Of note, the role of the nurse practitioner has been introduced in Japan to help meet the general care needs of patients especially in rural isolated areas due to the lack of medical physicians (Fukuda et al. 2014; Kondo 2013). This emerging advanced practice role is still being developed among the various national nursing organizations. The JANPU (2015) approved a primary care curriculum. Further, differentiation and clarification are being determined.

In 2015, an amendment to the law governing nursing obliged nurses who perform medical interventions specified in the law to be trained for the 38 interventions (JNA 2016). This new system will allow trained nurses to perform the interventions without waiting for physician decision-making. Completion of the training course with a certificate of completion and qualification is not a license and does not have a legal basis. How this new system will affect CNSs is unknown.

12.8 Credentialing: Regulatory, Legal, and Certification Requirements

In Japan, laws governing health professional scope of practice are national. National law stipulates the qualifications for licensure of Japanese healthcare professionals, such as nurses, midwives, public health nurses, physicians, and dentists. As a result, practice does not legally differ by prefecture. The law does not identify certification as a specialist, and there is no separate licensure for CNSs. The credentialing system by the JNA, which is socially recognized, certifies CNSs. However, not all institutions include CNS roles, and the activities may differ by institutional policy.

To obtain certification as a CNS, a nurse must complete a master's program at a graduate school, after obtaining a national nursing license, accumulate at least 5 years' experience as nurse, and then pass the credentialing examination given by the JNA. A graduate of a CNS program may sit for the exam 6 months after graduation (Dr. Mieko Tanaka, personal communication, 6/11/18). Certification is renewable every 5 years (JNA 2016).

The term "advanced practice nurse" (APN) does not have a universally agreed upon definition about which roles are included. The JANPU uses the term but not the JNA. Universities use the term because of the influence of the JANPU. The idea has arisen to make a new APN national license to differentiate advanced practice from registered nurse practice (Dr. Keiko Okaya and Dr. Mieko Tanaka, personal communication, 6/11/18.). The use of the APN term is dynamic and not settled yet. Consensus building is difficult when participants (i.e., different professional nursing organizations) hold divergent views, especially with the introduction of the nurse practitioner role.

12.9 Moving Forward: Challenges and Opportunities

Overall, in Japan, there is limited public recognition and understanding of CNS roles. Therefore, CNSs in Japan can take some specific steps to help increase the visibility and recognition of the role. First, the CNS/APN role will be most effective if it is designed to fit the social and healthcare system context and the population needs. The Goals of Healthy Japan 2021 (http://www.kenkounippon21.gr.jp/kenkounippon21/about/kakuron/) can provide a guide for action (Minarik and Chan 2014). Second, those practicing as CNS/APNs can collaborate with the emerging nurse practitioners to ensure that both APN roles demonstrate the true value of advanced practice by including the nursing perspective in care, making the care more holistic than care focused primarily on the medical model and procedures. Third, a national consensus on curriculum standards, core competencies, scope of practice, and minimum qualifications for recognition and practice as an APN have to be created so there is no ambiguity among the nursing profession, other health-care disciplines, the government, and the public about who APNs are and what they are capable of doing to help improve health outcomes of the population.

Fourth, careful attention should be given when creating scope of practice, titles, certification, and educational standards for APNs. Architects of these key components of APN practice and regulation need to write the scope of practice and standards for licensure, certification, and education in a broad enough way to apply to various situations where APNs practice as well as when changes in science and practice naturally evolve over time. It is difficult to change laws through legislation as this process is heavily influenced by politics. If professional nursing organizations create national standards of education, competencies, and certification, then the law should reference those national standards as being the standards by which APNs are recognized and have authority to practice.

Universities and hospitals can support novice CNSs with mentorship through transition-to-practice support programs to help them firmly establish themselves in work settings (Minarik and Chan 2014). Such support will enable them to increase their ability to provide clinical experiences for CNS students, necessary for increasing numbers of CNSs visible and in practice.

To gain more role recognition and to create the evidence that CNSs improve patient, population, educational, and healthcare system outcomes, CNSs need to implement and study large-scale innovations.

Japanese nursing leaders are poised to define the scope of practice and the model for a Japanese APN. We recommend a single scope of practice for both CNS and NP roles in Japan (Minarik and Chan 2014).

12.10 Envision the Future APN

The following are the steps proposed for designing the APN role of the future. The authors cannot say what the future Japanese APN will look like nor whether these steps are necessary in Japan. Japanese nursing leaders must create the Japanese APN to fit the Japanese context (Minarik and Chan 2014). The following are some recommended steps:

1. Define necessary competencies (i.e., knowledge, skills, and attitudes) and scope of practice.
2. Define and codify the core educational foundation, including required clinical hours during education. Adequate supervised clinical hours are vital during the educational program to provide a foundation for developing clinical expertise. Supportive programs such as transition-to-practice programs to help new graduate CNSs are essential for the success of individual CNS role development and the role overall (Minarik and Chan 2014). After certification, CNSs need further training from CNS experts to improve their clinical competency, especially in direct patient and family care.

3. Design outcome studies from the outset to measure the impact of the CNS/ APN. Outcomes should be selected for their importance to Japan, its healthcare system, and Japan's healthcare challenges (Minarik and Chan 2014). Evidence-based outcomes will result in CNS/APN effectiveness being visible to the public and other providers.

In a publication for a Japanese nursing audience, Minarik & Chan wrote "When providing advanced care, nurses bring a different perspective than their physician colleagues. They use the same scientific method (data, diagnosis, plan, treat, evaluate), obtain the same measurements of biopsychological data, including laboratory tests, and utilize many of the same interventions. However, the focus on active engagement of patient and family and adding health promotion and disease prevention strategies as central components of the plan of care as opposed to passive compliance with prescriptions and instructions is different as is the attention to environmental and resource factors in addition to medical symptoms and diagnoses. The APNs must include the nursing perspective otherwise, they will only become a mini-doctor and lose their nursing identity. Both CNSs and NPs can co-exist in the healthcare system since CNSs are specialists and NPs are generalists" (Minarik and Chan 2014: 46).

12.11 Conclusion

This chapter described and defined the Certified Nurse Specialist (CNS) role and practice in Japan from the history of the role's development to current challenges and opportunities. The CNS was the first graduate nursing role in Japan. The chapter includes a brief history of modern Japanese nursing since 1874 noting the first CNS practice in hospitals, modeled on the U.S. CNS, began in the early 1990s. A case exemplar described the practice of an expert Japanese psychiatric mental health CNS. In Japan, practice competencies for CNSs are jointly endorsed among three organizations: the Japanese Nurses Association (JNA), the Japanese Association of Nursing Programs in University (JANPU) and professional nursing specialty organizations. An example of psychiatric CNS outcomes research that demonstrated the effectiveness of psychiatric liaison CNSs, influencing health policy and research on CNS outcomes. Current issues in advanced practice nursing development have been reviewed in relation to challenges and opportunities for the future. In Japan, creating the future of APN roles importantly is done while respecting and building on past development of APN roles.

Exemplar: Psychiatric Mental Health Certified Nurse Specialist Practice
The CNS in psychiatric mental health nursing may work in psychiatric inpatient and outpatient settings with patients repeatedly hospitalized for psychiatric disorders, in general hospitals with patients who have undiagnosed

psychiatric disorders or problems in coping, or in ambulatory settings. Psychiatric CNSs provide psychotherapy to individuals, groups, and families and consult with nurses and other providers, educate nurses, coordinate care and ethical issues, and conduct research.

This case is an example of direct care and consultation by an expert CNS in psychiatric mental health nursing in Japan. This case involved a 34-year-old woman, Mrs. K, with a diagnosis of major depressive disorder and borderline personality disorder who was an inpatient in a psychiatric hospital. Her admission was due to self-harmful behavior of wrist cutting and overdose, behaviors labeled as acting out.

Her history included family stressors. She graduated from a university and then worked for 5 years as a city public officer. She married and had one daughter. After her husband died of cancer, she raised her child by herself. At 32 years old, she married again and had another child with her second husband. However, her husband was unable to help with childcare; she cared for both children by herself. The family moved to live closer to her husband's work. Following the move, she started to cut her wrist and overdose.

This third admission, due to acting out behavior (wrist cutting and overdose), was considered a repeat admission because it was within 3 months of discharge. At the unit, she expressed anger because nurses did not listen at night when she wanted a listener. And the multidisciplinary team was split and disagreed about both her treatment goals and treatment approach.

Prior to interaction with the CNS, Mrs. K's behavior included eating three to four meals daily, insomnia at night, and daytime sleeping. She was angry about nurses' behavior of not listening.

With the patient, the CNS implemented a theory-based approach to care (Psychoanalytic Systems Self-Care Therapy, PAS-SCT) that is designed to help difficult patients, who have acted out many times and have repeated admissions, to implement self-care with deliberate action. PAS-SCT is a self-care therapy developed by the CNS and her colleague Dr. Kotani [Usami and Kotani 2018]. The psychotherapy model was based on the Orem-Underwood self-care model, which is the foundation for psychiatric nursing care in Japan [Usami and Kotani 2018] and the psychoanalytic systems theory developed by Dr. Kotani [2018].

The CNS met with Mrs. K three times per week; psychotherapy focused on how to control her self-harmful behavior and improve her problems with overeating, her imbalance of activity and rest, and imbalance of solitude and social interaction. Using the theory-based psychotherapy (PAS-SCT), the CNS encouraged the patient to express her anger and clarify her unmet needs. The CNS and Mrs. K focused on setting self-care goals necessary for staying in the community. The goals set were to control food intake and develop activity and rest balance and solitude and social interaction balance.

With psychotherapy, Mrs. K gradually recognized she had been angry with her husband, because her husband complained about her money management and her lack of housekeeping. With therapy, Mrs. K came to control her impulsive self-harmful behavior and improved her self-care.

The CNS coached the primary nurse about the interventions for enhancing self-care. Following the coaching, the primary nurse used these interventions daily with the patient.

Addressing the multidisciplinary team, the CNS regularly shared information about Mrs. K's nursing care on the unit and informed the team of the psychodynamic assessment of Mrs. K. The shared information and focus on teamwork contributed to improved functioning of the team. The team was able to work together to set treatment goals for Mrs. K and determine the roles for each team member.

Then, the CNS provided psychoeducation and mental support for the husband. The CNS and Mr. K talked about how to respond to the patient and cope with her behavior. Gradually her husband understood her behavior and was able to cope with her.

In this case, CNS outcomes were improved self-care ability of patient and improvement of the teamwork and collaboration of the multidisciplinary team. In Japan, the role of the psychiatric CNS is to improve patients' self-care ability, provider teamwork, and the functioning of the organization or community. The CNS can facilitate discharge of challenging patients into successful community living.

References

Fukuda H, Miyauchi S, Tonai M, Ono M, Magilvy JK, Murashima S (2014) The first nurse practitioner graduate programme in Japan. Int Nurs Rev 61:487–490

Japanese Association of Nursing Programs in University (2015). http://www.janpu.or.jp/download/pdf/apn_e.pdf. Accessed 4 Aug 2018

Japanese Nursing Association (2016) Nursing in Japan. https://www.nurse.or.jp/jna/english/pdf/nursing-in-japan2016.pdf. Accessed 31 July 2018

Japanese Nursing Association (n.d.) Nursing education in Japan. http://www.nurse.or.jp/jna/english/nursing/education.html. Accessed 4 Aug 2018

Komatsu H (2010) Oncology certified nurse specialist in Japan. Jpn J Clin Oncol 40(9):876–880

Kondo A (2013) Advanced practice nurses in Japan: education and related issues. J Nurs Care S5:004. https://doi.org/10.4172/2167-1168.S5-004

Kotani H (2018) A psychoanalytic systems theory, We can change. Institute of Psychoanalytic Systems Psychotherapy Press, Tokyo

Kotani H, Usami S (2018) PAS self care therapy. Institute of Psychoanalytic Systems Psychotherapy Press, Tokyo

Kotani H, Usami S (2018): The First PAS Self Care Therapy Book in Honor of Patricia Underwood Institute of Psychoanalytic-Systems Psychotherapy, Printed in Japan

Minarik PA, Chan GK (2014) Advanced practice nursing in the United States and Japan: issues comparison, lessons learned and future directions for Japan. Advanced Practice Nursing, A bulletin of the Development of Postgraduate Education Program for Mid-Level Providers (Advanced Practice Nurses) and the Innovation of a Health Delivery Model 3(1):33–53

Minarik PA, Sato Y (2016) An introduction to psychiatric liaison nursing in Japan. ISPN Connections: Newsletter of the International Society of Psychiatric Mental Health Nurses, 19(3 Fall). https://www.ispn-psych.org/assets/docs/Newsletters/2016%20Fall%20Newsletter. pdf. Accessed 5 Aug 2018

Nozue K, Usami S, Fukuda N, Kuwahara T, Ishii M, Fukushima Y, Hayashida Y, Ando S, Ueno K, Shimokawa T (2016) Randomized controlled study evaluating the intervention effect of certified nurse specialist in psychiatric mental health nursing on depressive cancer patients. J Jpn Acad Nurs Sci 36:147–155. https://doi.org/10.5630/jans.36.147

Usami S (2014) A proposal for advanced practice nurses as core of new health care delivery system (5th symposium): from the perspective of a CNS in psychiatric mental health nursing and an educator of CNS: fusion of independent practice model and collaborative model. Advanced Practice Nursing, A bulletin of the Development of Postgraduate Education Program for Mid-Level Providers (Advanced Practice Nurses) and the Innovation of a Health Delivery Model 3(1):4–5. (Japanese)

Usami S (2015a) The realities and evaluation of certified nurse specialist. Japanese J JACNS 1:9–13

Usami S (2015b) Activities and evaluation of certified nurse specialists in transitional care. Nursing, 65(14), P23–27, 67(7), 78–90

Usami S, Fukushima Y, Nozue K, Okaya K, Hiyama M, Migita K, Hirata S, Kitasato M (2009) The effectiveness of psychiatric liaison consultation team for the people with physical illness in the general hospital. Bulletin of Kumamoto University, School of Health Sciences (Medicine) 5, 9-18. Retrieved February 27, 2009, from Kumamoto University repository system at http://hdl. handle.net/2298/11269

Usami S, Nozue K, Sachiko A, Ueno K, Fukuda N, Ishii M (2015) Evaluation research of CNS in psychiatric nursing for the patients with depression and anxiety among chronic illness. Journal of Japanese Association of Certified Nurse Specialist 1:1–7

Clinical Nurse Specialist Role and Practice in Mainland, China

13

Huaping Liu and Hu Yan

Abstract

Clinical nurse specialist has been introduced to China in the early 1990s and has developed rapidly in recent decades. But in comparison with other countries, the connotation of CNS is different in China; it is more likely to be the specialty nurse rather than the CNS in consideration of the nursing development in China. The training program, certificate issuing, registration, and management of SN are conducted by various institutions at different level; until now there is no existing law to regulate the conduct of SN in the clinic. In conclusion, we are still in the initial stage of development of CNS; in the future, more emphasis will be placed on the constructing a consistent definition and index of core competencies, improving training programs, and developing a national organization to manage the CNS, thereby promoting the development of CNS more efficiently.

Keywords

Clinical nurse specialist · CNS · Specialty nurse · China · APN · SN

This chapter has been written before the 2020 APN ICN guidelines were published and reflects the views of the authors.

H. Liu (✉)
School of Nursing, Peking Union Medical College, Beijing, China

WHO Collaborating Centre for Nursing Policy-Making and Leadership, Beijing, China

H. Yan
School of Nursing, Fudan University, Shanghai, China
e-mail: huyan@fudan.edu.cn

13.1   Brief History of CNS Role and Practice

In 1888, the first nursing school was founded in Fuzhou, China. Since then, the nursing development in China progresses in twists and turns; in 2004, we finally finished the construction of a comprehensive nursing education system including Vocational Education, Undergraduate Education, Graduate Education, and Doctoral Education. After the reform and opening-up policy, there were more academic communications between China and abroad, nursing has entered a period of rapid development, and abundance of new nursing philosophy has been introduced in China. But it was not until the early 1990s that the term "clinical nurse specialist" was introduced to China and applied nationally.

In the year of 2001, Guangzhou started the first training school of enterostomal therapist in China. In 2005, the Ministry of Health of the People's Republic of China issued the Outline of China's Nursing Development Plan (2005–2010), which initiated the development of CNS in China and published a list containing five core nursing specialties (emergency department nursing, organ transplantation nursing, operating room nursing, oncology nursing, and intensive care nursing). Training syllabus for nurses in specialist nursing field was published in 2007 by the General Office of the Ministry of Health of the People's Republic of China, which officially clarified the enrollment criteria of the CNS training program, the target, the length of training, the training content, and its evaluation standard. CNS's importance and development were addressed almost in every version of the Outline of China's Nursing Development Plan in 2005.

13.1.1 Definition of CNS

Currently, there is no consensus on the definition of CNS in China, though a lot of nursing scholars have researched to discuss and analyze it. Due to the fact that the proportion of nurses with bachelor's degree or above was only 14.6%, it is impossible to require every CNS to be a postgraduate as in developed countries. Therefore, the controversy is whether the CNS definition should be aligned with the specialty nurse (SN) or the clinical nurse specialist (CNS). The SN places a greater emphasis on basic nursing practice, while the CNS places more emphasis on advanced nursing practice (Chen and Li 2017).

In the latest research about the definition of CNS, most experts agree that in China, the CNS should lean toward specialty nurse, which has been used for a long time and is more suitable for the situation in China. They come to a conclusion that nurse specialist is a nurse who has been systematically trained in nursing practice and nursing theory in certain nursing specialty, passed the evaluation of SN, and obtained the certificate from the Medical and Health Administration; on the other hand, CNS should have clinical experiences (2–15 years) and be capable of providing high-quality nursing service to patients (Chen and Li 2017).

13.2   CNS Practice Competencies

The core competencies of specialty nurse have been widely discussed and studied in Mainland; different nursing specialties developed their own core competencies.

In 2017, Liang stated that the core competencies of SN should include professional values, professional development ability, specialty nursing practice skills, clinical teaching skills, clinical research ability, and ability to organize, manage, and cooperate (Liang 2017).

Gao conducted research to construct a competency model of interventional radiology nurses in 2015. This model consists of 17 competency elements and 5 dimensions. The five dimensions are personality characteristics (physical quality, sterile consciousness, inner concentration, confidence, sense of responsibility), the ability to provide direct clinical care (ability to analyze the condition of patients, radiation health knowledge, intervention surgical cooperation), communication and collaboration (verbal and communication skills, teamwork), emergency rescue (control, rescue skills, predictability, flexibility), and research and development (innovation, subject interest, professional learning skills).

13.3   Outcome Measures and Evaluation

The outcome measures and evaluation vary greatly between hospitals and institutions. In most cases, the exam items are inconsistent with the core competency index of a certain type of SN, and the evaluation is always conducted in the form of a qualification review, paper testing, an interview, and an objective structured clinical examination.

For instance, Guangdong province, the origin place of SN, states that the SN applicant should firstly go through the verification of the qualification, after which the applicant will take paper examinations, interviews, and skill tests (Peng and Chen 2011). In Sichuan province, the applicant only needs to finish the training session and successfully pass the paper examination and skill test, in order to obtain the Certificate of Specialty Nurse issued by Sichuan Nursing Association and the training base (Sichuan Nursing Association 2016).

Generally, there is no consistent certification process in China; in most cases, if the applicant finishes all the training session and passes the evaluation process, they can get the Certificate of Specialty Nurse (Chen and Li 2015).

13.4   CNS Education

In developed countries through years of development, they already have mature training program. Though our CNS training program has only been developed in recent years, we still achieved good effects. Now we mainly provide the Specialty Nurse education through two ways in China: on-the-job training and academic degree.

13.5 On-the-Job Training Program for SN

The length of training program for SN in Mainland ranges from 2 to 6 months depending on the training institution, which is shorter than the length of the training program for CNS in abroad, which always lasts for more than 6 months. At present in Mainland, China, the training programs are mainly developed by the Chinese Nursing Association, provincial and municipal nursing association, provincial and municipal nursing quality and control center, some medical schools, hospitals, specialist nurse training center, or some CNS training agency overseas in China. For example, the specialty nurse in Anhui province must finish 4–6 months of theoretical learning and clinical practicing in the clinic (Song et al. 2007).

13.6 Master of Nursing Specialist

In the year of 2010, Academic Degrees Committee of the State Council in China decided to establish the Master of Nursing Specialist (MNS), aimed at cultivating high-level and specialized nursing professionals and providing a new method to promote the development of SN (Yang et al. 2015). Until 2017, there were 86 colleges that enrolled MNS students in China, and the number of MNS students is growing every year. In China, though no consistent standard of core competencies of MNS has been established, clinical practice skills are widely agreed to be the most important competency that a MNS student should possess, but professional development ability, critical thinking skills, scientific research skills, clinical teaching skills, nursing management skills, communicating and cooperation skills, and ethical decision-making ability are also important (You et al. 2012; Xu et al. 2009).

13.7 Credentialing: Regulatory, Legal, and Certification Requirements

Currently, there are no national entry criteria for SN in China; it varies among different provinces. In Guangdong province, the entry criteria for SN are as follows: (1) registered nurse; (2) bachelor degree or higher; (3) more than 8 years of clinical nursing experience and more than 5 years of working experience in specialized nurse department; (4) certain level of English language (CET-4); (5) strong clinical observation, evaluation, and complex problem-solving abilities; and (6) valid theoretical foundation and skilled nursing expertise (Peng and Chen 2011). In Jiangsu province, their entry criteria for SN are nurses with college degree or above, have 10 ~ 15 years of clinical working experience, and have working experience in this specialized nursing field. SN certificate is issued by the national/provincial government or nursing associations or CNS organization (Wang et al. 2017).

After SN obtained their certificate, they still need to be evaluated and to register again several years later. In 2018, Shanxi Medical Academy constructed and published the national specialized nurse assessment standard for re-registration (Guo et al. 2018). In this standard, five aspects of evaluation were addressed as shown below (Table 13.1):

The roles of SN are as follows:

1. Clinical nurses should offer specialized nursing care and resolve complex clinical problems in the form of consultation.
2. Supporter and coordinator should be responsible for explaining and coordinating problems between colleagues or patients with nurses.
3. Educator should have sharp sensitivity and deep understanding of patient's problems, promoting patients' self-management as well as being a leader among peers in nursing theoretical teaching, skill training, and evaluation.
4. Researcher should pay close attention to the latest development in the specialized nurse field and apply the research finding in daily work.
5. Clinical leaders should actively engage in the promotion of the development of nursing (Wang et al. 2017).

Table 13.1 Specialized nurse evaluation for re-registration (Guo et al. 2018)

Aspect	Items
Job performance	Conduct consultation within institution for more than five times each year
	Attend specialist nurse clinic
	Join critically ill patient rescuing
	Participate in the formulation of regulation and standard of CNS within the hospital
	Work in the registered specialty field for more than 5 years
On-the-job learning	Participate at least one program of CNS training in other hospitals or institutions each year
	Participate at least one program of CNS training within the hospital every half a year
	Obtain certain credits in the registered nursing specialty field every year
	Catch up with the latest research and development of the registered nursing specialty, and report once every 4 months
Clinical teaching	Give a lecture at least once a year in other hospitals or institutions
	Give a lecture at least once every half a year within the hospital
	Organize the patient rounds in her/his department concerning the nursing specialty practice
	Evolved in the training for nurse specialist
Scientific research performance	At least applied one patent every year
	Publish at least one paper on national nursing journal every 2 years
	Successfully applied a scientific foundation in her/his specialty field within 5 years
Register criteria	If she/he leaves the specialty for more than 2 years, she/he needs to be evaluated and registered again
	Before registering, she/he must take examination of specialty knowledge test and skill examination

For the work arrangement of SN, some of the SN works in collaboration with the doctors. For example, in the endocrinology, gynecology, and obstetrics departments, the doctors will refer patients to the nurse clinic, while some nurse clinics, such as PICC or Wound Care Clinic, require patient to make an appointment. According to a survey, more than 30% of SN take the roles of SN and head nurse at the same time, and 80% of their time are spent administering the nursing department, indicating that we need to further clarify the division of responsibility and the role of positioning.

13.8 Moving Forward: Challenges and Opportunities

Through years of hard work, we have made huge progress in SN cultivation and management. In most hospitals across China, the leaders of medical institutions place ever-increasing importance on the SN, and every year, a large number of nurses will go to different institutions to attend the SN training program. The SN also established their own network (http://www.gc-nurse.com/) to share their experience and latest information about the development of SN both in China and abroad. Many nursing scholars are now conducting a lot of research about the training curriculum, evaluation, registration, and management of CNS.

But challenges remain in the way to the further development of SN in China. Firstly, until now, we do not have consistent definition of SN, which will lead to different levels of comprehension and threaten the possibility of national regulation and communication in nursing, thereby obstructing the development of specialist nurses. Secondly, in comparison with the large number of trainees, we still need more qualified training teachers. Thirdly, we need to improve the quality of training programs. Fourthly, in order to manage SN more efficiently, we need to establish a more unified qualification certification system and issue related laws to ensure the conduct of SN in clinic. Last but not the least, traditional Chinese medicine has been widely acknowledged for curing chronic and complex diseases, and as an old Chinese proverb goes, "three points treated seven point nursing." We should emphasize the development of traditional Chinese medicine SN in the near future (Wang et al. 2017).

13.9 Exemplar of Clinical Nurse Specialist Practice

13.9.1 Nurse-Led Clinics for Diabetic Patient

In nurse-led clinics in China, nursing practice is performed by a group of experienced, highly educated, and higher professionally ranked nurses. SN offer advanced practice in certain nursing areas. Their work is conducted independently or in collaboration with other healthcare workers. Rather than making diagnoses or providing treatment, SN in a nurse-led clinic will apply the holistic view as a nursing principle and cooperate with patients to meet the needs of the patients and their families, as well as maintain or promote the health condition of the patient.

In 2002, the first nurse-led clinic for diabetic patients in China was opened in Beijing. Since then, more hospitals opened nurse-led clinics for diabetic patients. SN in a nurse-led clinic for diabetic patients will provide health education in person, hold regular lectures in the clinic, and organize different forms of health education for diabetic patients, such as disseminating brochures, experience sharing with peers, family visiting, etc.

The work content of SN in the clinic includes informing the patients about the procedure, cooperation tips, the meaning of oral glucose tolerance test, medication knowledge, psychological consultation, feet caring, self-monitoring of blood sugar, how to give insulin injection, how to recognize the symptoms of hyperglycemia and hypoglycemia, etc.

During the work of SN in the nurse-led clinic for diabetic patients, problems still exist, for example, the SN works in the nurse-led clinic as well as in other depart-ments, there are only a few hospitals equipped with such institution, a unified man-agement scheme has no consensus on clinic working time, SN's qualification, nursing procedure, work scope, etc. Their contributions to the clinic are under no connection with their work performance, which means the billing is directly charged from the doctors' registration fees rather than individual nursing fees.

References

Chen FJ, Li JP (2015) The introduction of specialist nurses in China and abroad and its enlighten-ment. J Nurs Training 30(3):209–211

Chen FJ, Li JP (2017) Analysis of related problems of specialist nurses in China. J Nurs Sci 24:68–71

Gao SQ (2015) Study on the competency model of nurses in the intervention operation room. The Second Military Medical University, Shanghai

Guo HL, Zhang XH, Cui LP et al (2018) Construction of assessment criteria for national profes-sional nurses after qualification certification. Nurs Res 02:256–258

Liang L (2017) Construction of competency factor system for specialist nurses. People's liberation army Journal of nursing 21:20–3

Peng GY, Chen WJ (eds) (2011). Standard of nursing management. Guangzhou, pp 17–63

Sichuan Nursing Association (2016) Enrollment Guide for training programs of specialist nurses. http://schl.scyx.org.cn/news-pxl.asp. Accessed 21 July 2018

Song GQ, Fang T, Zhu XQ et al (2007) Experiences of training program for specialist nurses in emergency department. Chin Nurs Res 21(4):1027–1029

Wang JF, Han L, Guo HL et al (2017) Development status of specialist nurses at home and abroad and its enlightenment to the development of TCM nursing specialist. J Nurs Sci 11:93–97

Xu J, Shang LP, Wang BQ et al (2009) Construction of nursing master's degree education in line with CNS. Nurs Res 4:1103–1105

Yang JY, Jia NF, Li GX et al (2015) Problems and reflection in the training and certification of specialized nurses in China. Chinese J Modern Nurs 6(21):635–636

You LM, Wan LH, Yan J et al (2012) Training status of specialist nurses and its enlightenment to professional master's degree training. Chinese J Nurs Educ 5(9):211–214

The Role and Practice of Clinical Nurse Specialist in Taiwan

14

Li-Min Wu, Yao-Mei Chen, Chin-Mi Chen, and Yvonne Yueh-Feng Lu

Abstract

The objectives of this chapter are to help readers to (1) trace the historic development of advanced nursing practice in Taiwan; (2) identify the conceptualization and cooperative teamwork model of advanced nursing practice in Taiwan; (3) describe the core competencies of advanced practice nursing, the outcomes measures, and evaluation of competencies in different healthcare facilities; (4) distinguish the educational preparation and practice roles; (5) explore challenges and future opportunities in advanced nursing practice development; and finally (6) discuss a brief case of the impacts of advanced practice nursing in significantly reducing the rate of ventilator-associated pneumonia in a large acute hospital setting in Taiwan.

This chapter has been written before the 2020 APN ICN guidelines were published and reflects the views of the authors.

L.-M. Wu (✉)
School of Nursing, Kaohsiung Medical University, Kaohsiung, Taiwan
e-mail: painting@kmu.edu.tw

Y.-M. Chen
School of Nursing, Kaohsiung Medical University, Kaohsiung, Taiwan

Superintendent Office, Kaohsiung Medical University Hospital, Kaohsiung, Taiwan

Taiwan Nurses Association, Taipei, Taiwan
e-mail: ymchen@kmu.edu.tw

C.-M. Chen
Department of Nursing, Fu Jen Catholic University, New Taipei City, Taiwan
e-mail: 128135@mail.fju.edu.tw

Y. Y.-F. Lu
School of Nursing, Kaohsiung Medical University, Kaohsiung, Taiwan

Department of Science of Nursing Care, School of Nursing, Indiana University, Indianapolis, IN, USA
e-mail: yuelu@iu.edu

© Springer Nature Switzerland AG 2021
J. S. Fulton, V. W. Holly (eds.), *Clinical Nurse Specialist Role and Practice*, Advanced Practice in Nursing, https://doi.org/10.1007/978-3-319-97103-2_14

Keywords
Nursing · Career · Clinical ladder · Clinical nurse specialist · Advanced practice nursing · Professional competencies · Health assessment

14.1   Brief History of Clinical Nursing Specialists' Roles and Practice in Taiwan

Taiwan is a small country in eastern Asia with a population of 23.6 million (Department of Statistics 2018a). Its economy has developed rapidly in the last 60 years, with rapid transition from an agricultural to an industrial basis. Taiwan adopted a government-administrated, insurance-based national healthcare system in 1995. Life expectancy in the country has reached a record high of 80.0 years. People aged 65 years and older accounted for 13.2% of the population in 2016, and this proportion will reach 38.9% by 2050 (Department of Statistics 2018b; National Development Council 2016). The changing demands of this growing aging population, the rapid expansion of knowledge underlying practice, and the complexity of Taiwan's healthcare environment require healthcare practitioners to have a high level of scientific knowledge and practice expertise to ensure high-quality patient outcomes. Thus, the reconceptualization of clinical nursing practice competencies and educational programs to prepare professional nurses is essential.

In 1992, the Taiwan Nurses Association (TWNA) developed the Clinical Ladder System (CLS), which aimed to (1) create stability for nurses in the workplace, (2) meet the professional needs of nurses, and (3) promote high-quality nursing care. In the CLS, nurses are ranked using four practice levels from novice (level I, N, N1) to expert (level IV, N4; Fig. 14.1). Progression through the CLS system has been considered to be preliminary training for advanced practice nursing (APN). Since 1996, the CLS has been utilized increasingly in healthcare settings such as medical centers, regional hospitals, and home care and long-term care organizations (TWNA 2017b).

In 2012, the TWNA established the Advanced Nursing Practice Committee to promote APN certification development (TWNA 2017a). Taiwan's Ministry of Health and Welfare also proposed the nursing reform program to redefine the scope of nursing practice, enhance nursing practice with interprofessional and cooperative care, and improve professional nursing tasks (Chen et al. 2016). In February 2016, the TWNA defined the core competencies and scopes of APN and revised the CLS (Fig. 14.1) (Wang et al. 2017a).

14.2   Definition of APN

Advanced practice nurses integrate knowledge from the humanities and science; apply technology and information systems to conduct interprofessional cooperation; develop, implement, and evaluate advanced nursing interventions; enhance the

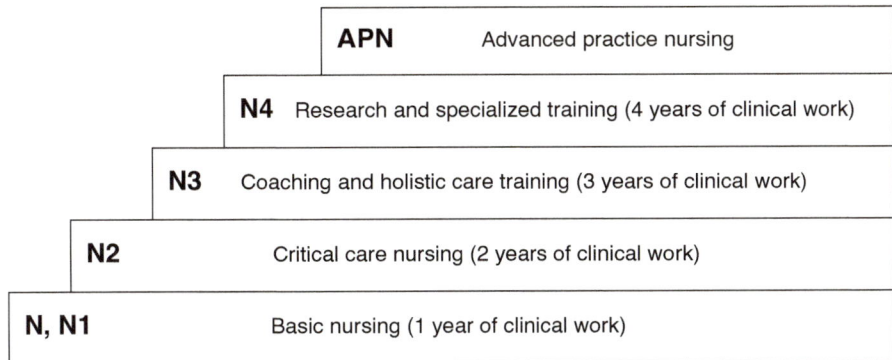

Fig. 14.1 The Clinical Ladder System for nursing in Taiwan

quality of care; promote the health of individuals, families, and groups; and advocate strategies to promote fairness and healthcare policy. Therefore, the definition of clinical APN is advanced nursing with the use of professional knowledge to manage complex situations, make decisions, and expand professional competencies. Advanced practice nurses function as expert clinicians and leaders in advancing nursing practice by caring, teaching, consulting, coordinating, leading, and researching (Wang et al. 2017a).

14.3   Conceptualization and Model of APN

The missions of the Advanced Nursing Practice Committee include definition of the scope of APN, facilitation of its professional development, hosting of APN-related education and training, and promotion of advanced nursing practices and policies at the national level (TWNA 2012). A national survey funded by Taiwan's Ministry of Health and Welfare was conducted in 2014 with a sample of 500 nursing experts (nursing educators, researchers, and administrators and experienced clinical nurses) (Chen et al. 2016). The research team conceptualized APN using a cooperative teamwork model, which involves collaboration with registered nurses (RNs) and nurse aides (NAs) to provide nursing care at different levels (Fig. 14.2). NAs provide basic physical care and assist with activities of daily living and logistics, whereas RNs facilitate the nursing process, health promotion, and disease prevention and communicate and coordinate with the medical team to assure high-quality care delivery. Master-educated APNs act as system leaders, (1) providing higher levels of direct care to patients with complex and difficult needs; (2) working as consultants, coaches, and coordinators for the medical teams and clients; and (3) conducting research and innovation projects to achieve effective care and evidence-based practice, thereby assuring the quality of care and patient safety.

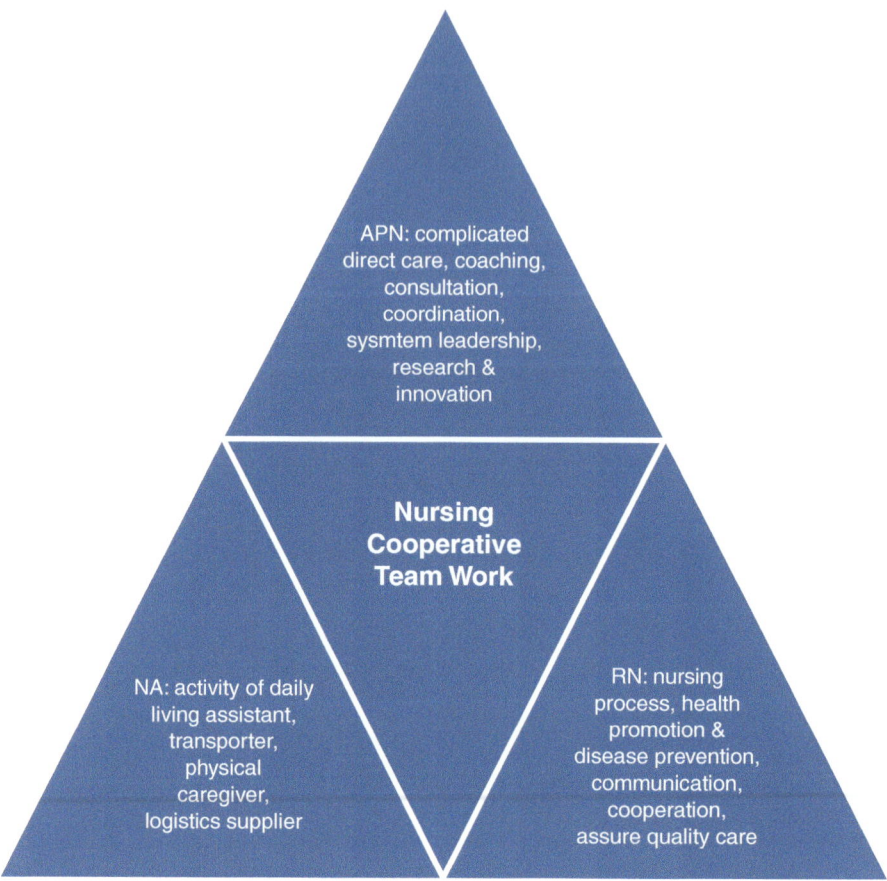

Fig. 14.2 The model of cooperative nursing teamwork (modified from Chen et al. 2016)

14.4 APN Competencies

APN has six core competencies, described as follows (TWNA 2017a):

- **Direct care competence:** Develop and participate in clinical care treatment; manage complex, special, or difficult patients; and provide individual care through using advanced and integrated assessment skills.
- **Coaching competence:** Provide health education guidance for patients and primary caregivers to enhance awareness and self-efficacy in care and health promotion. Provide professional education/or training within medical teams to promote professional academic exchanges.
- **Consultation competence:** Provide professional consultations for patients, primary caregivers, and medical teams, and develop and maintain therapeutic partnerships with patients in order to solve medical care issues together.

- **Coordination competence:** Focus on client-centered care, integrate medical resources, conduct multidiscipline communication and cooperation, and provide consistent high-quality care plans and a safe medical environment.
- **System leadership competence**: Engage in lifelong learning, promote quality care, and manage crisis events to facilitate holistic care in person, family, medical team, and community care system.
- **Research and innovation competence:** Use scientific analysis, discover clinical problems, conduct clinical research based on evidence-based studies, and develop innovative care and standards.

14.5   Outcome Measures and Evaluation

APN performance and outcomes should be evaluated according to the six core competencies recognized by the TWNA (2012). The direct care, coaching, consultation, coordination, system leadership, and research and innovation are performed in a wide variety of healthcare systems, with outcome measures differing, sometimes markedly, among care settings. For example, the first nurse-led peripherally inserted central venous catheter team successfully provided services, ensuring safe and comfortable delivery of chemotherapy, to patients with cancer (Chang and Wang 2004). A neonatal ward employed a nurse specialist as a case manager for low birth weight infants, successfully reducing hospitalization rate after birth (Lee and Wu 2005). Recently, advanced practice nurses have provided evidence-based appraisals and clinical recommendations (Sun et al. 2018). APN core competencies are presented collectively in the practices. However, APN roles in Taiwan are newly developed, and many obstacles have challenged the profession (Chen et al. 2007; Wang et al. 1995). More research is needed to clearly define outcome measures and evaluate the impact or contribution of APN in Taiwan.

14.6   APN Education

Advanced nursing education in Taiwan has comprised master's and doctoral programs for decades. The master's education program was initiated in 1979. Currently, 19 universities and colleges provide master's programs for such APN roles as clinical nurse specialist, advanced community health nurse, nurse practitioner (NP), clinical research nurse, and nurse midwife. The PhD program was initiated in 1997 and is currently offered by 11 universities in Taiwan (Wang et al. 2017b). Societal changes affecting healthcare needs have provided opportunities for the development of new APN roles. A position statement for master's education was endorsed by the TWNA, Taiwan Nurse Practitioner Association, and Taiwan Nurses Education Association in 2017 (TWNA 2017a). The aim of this master's education is to cultivate registered nurses with advanced clinical competencies to meet the healthcare needs of the society. Students should be able to integrate knowledge from the humanities and sciences, apply technology and information systems, participate in multidisciplinary collaboration, and advocate strategies for the development of healthcare policies reflecting justice and equality. The master's programs cultivate the six APN core competencies. The APN curriculum in master's education has three domains (TWNA 2017a):

1. Advanced professional domain knowledge, including advanced pathophysiology, advanced theory, and concept courses in the specialty area
2. Research, including methodologies for evidence-based healthcare and clinical decision-making, as well as a 6-credit hour thesis
3. Clinical practicum hours, including sufficient advanced clinical practicum hours (at least 288 hours for non-NP programs and 504 hours for NP programs, according to Taiwan's NP accreditation law)

A total of 36 credit hours of coursework, including domain knowledge, research, and clinical practicum, is required for graduation.

The main developmental differences between NP and advanced APN in Taiwan are presented in Table 14.1. NPs receive training in specific certified teaching hospitals for 6 months, and the training program consists of 184 hours of lectures and 504 hours of clinical practicum. The NP training lectures focus on differential diagnosis, pathophysiology, and medical treatments. The certification of teaching hospitals for NPs is accredited by the Ministry of Health and Welfare in Taiwan. The main role of NPs is to cooperate with physicians in implementing medical treatments and working in a specific specialty focusing on patients and families in hospitals. APNs are required to complete graduate nursing programs on developing system skills and emotional and intellectual competency. The expectations of APNs are to develop expert competence in self-awareness, resilience, handling difficult information, active coaching and mentoring, and participation or cooperation on interprofessional teams within organization(s) to address ethical risk issues and inform patients of the risks and benefits and the outcomes of healthcare.

14.7 Moving Forward: Challenges and Opportunities

APN in Taiwan is still evolving. APN education programs and credentialing regulations are in place, with some challenges ahead and emerging opportunities.

14.7.1 Challenges

Undergraduate nursing education programs vary in terms of the qualification, maturity, and humanistic literacy of students, with differences in curriculum designs (Chao 2008; Chao et al. 2010). Furthermore, the RN licensure examination has had a low passing rate of around 50% (Ministry of Examination 2017). These students are APN program candidates. RNs should have soundly developed basic nursing competencies before moving toward advanced roles.

Table 14.1 Description of the developmental differences between NP and APN in Taiwan

Developmental differences	Nurse practitioners (NP)	Advanced practice nurses (APN)
Criteria	• Licensed as a professional registered nurse • At least an Associate Degree of Nursing • At least 3 years of nursing clinical experience • Must attend a training program provided by specific certified teaching hospitals for 6 months and accredited by the Ministry of Health and Welfare in Taiwan • Training consists of 184 hours of lectures and 504 hours of clinical practicum	• Licensed as a professional registered nurse • At least a Master's Degree of Nursing • At least 5 years of nursing clinical experience • At least nursing clinical ladder 4 (N4) level • Completed at least 288 hours of advanced clinical nursing practicum • Member of the Taiwan Nursing Association
Certification	• Passed the National State Board written exam and Objective Structured Clinical Exam within 2 years • Certified by the Taiwan National State Board	• No National State Board exam required • Certified by the Taiwan Nursing Association
Credential	• Recognized and approved by the Taiwan National State Board • 120 contact hours of continued education required for the renewal of NP license every 6 years	• Recognized and approved by the Taiwan Nursing Association • 120 contact hours of continued education required for the renewal of APN license every 6 years
Clinical expertise	• Competency and excellence with patients and families by assisting physician in medical assessment and differential diagnosis and implementing some medical treatments (wound care, physical assessment, some symptom treatment)	• Hands-on direct care • Excellence with patients, families, and related system-level initiatives
System skills	Communication bridge between physician and nurse	Role models skills to other nurses, coaches development of skills; collaborates with and provides consultation to other members of the healthcare team
Practice setting	• Hospitals	• Hospitals • Community settings • Home care agencies • Long-term care facilities • Nursing homes • Assisted living facilities • Rehabilitation facilities

(continued)

Table 14.1 (Continued)

Developmental differences	Nurse practitioners (NP)	Advanced practice nurses (APN)
Clinical focus	Within a specialty unit (e.g., medical, surgical, pediatric, psychiatric or obstetrics and gynecology)	Within specialty organizations/systems and populations: critical care, medical, surgical, pediatric, clinical research, clinical nursing education, infection control, oncology, hospice care, diabetes educator, gerontology nursing care, quality assurance, long-term care and others

Note: NP can be also considered as APN, if NP completed the master's education program and met the criteria of APN

The state-issued APN credential and the APN license are not officially required by the Taiwanese government (Chao et al. 2010), but the TWNA accredited the APN certification in 2016. As APN is in an early phase of development, institutions (e.g., medical centers) have created few APN positions, and the information about the impact of APN on the quality of care is limited (Chang et al. 2003; Feng et al. 2015). Thus, more evidence-based knowledge regarding the impacts of APN on the quality of care, patient outcomes, and healthcare costs is critically needed.

14.7.2 Opportunities

In Taiwan, emerging needs promote advanced nursing education and the enhancement of evidence-based clinical practice in various healthcare settings. The country's Ministry of Education has promoted nursing education reform by establishing the Taiwan Nursing Accreditation Council (TNAC) in 2006 and by overseeing peer-reviewed evaluation of various nursing education programs (Chao et al. 2010). The aims of the TNAC are to identify strategies to minimize the gap between nursing educational programs and clinical practice (Chao et al. 2010). Following recommendations for reform, many nursing schools have consolidated their programs to focus on the translation of scientific knowledge and research findings and the implementation of evidence-based nursing practice and research (Chen 2014). Preparing nurses to perform evidence-based clinical practice, promote healthcare quality, improve patient outcomes and safety, and promote the cost effectiveness of services is crucial.

As the world and its economies are becoming increasingly globalized, with extensive international travel and commerce, global health plays an increasingly crucial role in global security and the security of Taiwan's population. Infectious disease emergencies (e.g., severe acute respiratory syndrome [SARS] outbreak) and other health threats in the world must be minimized or prevented. For example, the majority of public health nurses reported lacked of confidence in implementing extensive quarantine policies (Hsu et al. 2006). With advanced competencies, APN has full capabilities to work with medical team for pandemic control. Thus, the integration of various global education components into an APN program is critically needed. Fostering of the APN capability to manage any global health-related issue is important. The development of APN clinical competence to lead and cooperate with interdisciplinary teams in dealing with such issues, maintaining the security of the global population and that of Taiwan, is also important.

14.8 APN Case Example

In the pilot case study described here, advanced practice nurses led an interdisciplinary team in executing a revised bundle care protocol to reduce the rate of ventilator-associated pneumonia (VAP) among patients in a surgical intensive care unit (SICU) in northern Taiwan. In February 2013, these nurses identified an increase in the VAP rate from 2.6 to 9.7% among SICU patients after the implementation of the initial standardized bundle care in January 2013. After identifying this poor outcome (American Thoracic Society, & Infectious Diseases Society of America 2005; Wip and Napolitano 2009), they led an interdisciplinary team (including a physician, an infection control team, a respiratory therapist, and clinical nurses) in a project to reduce the VAP rate in this patient population from April to December 2013 by using the following strategies: (1) identifying the factors associated with the increase in the infection rate, (2) evaluating each component of the initial standardized bundle care, (3) integrating the evidence-based practice findings to support or modify initial bundle care components (e.g., revising the oral care guidelines and inspection methods, using hand washing tips and marking labels, and elevating the heads of patients' beds to 30–45° angles), (4) training clinical nurses and the respiratory therapist to apply the revised bundle care protocol for SICU patients and developing the modified bundle care protocol, and (5) evaluating the outcomes of modified bundle care protocol implementation. These advanced practice nurses showed that these measures significantly improved outcomes, increasing the rate of proper implementation of revised bundle care from 48.3 to 93.3% and reducing the VAP rate in the SICU from 9.7% to 0% (Chen et al. 2017).

 This case study illustrated several APN competences mentioned above. The APN detected the reasons of poor outcome and effectively reduced VAP rate to present direct care and research competence. Additionally, they managed an interdisciplinary team to solve problems resulting in VAP to demonstrate leadership, consultation, collaboration, and coaching competence.

References

American Thoracic Society, & Infectious Diseases Society of America (2005) Guidelines for the management of adults with hospital-acquired, ventilator-associated, and healthcare-associated pneumonia. Am J Respir Crit Care Med 171(4):388–416

Chang LL, Wang SC (2004) A nurse-led PICC insertion service in a cancer center. J Oncol Nurs 49(2):35–41

Chang LL, Chang P, Tsai JS, Yu LH (2003) Clinical nurse specialist in cancer care. Med Educ 7(2):179–190

Chao YM (2008) Nursing education in Taiwan. In: Wang HH (ed) Nursing care in Taiwan, 1st edn. Department of Health, Executive Yuan, Taiwan, ROC, Taipei, pp 21–30

Chao YM, Dai YT, Yeh MC (2010) Perspectives on nursing education, licensing examinations and professional core competence in Taiwan in the context of globalization. J Nurs 57(5):5–11

Chen CH (2014) Nursing education in Taiwan: the current situation and prospects for the future. Kaohsiung J Nurs 31:6–9

Chen Y, Chen S, Tsai C, Lo L (2007) Role stress and job satisfaction for nurse specialists. J Adv Nurs 59(5):497–509

Chen YM, Wang HH, Kao CC, Chan SC, Chang TY, Tseng HC, Huang IC (2016) The facilitation and prospects of schematization of skill-mixed nursing care model in Taiwan. J Taiwan Nurs Pract 2(1):5–12

Chen YT, Lai HF, Lee CC, Lin JP (2017) To increase the implementation rate of ventilator-associated pneumonia bundle care in a surgical intensive care unit. J MacKay Nurs 11(2):48–59

Department of Statistics, Ministry of the Interior, Taiwan, ROC (2018a) Household registration. https://www.ris.gov.tw/en/web/ris3-english/home. Accessed 3 May 2018

Department of Statistics, Ministry of the Interior, Taiwan, ROC (2018b) Monthly bulletin of interior statistics. https://www.moi.gov.tw/files/site_stuff/321/1/month/month_en.html. Accessed 3 May 2018

Feng RC, Lee YL, Lee TY (2015) The role development of informatics nurse specialists in Taiwan. J Nurs 62(3):23–29

Hsu CC, Chen T, Chang M, Chang YK (2006) Confidence in controlling a SARS outbreak: experience of public nurses in managing home quarantine measures in Taiwan. Am J Infect Control 34(4):176–118

Lee YH, Wu CH (2005) Promote the model of premature and the family care by nurse specialists. VGHN J 22(1):30–40

Ministry of Examination, Taiwan, ROC (2017) Various exam statistics. http://wwwc.moex.gov.tw/main/ExamReport/wFrmExamStatistics.aspx?menu_id=158. Accessed 22 Dec 2017

National Development Council, Taiwan, ROC (2016) Population projections for R.O.C. (Taiwan): 2016~2060. https://www.ndc.gov.tw/Content_List.aspx?n=84223C65B6F94D72. Accessed 3 May 2018

Sun WN, Su JW, Shen ZP, Hsu ST (2018) Effect of oral glutamine on chemotherapy-induced peripheral neuropathy in cancer patients: an evidence-based appraisal. J Nurs 65(1):61–69

Taiwan Nurse Association (2017a) Advanced practice nurse certification program development. https://www.twna.org.tw/frontend/un10_open/welcome.asp#. Accessed 22 Dec 2017

Taiwan Nurse Association (2017b) The clinical ladder system. https://www.twna.org.tw/frontend/un10_open/welcome.asp#. Accessed 22 Dec 2017

Taiwan Nurses Association (2012) The missions of TWNA committees. http://www.ngo.e-twna.org.tw/about_4.php. Accessed 24 Apr 2018

Wang J, Yen M, Snyder M (1995) Constraints and perspectives of advanced practice nursing in Taiwan, Republic of China. Clin Nurse Spec 9(5):252–255

Wang KY, Tsay SL, Chou FH (2017a) Taiwan nursing master education joint statement. http://www.twna.org.tw/frontend/un09_news/news_newsdetail.asp?t_id=6551&sector. Accessed 22 Dec 2017

Wang KY, Wang HH, Hwang LH, Tzeng WC, Chang HY, Chuang TS (2017b) The report on 18th ICN Asia Workforce Forum (AWFF) & 14th Alliance of Asian Nurses Association (AANA). 14–16: p 24

Wip C, Napolitano L (2009) Bundles to prevent ventilator-associated pneumonia: how valuable are they? Curr Opin Infect Dis 22(2):159–166

Part V

Africa and Middle East

The Role and Practice of Clinical Nurse Specialist in Turkey

15

Sultan Kav

Abstract

Clinical nurse specialists play an essential role in delivering care in a variety of settings. In Turkey, areas of specialization in nursing show a parallel development in the progress and demand for healthcare and the nursing profession. The term "nurse specialist" has become an officially recognized title in nursing practice in Turkey, following the new arrangements in nursing law. This chapter will address the history of nursing education, roles and practice, regulations, available programs, challenges, and the future of clinical nurse specialist in Turkey.

Keywords

Specialization · Clinical nurse specialist · Certificate programs · Nursing education · History · Nursing roles · Turkey

15.1 Brief History of the Role and Practice of CNS in Turkey

The works of Florence Nightingale during the Crimean War is often cited as the beginning of modern nursing; however, nursing did not begin in Turkey until the Balkan War in 1912. In 1920, the Admiral Bristol Nursing School began a two-and-a-half-year nursing education program to train nurses for the American hospital,

---

This chapter has been written before the 2020 APN ICN guidelines were published and reflects the views of the authors.

S. Kav (✉)
Baskent University Faculty of Health Sciences, Ankara, Turkey
e-mail: skav@baskent.edu.tr

© Springer Nature Switzerland AG 2021
J. S. Fulton, V. W. Holly (eds.), *Clinical Nurse Specialist Role and Practice*,
Advanced Practice in Nursing, https://doi.org/10.1007/978-3-319-97103-2_15

203

which was followed in 1925 by the 2-year Society of Kizilay Nursing School, established through the efforts of the Mustafa Kemal Atatürk, the founder of the Republic of Turkey (Dal and Kitiş 2008; Can 2010; Terzioglu 2011).

Turkey was the first European country to provide facilities for undergraduate nursing education, followed by the UK (Smith 2006). The first Turkish University School of Nursing opened in 1955 at Ege University. There was no master's program for nursing until 1968.

The Master of Science in Nursing Program initiated in 1968, followed by the Nursing Doctoral Education Program in 1972 in Hacettepe University (Dal and Kitiş 2008; Bahçecik and Alpar 2009; Terzioglu 2011) (Table 15.1).

The International Council of Nursing identified specialties in nursing in 1992 and started to study the integration of these specialties. The Council of National Nursing and Nursing Education of Turkey started a project in 2005 titled "Study of National Specialization for Nursing and Midwifery." The following criteria have been determined for specialization (Adibelli et al. 2017):

- Specialization must be at the national level.
- It must be appropriate for the aim, function, and ethical standards of nursing/ midwifery.
- Specialization must be specific in identified areas of nursing/midwifery.
- It must cover the areas of society needs.
- It must be concentrated on core education of nursing and midwifery.
- Specialty practice must be achieved with professional development and continuing education, including both formal and informal education.

Table 15.1 Historical developments influencing nursing education in Turkey

Historical developments	Year
Introduction of a 6-month course to train voluntary medical attendants, with Dr. Besim Omer Pasha's advice to the Red Crescent Association regarding the inadequacy of healthcare services	1912
Admiral Bristol Nursing School introduced in Istanbul within an American hospital as caregiver course (a two-and-a-half-year nursing education program)	1920
Kizilay Nursing School opened in the Republic period as the first Turkish nursing school	1925
Turkish Nurses Association (TNA) was established	1933
The Ministry of Health founded the nursing schools, as a 3-year program; then extended to 4 years in 1958	1946
Ege University School of Nursing was the first academy in Turkey that offered university-level education (4 years Bachelor in Nursing Program)	1955
Hacettepe University initiated the Master of Science in Nursing Program	1968
The Doctorate in Nursing Program was initiated at Hacettepe University	1972
Foundation of associate programs (2 years university education)	1988
Health vocational high schools were assigned to universities to transform undergraduate nursing education	1992
Revision of the nursing law was confirmed	2007

15.2   Definition of CNS

Specialization in nursing, in Turkey, was legally defined in 2007. According to the "Nursing Law," nurses who completed their postgraduate education in the field of nursing were entitled as specialist nurse. "Expert (specialist) nurse: A nurse who specializes in post graduate education related to her profession and whose diploma is registered by Ministries'.

Item 8-Nurses who have specialized by completing postgraduate programs related to their profession and whose diplomas are registered by Ministry of Health and nurses who are graduated from these programs abroad and whose diplomas are approved as equivalents work as specialist nurse" (Law No: 5634 RG: 2.5.2007/26510).

Nurses who hold a baccalaureate degree in nursing can work as a "specialist nurse" after they completed graduate education and specialize in a given clinical area. Following graduation from a baccalaureate program, nurses receive an authorization document that allows them to practice within a given framework of standards determined at the unit level, based on the care required by patients in a specific unit, for example, intensive care, oncology, emergency care, stoma care, and diabetes care, as determined by the Ministry of Health. The revised law also states that nurses' authority and responsibility will be determined by their educational level (Nursing Regulation, Official Gazette Date 8.03.2010. Number: 27515).

15.3   CNS Practice Competencies

Under the Law on Amending the Regulation of Nursing, promulgated in 2011, specialization has acquired legal grounds. In this regulation, the following items were included:

- "Nurses makes comprehensive health assessments related to the area of specialization. Plans, implements and manages nursing care plan. In case care goals cannot be achieved, new strategies are developed.
- In critical situations related to the medical diagnosis and treatment procedures, counsel to the nurses in order to make appropriate decision and help to the nurses in terms of their professional development.
- Plan the education of the patient and his / her family. Inform patients about the possible side effects with their care and treatment methods. Provides means for patients to access to up-to-date and reliable health information.
- Provides consultancy and expertise to individuals, institutions and organizations related to the field of expertise and ethical issues. Can take part in the ethics committee on research in the institution."

Definitions of the duties, authorities, and responsibilities of the nurses according to the unit/service/areas of working were listed/published in the official gazette on 19 April 2011, No. 27910. These were:

- Intensive care nursing
- Emergency care nursing
- Medical nursing (diabetes educator nurse, oncology nurse, rehabilitation nurse, endoscopy)
- Surgical nursing (operation room nursing, ostomy and wound care nurse)
- Mental health nursing (psychiatric clinic nurse, child and adolescent psychiatric nurse, consultation-liaison psychiatry nurse, alcohol and substance abuse center nurse)
- Pediatric and neonatal nursing
- Women health and obstetric nursing
- Community health nursing (home care nurse, Mother and Child Health and Family Planning Center nurse, Community Mental Health Center nurse, occupational health nurse, school health nurse, Criminal and Detention House nurse)

Nursing interventions list included an annex and checked whether nurses can do/decide independently, with physician orders or jointly.

Professional specialization enables members of a profession to acquire in-depth knowledge regarding a special field, perform qualitative research, and enhance their scientific knowledge. A nurse with adequate knowledge and skills with respect to his or her special field will undoubtedly have the power and competency to make decisions (Baykara and Şahinoğlu 2014).

15.4   CNS Education

Initial education for nursing must be offered in an undergraduate program within a university. In Turkey, there are different types of university-level nursing schools: school of health, school of nursing, faculty of health sciences, and faculty of nursing. Although the names of schools are different, curricula of these schools are based on the regulations prepared by the Turkish Higher Education Council. According to these regulations, nursing education must be at least 4 years or 4600 hours in theoretical course and clinical practice. Theoretical classroom education must be at least one-third, and clinical practice must be half of the total education. The minimum requirement for admission to nursing education is a high school diploma (Can 2010; Güner 2015). In the 2017–2018 academic year, 124 undergraduate nursing programs are present, 90 of them were state and 34 foundation universities (https://yokatlas.yok.gov.tr/lisans-anasayfa.php).

The Turkish Higher Education Council (CoHE) controls all undergraduate and graduate education. Specialist nursing education is provided via Master's and Doctoral programs (Table 15.2). The National Qualifications Framework for Higher

Table 15.2   Master and doctorate programs in nursing

Master programs in nursing	Doctorate programs in nursing
Master of Science in Nursing	Doctorate in Nursing
Fundamentals of Nursing	Fundamentals of Nursing
Pediatric Nursing	Internal Medical Nursing
Public Health Nursing	Pediatric Nursing
Surgical Nursing	Public Health Nursing
Nursing Education	Nursing Education
Nursing Management	Nursing Management
Internal Medical Nursing	Surgical Nursing
Women Health and Obstetric Nursing	Women Health and Obstetric Nursing
Mental Health and Psychiatry	Mental Health and Psychiatry Nursing
Critical Care Nursing	
Gerontology Nursing	
Oncology Nursing	

Education in Turkey developed with reference to the Qualifications Framework of the European Higher Education Area and the European Qualifications Framework for lifelong learning was adopted by the CoHE in 2010 (http://www.yok.gov.tr/en/web/cohe/higher-education-system).

Admission requirements for postgraduate programs include Bachelor's Degree in Nursing for master's degree and master degree for the doctorate program, satisfactory scores on the Academic Graduate Studies Entrance Exam and the English-language proficiency test, and a test of general nursing knowledge that is administered by each school (Can 2010).

Master programs consist of two stages: completing a number of courses and conducting research in related subject. Students are required to take 21 credits (120 ECTS: European Credit Transfer System) minimum in two semesters. The students have to complete all the requirements for an MSc degree in four semesters.

Doctoral education in nursing in Turkey began as a single topic nursing program; today it is divided into eight: Fundamentals of Nursing, Medical Nursing, Surgical Nursing, Women's Health and Obstetrics, Children's Health and Diseases, Mental Health and Psychiatry, Public Health, and Education in Nursing (Yavuz 2004). In 2001, 6 universities provided nursing doctoral education while 20 universities provided nursing doctoral education in 2015. 44 universities now offering doctoral programs (Fig. 15.1).

In Turkey, the doctoral education in nursing is carried out with a Doctor of Philosophy in Nursing (PhD) via the Health Sciences Institutes doctoral programs and takes about 4 years. Students are required to take a minimum of 24 credits (120 ECTS for compulsory and elective courses and 120 ECTS for PhD thesis study) in doctoral programs. If students complete the courses successfully, they make their research in the area chosen by them with their supervisor. After the completion of the thesis, it is defended against a jury consisting of five faculty members, and, if successful, students are awarded with a PhD degree. A distinct difference from the master program, students of the doctorate program need to take a comprehensive/qualifying examination (comprehensive written and oral examination conducted by

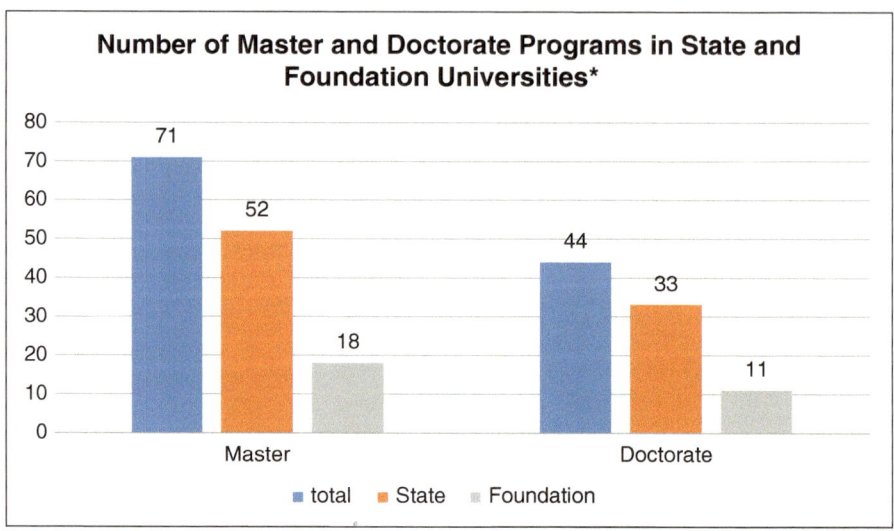

Fig. 15.1 Number of master and doctorate programs in nursing. *Based on universities' website*

a committee of five examiners, at least one of whom is external to the university) to pursue PhD thesis work (Can 2010).

The Council of Higher Education organized a workshop on undergraduate education in nursing in order to increase the quality of education in nursing undergraduate programs and raise the standards of these undergraduate programs in November 2017. In this workshop report, it was documented that there are total of 79,054 students, of which 71,538 are undergraduate students, 6157 are postgraduate students, and 1359 are doctoral students in nursing programs. The number of academic staff is 1562. There are a total of 694 faculty members, of which 125 are professors, 140 are associate professors, and 429 are assistant professors. The number of staff other than faculty members is 868 (A report of the Council of Higher Education workshop on undergraduate education in nursing 2017).

According to the Report on Health Education and Workforce in Turkey (Ministry of Health Statistics Year Book 2016), a total of 871,334 healthcare professionals, of which 144,827 are medical doctors, 26,674 are dentists, 27,864 are pharmacists, 152,952 are nurses, 52,456 are midwives, and 144,609 are other health personnel, are currently working in Turkey.

15.5   Credentialing: Regulatory, Legal, and Certification Requirements

In Turkey, nurses are working under the law of civil servants numbered 657 or the labor law numbered 4857. The Nursing Law numbered 6283 and dated February 25, 1954, and its amendment dated April 25, 2007, acknowledged that nursing practice could only be offered as an undergraduate degree, which revised the definition of

Table 15.3 Current certification programs for nurses

Areas	Year	Theory[a]	Practice[a]	Total[a]
Hemodialysis and peritoneal dialysis nursing	2014	26	454	480/60
Intensive care nursing	2015	120/15	120/15	240/30
Oncology nursing	2015	56/7	64/8	120/15
Palliative care nursing	2015	35/5	80/10	115/15
Diabetes nursing	2015	88/11	72/9	160/20
Ostomy and wound care nursing	2015	80/10	160/20	240/30
Nutrition nursing	2015	80/10	80/8	160/18
Home healthcare services nursing	2015	52/7	108/13	160/20
Operating room nursing	2015	96/12	80/10	176/22
Pediatric intensive care nursing	2016	80/10	120/15	200/25
Emergency care nursing	2016	120/15	120/15	240/30
Infection control nursing	2017	35/10	120/15	155/25
Pediatric emergency care nursing	2017	80/10	120/15	200/25
Neonatal intensive care nursing	2017	66/10	120/15	186/25
Psychiatric units nursing	2017	94/12	156/20	250/32

[a]Study hours/working days

nurse as a title granted to those graduating from universities offering undergraduate degrees. Another amendment to this law made it possible for nurses to be granted authorization certificates in their field and also for those nurses doing a graduate degree to be given the title of specialist nurse. Dialysis nursing, infection control nursing, diabetes nursing, ostomy and wound care nursing, chemotherapy nursing, and intensive care nursing certification programs started much earlier and are revised and extended based on the certification requirement set by the Ministry of Health. In Table 15.3, current certification education programs are listed.

In our country, branching can still be used for both "specialist training" and "certificate training." Specialist education is provided by graduate programs in universities, while the Ministry of Health and institutions provide certification programs. Certification programs are not academic; duration, content, and adequacy level vary (Table 15.3). Specialist Nursing Associations and universities are also collaborated to organize such programs.

15.6 Moving Forward: Challenges and Opportunities

Although nursing has started since the 1960s, "nurse specialist" title has gained ground on a proper legal recognition with the new arrangements in nursing law. However, no expert/clinical nurse specialist title has been legally used in the field of work or nurse employment. Until now, the only environment where nurses can use their specialization areas is the universities (Oflaz 2011; Ustun 2016).

Nurses with an additional training remain only recognized as a general nurse even though they have achieved, often significant, further specialization. Although nursing specialization and expertise are legally defined, nurses work in many units of healthcare services (ambulances, emergency service, intensive care, internal diseases, polyclinics, etc.). However, they are unable to acquire a title of specialization or expertise that is particular to those units. This situation prevents them from choosing a field in which to specialize. In addition, working in a specialist area leads to a relevant wider knowledge base but does not lead to being a specialist nurse. Nevertheless, the nurses who specialize through master's and doctoral programs in accordance with the regulation cannot be employed in health services according to their fields of expertise (Çelik et al. 2011; Oflaz 2011; Ustun 2016).

In a study conducted by Adibelli et al. (2017) to determine opinions and suggestions of nurses on specialization, including 458 nurses working in public hospitals, nurses reported problems concerning specialization. Some statements by nurses were as follows: training is not practical and not used during working life (77.5%); nurses are charged with non-nursing tasks in order to relieve the workload of doctors (73.8%); there are not enough associations and institutions protecting the nursing profession (52%); and nurses have inadequate authority and responsibilities (39.5%).

15.7   Future of Specialist Nursing

Specialization will contribute to nursing in several ways: an increase in quality of service and care, a decrease in practical errors, and an increase in job loyalty and satisfaction (Hacihasanoglu Asilar 2017). As the world's largest healthcare professional workforce, providing over 70–80% of healthcare globally, nurses influence the care of patients, families, communities, and healthcare systems (World Health Organization 2015). Aging population indicates an increase in chronic conditions, suggesting potential increase in healthcare demand for complex, integrated, and long-term condition management. Turkish Private Healthcare Sector has grown in parallel with the development of healthcare services across Turkey over the years and is expected to continue to maintain this strong position in the upcoming period and transitions of qualified health personnel from public to private industry.

In today's health system, the necessary nursing services can be provided in a qualified and sufficient way only after specialization. However, studies on effectiveness and contributions into patient care of the clinical nurse specialist in Turkey are scarce (Ardahan and Ozsoy 2015). Clinically oriented graduate programs are needed, and nurses should be employed according to their fields of expertise. Legalization of specialization and nursing specific central examination for its recognition by all other disciplines are required rather than the current system of postgraduate education and certificate programs.

References

Adibelli D, Turan GS, Çinar H (2017) A new system for nursing specialisation: the thoughts and opinions of nurses. J Res Nurs 22(5):354–369

Ardahan M, Ozsoy S (2015) Nursing research trends in Turkey: a study on postgraduate and doctorate theses. Gümüşhane Univ J Health Sci 4(4)

Bahçecik N, Alpar SE (2009) Nursing education in Turkey: from past to present. Nurse Educ Today 29(7):698–703. https://doi.org/10.1016/j.nedt.2009.05.008

Baykara ZG, Şahinoğlu S (2014) An evaluation of nurses' professional autonomy in Turkey. Nurs Ethics 21(4):447–460. https://doi.org/10.1177/0969733013505307

Can G (2010) Nursing education in Turkey. Nurse Educ 35(4):146–147

Çelik S, Keçeci A, Bulduk S (2011) Is nursing a profession in Turkey? Hosp Top 89(2):43–50. https://doi.org/10.1080/00185868.2011.587735

A report of the Council of Higher Education workshop on undergraduate education in nursing. 2017. http://www.yok.gov.tr/web/guest/hemsirelik-lisans-egitimi-calistay-raporu-yayimlandi. Accessed 8 June 2018

Dal U, Kitiş Y (2008) The historical development and current status of nursing in Turkey. OJIN: Online J Issues Nurs 13(2). https://doi.org/10.3912/OJIN.Vol13No02PPT02

Güner P (2015) Preparedness of final-year Turkish nursing students for work as a professional nurse. J Clin Nurs 24(5–6):844–854. https://doi.org/10.1111/jocn.12673

Hacihasanoglu Asilar R (2017) Specialisation trends in nursing. International congress of Black Sea nursing education (ICOBNE) abstract book, October 12–13, 2017, Samsun, Turkey, p 30. https://www.icobne.com/bildiri-kitabi/. Accessed 8 June 2018

Law on Amending the Regulation of Nursing (n.d.) Official Gazette Date 19.04.2011, Number: 27910. http://www.resmigazete.gov.tr/eskiler/2011/04/20110419-5.htm. Accessed 8 June 2018

Ministry of Health Health Statistics Yearbook (2016). http://ohsad.org/wp-content/uploads/2017/12/13160.pdf. Accessed 8 June 2018

Nursing Law (n.d.) Law No: 5634 RG: 2.5.2007/26510. www.saglik.gov.tr/TR/dosya/1-46937/h/hemsirelikkanunu.doc. Accessed 8 June 2018

Nursing Regulation (n.d.) Official Gazette Date 8.03.2010. Number: 27515. http://www.resmigazete.gov.tr/eskiler/2010/03/20100308-4.htm. Accessed 8 June 2018

Oflaz F (2011) Specialization in nursing: in the world and Turkey. SENDROM 23(4):97–100

Smith JP (2006) Higher education and nursing. J Adv Nurs 53(3):259

Terzioglu F (2011) The history of nursing in Turkey. Nurs Hist Rev 19:179–182

Ustun B (2016) Psychiatric nursing in Turkey real or a myth? J Psychiatr Nurs 7(3):157–162

World Health Organization (2015) Options analysis report on strategic directions for nursing and midwifery (2016–2020). http://www.who.int/hrh/nursing_midwifery/options_analysis_report.pdf?ua=1. Accessed 8 June 2018

Yavuz M (2004) Nursing doctoral education in Turkey. Nurse Educ Today 24:553–559

The Role and Practice of Clinical Nurse Specialists: An International Focus on Saudi Arabia

16

Denise Hibbert

Abstract

The roles of clinical nurse specialists (CNS) have been evident in Saudi Arabia since the 1980s. Despite this, and the fact that nurse education has moved from diploma level to university baccalaureate level, the advancement of nursing practice is hampered by the poor image of clinical nursing, leading to poor recruitment into nursing colleges. The slow pace to the Saudization of nursing delays the development of higher education programs aimed at specialist and advanced practice nursing, which in turn prevents legitimization of the CNS role. The Saudi Commission for Health Specialties (SCFHS) registers nurses to practice in Saudi Arabia and has a Nursing Scientific Committee, but does not regulate nursing practice or protect nursing titles. Today, the consequences are clear: there is a shortage of experienced clinical nurses in CNS roles. It is hoped that the Saudi Government's 2030 vision for healthcare, including high reliability organizations, will push the advanced practice nursing (APN) agenda forward.

Keywords

Saudi Arabia · Nurse specialist · Clinical nurse specialist · Advanced practice nurse · Specialty practice

---

This chapter was written before the 2020 APN ICN guidelines were published and reflects the views of the author.

D. Hibbert (✉)
KAAUH, Riyadh, Saudi Arabia

Princess Nourah bint Abdulrahman University, Riyadh, Saudi Arabia

Annals of Saudi Medicine, Riyadh, Saudi Arabia

© Springer Nature Switzerland AG 2021
J. S. Fulton, V. W. Holly (eds.), *Clinical Nurse Specialist Role and Practice*,
Advanced Practice in Nursing, https://doi.org/10.1007/978-3-319-97103-2_16

16.1 Brief History of the Role and Practice of CNS

Nurse training in Saudi Arabia commenced in the mid-1950s (El-Sanabary 1993), and there is evidence of nurses caring for specialist patient populations, in clinical nurse specialist (CNS) roles, since the 1980s. Advanced practice nurse (APN) job descriptions first appeared in the 1990s, while a clinical grading ladder aimed at developing CNS in advanced practice was first approved at a hospital level in 2008. Despite this, employment of CNS as APN is uncommon, most likely due to the low number of Saudi nurses and the poor image of clinical nursing (Hibbert et al. 2012, 2017; Kleinpell et al. 2014). In 2016, the Ministry of Health (MOH) reported a total of 470 hospitals in Saudi Arabia, with 70,844 beds and 2259 primary care centers, serving a population of 31,742,308. At the same time, they reported a low nurse-to-population ratio, 57 nurses to 10,000 of the population. Saudi nurses are reported to make up 49% of the nursing workforce, an increase from 29% in 2008. However, only 14.9% are reported to be employed in tertiary referral centers where CNS are most likely needed (MOH 2008, 2016). For example, the author estimates that there are presently only 12 qualified enterostomal therapists (ostomy, wound, and continence nurses) employed in the Kingdom of Saudi Arabia.

CNSs in Saudi Arabia have traditionally worked with chronic and complex patient populations such as those with stomas, wounds, incontinence, pain, chronic renal failure, in infection control, and palliative care. These CNS are evident in specialist centers but not common in MOH hospitals, general practice, or community settings. They work toward meeting patient population needs, which are similar to those reported internationally and include nurse-led clinics. They commonly include easy access to a knowledgeable key professional; expert care and coordination across the continuum; access to evidence-based information, standards, and resources; and advocacy within the multidisciplinary team and across organizations. They are also involved in education, leadership and research related to their specialty knowledge (Hibbert et al. 2012).

16.2 Definition of CNS

Officially, Saudi Arabia is yet to formerly define APN or the role and scope of the CNS; unofficially, the International Council of Nursing's Definition is commonly quoted; a masters-prepared nurse who works at a higher level than an RN and has more responsibility and accountability. Consequently, there are no standardized or protected job titles or descriptions. The SCFHS assigns non-job-related titles to nurses when registering their qualifications, without consideration of role, level, or scope of practice. The title Nurse Specialist is allocated to all nurses who have a BSN, Senior Specialist to those who have an MSN, and Nurse Consultant to those with a PhD. Unofficially, the title CNS or Clinical Specialist has been utilized in job descriptions to capture the role of clinical nurses working with specialty or subspecialty populations, at a higher level and with more accountability than staff nurses. A higher level of knowledge, skill, and expertise within the specialty is expected along with the ability to utilize evidence-based practice (EBP), manage resources, maintain standards and quality of care, educate others, and develop or integrating services based on population needs (Hibbert et al. 2012, 2017; Kleinpell et al. 2014; SCFHS 2017).

16.3   Conceptualizations/Model(s) of CNS Practice

Although there is not a nationally agreed CNS model, Hibbert et al. (2012) discussed a conceptualized model based on holistic patient-centered care, the four domains for nurse consultants in the United Kingdom (expert clinical practice, education, research, and leadership), and specialist nurse-physician collaboration. The masters-prepared colorectal CNS and colorectal surgeons, represented in this model, work on behalf of the patient toward excellence in patient-centered care. They utilize overlapping specialist knowledge and skills, complemented by their distinct professional knowledge, respecting each other's professional opinion, which is underpinned by equality in decision-making (Fig. 16.1). CNS may or may not work at an advanced level, depending on their qualifications, experience, and the privileging framework within the hospital. Despite the lack of national agreement the role is comparable to other countries (Hibbert et al. 2012).

- **Expert clinical practice:** CNSs in Saudi Arabia tend to care for specialty populations with chronic and complex conditions, providing holistic and individualized patient-centered care across settings. They utilize critical thinking and autonomous decision-making skills during assessment, diagnosis, treatment planning, and evaluation for specialty populations in acute care areas and in nurse-led clinics. They are involved in direct care, health promotion and disease prevention, rehabilitation, and self-care promotion. They are skilled at building therapeutic relationships, in advocacy, education, and counseling. They tend to be the key, accessible healthcare professional across settings and specialties and so are involved in care coordination.
- **Leadership:** CNSs collaborate with multidisciplinary teams (MDT) and patients and their families to ensure good communication and advocacy in the provision of patient-centered care. They use innovative and cost-effective methods for sourcing, acquiring, and utilizing resources. They utilize evidence-based practice (EBP) to optimize patient outcomes and develop, maintain, and standardize care paths and guidelines. They are responsible for the quality, safety, and effectiveness of care and are role models for change management. They are instrumental in assessing patient population needs and in developing and restructuring patient

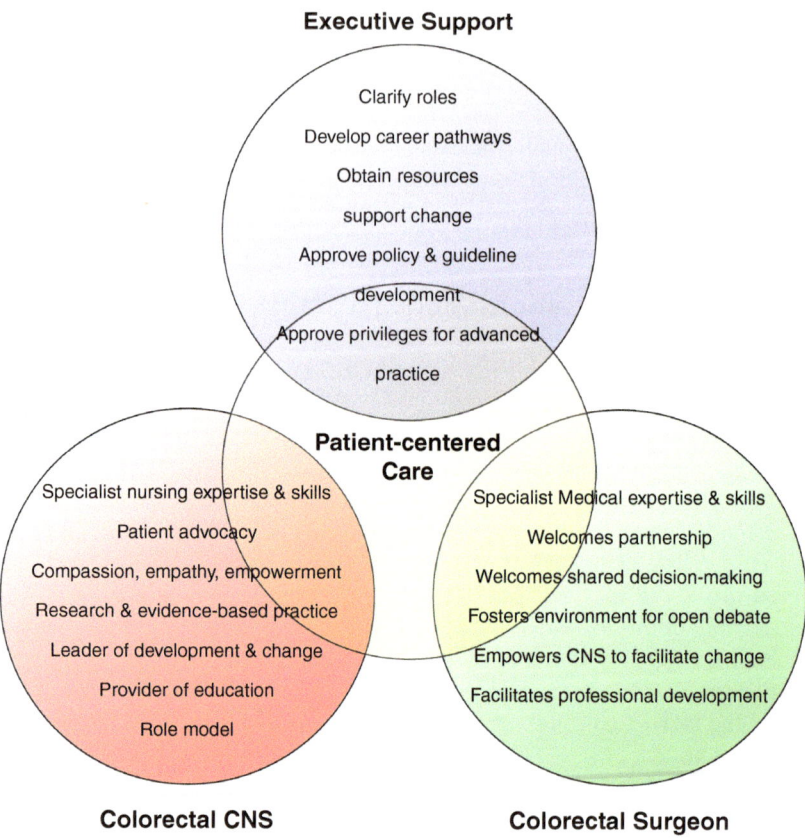

Fig. 16.1 Colorectal model for specialist nurse-physician collaborative care

services. They are required to be knowledgeable about how their patient population may be affected by organizational, political, or economic change.

- **Research:** CNSs are expected to be involved in the development and dissemination of new knowledge and to be experts at knowledge translation and implementation of evidence.
- **Education**: They are required to provide both formal and informal education in the development of staff and in clinical supervision and coaching.

Although not a national standard, several hospitals have instituted a CNS career ladder (Fig. 16.2) to ensure the nurses' scope of practice remains within the development of skills, experience, and higher education. This clinical career ladder works within a collaborative model (Fig. 16.1) and was first implemented in the King Faisal Specialist Hospital and Research Center, Riyadh, in 2008 for the care of patients with colorectal conditions (Hibbert et al. 2012, 2017).

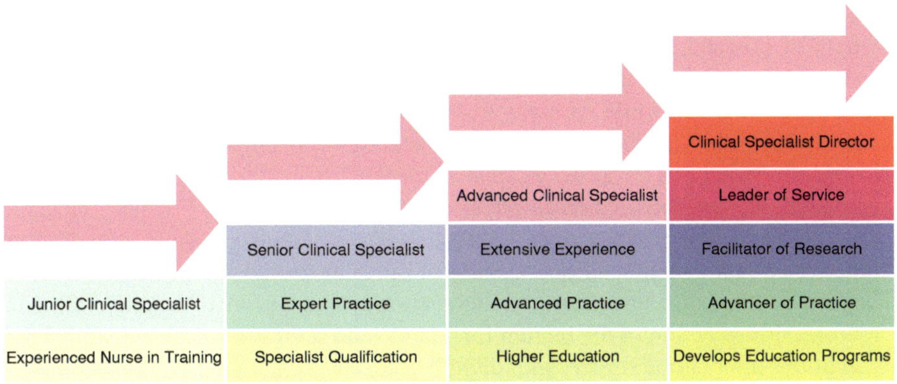

Fig. 16.2 Career pathway-clinical grading ladder

16.4 CNS Practice Competencies

Presently there is no national framework for assessing competency for clinicians; each hospital uses its own methods. The large tertiary referral center, where the author is employed, utilizes a competency framework for onboarding of all new staff. In addition, nurses who are advancing their practice are expected to meet additional competencies specific to their role. Due to the lack of APNs, it is common for consultant physicians within the same specialty to act as clinical supervisors, with nursing input from senior nurse educators and leaders. CNS, with their supervisors and managers, are responsible for identifying the competencies necessary for the specific role. Competency is developed via clinical supervision in practice and in coaching sessions, knowledge, procedural skills, and critical thinking and decision-making skills are formally assessed. Common competency assessments are for nurse-led clinics, invasive or diagnostic procedures, advanced assessment skills, and prescribing. A logbook is signed by both CNS and clinical supervisor, before applying for privileges via a privileging committee. Experienced APNs, who have already been practicing outside of the facility, undergo a review of credentials and privileges by a privileging committee in collaboration with a clinical supervisor (Hibbert et al. 2017).

16.5 Outcome Measures and Evaluation

Measures of patient outcomes are not standardized for CNS, even at an organizational level, and results are not shared nationally. Some organizations include indicator data, based on organizational goals and objectives, which are reviewed during employee performance management and evaluation, expectations are generally based on role and level or grade. Productivity data, patient safety and quality indicators such as pressure injury, patient satisfaction, emergency room visits and length of hospital stay are all common, while cost-benefit is less common. Unit-based CNSs may find it easy to demonstrate their influence in accordance with a unit's performance, while specialty population CNSs find it more difficult to measure their worth. The APN committee at the authors' facility has recently managed to add nurse-led clinics to the hospitals' measure of patient satisfaction, where it compares well to satisfaction in physician clinics. The author and her colleagues have also added several specialty-specific patient outcome measures to their computerized documentation. Global quality of life is measured along with fecal incontinence, constipation, and obstructed defecation scores, a score of function following low anterior resection of the rectum for cancer, and scores to assess peristomal skin conditions after stoma surgery in individuals at each visit. Outcome data are not yet available.

16.6 CNS Education

There is presently no provision of university education for either unit-based or population-based CNS in Saudi Arabia. One university offers an APN education program, but none offer higher education for specialty practice. In 2010, the SCFHS approved the first training program aimed at providing nurses with the necessary advanced knowledge, skills and competence to care for individuals with stoma, wound and continence conditions including nurse-led clinics. This was a 12-month, fulltime diploma program offering both theory and supervised clinical practice. The program ran until 2016, having graduated only seven nurses, when the SCFHS advised that the feasibility of a fulltime 24-month Advanced Diploma Program should be considered. Unfortunately, expatriates working full time cannot take advantage of these opportunities. Distance and web-based learning is not recognized in any format by the SCFHS, and recently the Ministry of Education has announced that part-time education will not suffice for promotional opportunities. Saudi nurses are supported by scholarship to travel to countries such as the United States, the United Kingdom, and Australia. As each of these countries graduate CNS and APN via a variety of pathways, without national legislation, regulation, or credentialing of APN in Saudi Arabia, it remains difficult to develop protected titles with standardized qualifications (Hibbert and Al-Dossari 2015; Hibbert et al. 2017).

16.7 Credentialing: Regulatory, Legal, and Certification Requirements

AP nursing is not presently legislated or regulated in Saudi Arabia; therefore, there is no official stance on credentialing or privileging. The recent development of an ANP program at a local university, and the support for developing community NPs by the SCFHS, will hopefully ignite a conversation on qualifications, credentialing, and privileging at a national level. Some hospitals specify in job descriptions the level of education required including specialty certifications. If the specific role requires advanced assessment, invasive procedures, or prescribing, the CNS may be expected to undergo clinical supervision and apply for credentialing and privileging via a multidisciplinary committee (Hibbert et al. 2017).

16.8   Moving Forward

"care for patients today while laying solid foundation for our APNs of the future".
   (Hibbert et al. 2017)

The governments' 2030 vision for Saudi Arabia aims to improve health awareness and disease prevention, to improve quality of care and provide better access, to optimize health resources, and to reduce waiting times for specialist treatment. It is hoped that this will highlight the need for highly educated, experienced, and motivated nursing experts to work in CNS roles (Government of KSA 2018).

Challenges
- Poor image of clinical nursing
- Low numbers of Saudi nurses in clinical practice
- Lack of qualified CNS to meet population needs
- No university education programs, no professional development
- No nationally agreed model of APN to meet Saudi needs and available resources
- No legislation
- No regulation
- No protected titles
- No structure for clinical academics for mentoring APNs
- Lack of awareness and understanding of APN roles
- No national guidelines for credentialing or privileging

Opportunities
- The Government of Saudi Arabia's 2030 vision, including improvements in education and healthcare, will demonstrate the need for nurses to work at a higher level of practice.
- Continued Saudization of nursing, improving the image of clinical nursing.
- Saudi APNs as role models.
- The SCFHS's support of APN, in theory.
- The SCFHS's Advanced Diplomas.
- The first university-based APN program in Riyadh.

16.9 Exemplar of Clinical Nurse Specialist Practice

In 2008, a masters-prepared CNS led the development of a clinical grading ladder for the advancement of specialty nursing practice at the King Faisal Specialist Hospital and Research Center in Riyadh Saudi Arabia (Fig. 16.2). At the top of the ladder, the colorectal CNS provides oversight for all specialist nurses caring for patients with colorectal conditions. The patient population includes all individuals admitted for colorectal surgery, individuals with colorectal cancer including hereditary tumors, patients with inflammatory bowel disease when medical treatment has failed, all patients with stomas, and individuals with disorders of defecation and bowel dysfunction when surgery is not required and when general dietary and medication modification has failed (Hibbert et al. 2012, 2017).

Patients commonly require information, education, advocacy, advice, counseling, and care coordination, throughout the trajectory of their investigation, treatment, and follow-up. Families with hereditary tumors additionally require genetic education and counseling, family conferencing, case finding, screening, and registration. Patients with stomas are cared for in the acute phase and in nurse-led clinics for prevention, assessment, diagnosis, and management of stoma or peristomal dermatological complications and complaints such as constipation, high output ileostomy, and parastomal hernia. CNS also provides expert advice during consultation for all patients with enterocutaneous fistula. They may provide direct care when necessary, which usually involves education and skill building with other team members, and are also key experts in relation to wound healing, containment of effluent, fluid and electrolyte balance, and nutritional management (Hibbert et al. 2015).

Patients with disorders of defecation or bowel dysfunction may present with fecal incontinence, obstructive defecation, constipation not responding to medical management, or unrelieved anal or rectal pain. The origin of these conditions may be congenital (neurogenic conditions, imperforate anus, cloacal abnormality), iatrogenic (rectal resection and radiation for cancer, proctocolectomy and ileoanal pouch for familial polyposis or ulcerative colitis, anal surgeries), and traumatic (obstetric injury, impaling injury). But it may also have behavioral foundations related to a significant psychological trauma, such as, but not limited to, sexual abuse (dyssynergia due to paradoxical puborectalis or lack of relaxation of the pelvic floor during defecation). Complications of some of these conditions can lead to chronic pelvic floor problems such as significant pelvic floor descent, rectocele, cystocele, omentocele, enterocele, rectoanal intussusception or rectal prolapse, solitary rectal ulcer syndrome, and urinary or fecal incontinence. These conditions have major long-term implications for QOL (Rao and Patcharatrakul 2016). These patients are cared for holistically by CNS in a therapeutic relationship. Cure is not usually possible in most cases; the aim is to reduce symptoms and improve QOL by facilitating adaptation and developing and improving healthy coping mechanisms. Patients undergo:

- In-depth, specialty focused history and physical assessment
- Anorectal physiology and radiological tests

- Assessment of lifestyle including nutrition
- Assessment of education level and education needs and cognitive ability
- Assessment of emotional, psychosocial, sexual, and spiritual concerns
- Patient empowerment, health promotion and behavior modification via the provision of information and education (anatomy and bodily function, including the effect of diet, fluids, exercise, medication, and psychological effects)
- Modification of diet and medications
- Exercises aimed at isolating pelvic floor, anal sphincter and abdominal oblique muscles (building strength and endurance, improving rectal sensation and capacity)
- Advice and counseling, referral to psychiatry as necessary
- Behavioral therapy and positive reinforcement with biofeedback
- Facilitation of referral as necessary (dietitian, psychiatry, colorectal surgeon)

(Hibbert et al. 2012; Hibbert and Rafferty 2015)

The Kingdom of Saudi Arabia did not provide comprehensive services for patients with disorders of defecation until 2010. Patients who could not be helped with surgery, medical intervention or physical therapy were either left to cope with their chronic condition or sent abroad, at great expense, to centers of excellence in the United States or the United Kingdom. In 2010 the results of the collaboration between a masters-prepared CNS and colorectal surgeon were realized. Between 2008 and 2010, the CNS was supported to travel abroad to centers of excellence to gain an insight into models of care and the infrastructure and resources required to build a center of excellence in Saudi Arabia. The CNS also acquired the knowledge and skills to be instrumental in developing the service and in setting up the nurse-led clinics and anorectal physiology laboratory in a purpose-built unit, including the sourcing and acquisition of the latest equipment and medical supplies. Back in Saudi Arabia, colorectal surgeons provided clinical supervision, and the CNS was assessed for competency in specialty physical examination and history-taking and in digital rectal and pelvic floor examination and proctoscopy; for acquisition and interpretation of data and diagnostic reporting for anorectal manometry, EMG-pudendal nerve terminal motor latency, and endorectal ultrasound; and for the provision of biofeedback. The CNS has since provided nurse-led services autonomously for this patient population, utilizing the clinical supervisory process as needed (Hibbert et al. 2012; Hibbert and Rafferty 2015).

The CNS has been responsible for the recruitment, training and retention of additional staff, including a second AP CNS and a senior clinical specialist. The development and implementation of an EB guideline for investigation and referral criteria has improved patient flow and enables a form of one-stop shop patient experience. Recent evidence that biofeedback is optimal if provided every 1–4 weeks for at least six sessions in the management of obstructive defecation has spurred the CNS to lead a performance improvement project aimed at reducing waiting times and meeting these requirements. Positive outcomes were achieved within the first three quarters with good patient satisfaction results (Cadeddu et al. 2015; Hibbert and Rafferty 2015).

The CNS developed and has directed the Saudi Enterostomal Therapy Diploma Program since 2009. This program provides both the theoretical knowledge and clinical experience for specialist nurses to not only practice within the specialty but to build similar services in other facilities. So far five facilities in three cities have benefited. The CNS has also been involved, as a clinical supervisor, on the Colorectal Surgery Fellowship and has been involved in the development of more than 16 colorectal surgeons. She is also a senior lecturer at a Medical College where she teaches Surgical Interns.

The CNS is involved in both nursing and collaborative research and was an expert panel member in the development of the Saudi Guidelines for Colorectal Cancer Screening. She has authored several publications within her specialty and is considered an expert at an organizational, national, and international level. She is an editorial board member of *Saudi Medical Journal* and sits on the Executive Board of both a national and international association. She is involved in the annual National Specialty Conferences and Public Awareness Days. She has been invited as a speaker both nationally and internationally. Additionally, she chairs an Education Committee for a global charitable organization that aims to ensure the provision of evidence based care for patients with stomas, wounds, and continence conditions. To this end, she is involved in the provision of education internationally and in the development of educational resources such as webinars, books, and guidelines.

As mentioned previously, there are several competencies specific to this patient population:

- History and physical exam including digital rectal and pelvic floor
- Proctoscopy
- Nurse-led clinics within specialty (including reading and interpreting specialty-specific radiology and laboratory reports)
- Acquisition, editing, and reporting ARM and balloon expulsion
- Acquisition and reporting PNTML and EMG
- Endorectal ultrasound
- Biofeedback
- Non-physician prescribing

The following are the typical outcomes of CNS practice in the specialty:

- Improved access to care
- Improved patient flow
- Informed and empowered patients
- Reduction or improvement in symptoms
- Adaptation and improved coping skills
- Improved patient satisfaction
- Improved QOL
- Reduced costs
- Better utilization of colorectal surgery services

- Increased public awareness
- Increase in specialty services, treatment nearer to home
- Improved image of clinical nursing
- Advancement of nursing practice

16.10 Summary

The role, scope, and level of practice for CNS have not yet been decided upon in Saudi Arabia. In "caring for patients today while planning for the future" nurses with specialist knowledge, skill and competence are filling the gap. It is hoped that the government's 2030 vision and an increase in Saudi Nurses will lead to an improved image of clinical nursing and the advancement of nursing practice.

References

Cadeddu F, Salis F, De Luca E, Ciangola I, Milito G (2015) Efficiency of biofeedback plus trans-anal stimulation in the management of pelvic floor dyssynergia: a randomized controlled trail. Tech Coloproctol 19(6):333–338. https://doi.org/10.1007/s10151-015-1292-7

El-Sanabary N (1993) The education and contribution of women health care professionals in Saudi Arabia: the case of nursing. Social Sci Med 37(11):1331–1343

Government of KSA (2018) Vision 2030 Kingdom of Saudi Arabia. http://vision2030.gov.sa/en

Hibbert D, Al-Dossari RR (2015) Developing enterostomal therapy as a nursing specialty in Saudi Arabia: which model fits best? Gastrointest Nurs 13(3):41–48. https://doi.org/10.12968/gasn.2015.13.3.41

Hibbert D, Rafferty L (2015) The development of nurse-led bowel dysfunction clinics in Saudi Arabia: against all odds. Gastrointest Nurs 13(5):33–40. https://doi.org/10.12968/gasn.2015.13.5.33

Hibbert D, Al-Sanea NA, Balens JA (2012) Perspectives on specialist nursing in Saudi Arabia: a national model for success. Ann Saudi Med 32(1):78–85. https://doi.org/10.5144/0256-4947.2012.78

Hibbert D, Aboshaiqah AE, Sienko KA, Forestell D, Harb AW, Yousuf SA, Kelley PW, Brennan PF, Serrant L, Leary A (2017) Advancing nursing practice: the emergence of the role of advanced practice nurse in Saudi Arabia. Ann Saudi Med 37(1):72–78. https://doi.org/10.5144/0256-4947.2017.72

Kleinpell R, Scanlon A, Hibbert D, Ganz F, East L, Fraser D, Wong F, Beauchesne M (2014) Addressing issues impacting advanced nursing practice worldwide. OJIN 19(2):5. https://doi.org/10.3912/OJIN.Vol19No02Man05

Ministry of Health (2008) Kingdom of Saudi Arabia: statistical year book. www.moh.gov.sa

Ministry of Health (2016) Kingdom of Saudi Arabia: statistical year book. www.moh.gov.sa

Rao SC, Patcharatrakul T (2016) Diagnosis and treatment of dyssynergic defeaction. J Neurogastroenetrol Motil 22(3):423–435. https://doi.org/10.5056/jnm16060

Saudi Commission for Health Specialties (2017) The executive regulations for professional classification and registration for health practitioners. Saudi Arabia. www.scfhs.org.sa

The Role and Practice of Clinical Nurse Specialist in Nigeria

17

Chidiebele Constance Obichi, John Emenike Anieche, Eunice Ogonna Osuala, and Ukamaka Marian Oruche

Abstract

Although the clinical nurse specialist was recognized as an expert practitioner in the United States for 50 years, there is an absence of a framework for the clinical nurse specialist role in Nigeria. There are three pathways through which the federal government, state government, and private sector provide specialist education and training for nurses in Nigeria. Nurses who have received graduate education should practice to the full extent of their education and training. Also, nurses who have their practice expanded in the treatment of communicable diseases and reproductive, maternal, newborn, and childcare should be appropriately recognized. This chapter explores challenges to developing the clinical specialist nurse role in Nigeria and the extent to which the clinical nurse specialist role is evolving in Nigeria through specialist education and training for nurses. Regardless of the pathway, setting, or specialty, Nigerian nurses may have achieved many clinical nurse specialist core competencies without a formal master's education. Hence, Nigeria is long overdue for the development,

This chapter has been written before the 2020 APN ICN guidelines were published and reflects the views of the authors.

C. C. Obichi (✉)
Indiana University Northwest School of Nursing, Gary, IN, USA

J. E. Anieche · E. O. Osuala
Department of Nursing Science, Faculty of Health Sciences and Technology, Nnamdi Azikiwe University, Nnewi, Anambra State, Nigeria
e-mail: je.anieche@unizik.edu.ng; eo.osuala@unizik.edu.ng

U. M. Oruche
Indiana University School of Nursing, Indianapolis, IN, USA
e-mail: uoruche@iu.edu

© Springer Nature Switzerland AG 2021
J. S. Fulton, V. W. Holly (eds.), *Clinical Nurse Specialist Role and Practice*, Advanced Practice in Nursing, https://doi.org/10.1007/978-3-319-97103-2_17

recognition, and legal inclusion of the clinical nurse specialist role and practice in the career structure of nurses at all levels of the Nigerian health system.

Keywords
Nigeria · Specialist nurses · Clinical nurse specialist · Advanced nursing practice · Nursing education · Midwives

17.1   The Clinical Nurse Specialist

Although the clinical nurse specialist (CNS) was recognized as an expert practitioner in the United States for about 50 years (National Association of Clinical Nurse Specialists 2004; Hamric et al. 2009), there is an absence of a framework for the CNS role and practice in Nigeria. The CNS role is one of the four advanced practice registered nurse roles in the United States which has evolved as a result of the societal need to address the increasing complexity of patients that require specialized acute nursing care and to improve access to quality and affordable care at primary care clinics (Gordon et al. 2012; Dunn 1997).

According to the US National Association of Clinical Nurse Specialists, CNSs are registered nurses with graduate or postgraduate certification from an accredited program prepared to practice for a specialty population and are clinical experts in the diagnosis and treatment of illness, delivery of evidence-based nursing interventions, and advancement of nursing practice and improvement of outcomes and may act as independent licensed provider, which includes prescribing medications (National Association of Clinical Nurse Specialists 2004). A clinical nurse specialist's specialty may be defined by population (pediatrics, geriatrics, women's health), setting (critical care, emergency room), disease or medical subspecialty (diabetes, oncology), type of care (psychiatric, rehabilitation), or type of problem (such as pain, wounds, stress) (National Association of Clinical Nurse Specialists 2004).

This chapter explores the challenges to developing the clinical nurse specialist role and practice and the extent to which the clinical nurse specialist role is evolving in Nigeria through specialized education and training for nurses and nurse midwives.

17.2   Brief History of Nursing Education and Training in Nigeria

Nursing education in Nigeria is either university-based or hospital-based (apprenticeship) and is provided by the federal and state governments and the private sector (missionary and individual organizations). The majority of nurses in Nigeria obtain their education through hospital-based nursing programs which began in 1949. These programs offer generic nursing or basic nursing education and training in the hospital setting. Nigerian hospitals do not award academic qualifications; hence, graduates of hospital-based programs earn a higher national diploma certificate and are registered and licensed upon graduation. The majority of these RNs work in acute care hospitals and community health centers (Ayandiran et al. 2013; University of Nigeria Teaching Hospital 2018; Agbedia 2012).

The preparation of nurses with Bachelor of Nursing Science (BNSc) degree began in 1965 with the approval by the National Universities Commission (NUC) and the Nursing and Midwifery Council of Nigeria (N&MCN). However, graduates of these undergraduate programs were very few that in 1999, the federal government approved private baccalaureate nursing programs to increase the number of BNSc-prepared nurses (Ojo and Onasoga 2009). Graduates of all nursing programs are professionally registered and licensed by the N&MCN to work in hospital and community settings such as schools, health centers, and manufacturing industries (Ayandiran et al. 2013; University of Nigeria Teaching Hospital 2018; Agbedia 2012). These nurses are expected to:

- Utilize the nursing process in providing care.
- Assist patients with coping with the biological and environmental changes experienced during hospitalization.
- Ensure safety and implement nursing interventions in collaboration with the healthcare team.
- Conduct and participate in research toward improvement of patient care and growth of the nursing profession.
- Participate in effective budgeting and auditing of the unit.
- Participate in evidence-based nursing practice.
- Participate in architectural design of Clinical Services Department to effect efficiency and quality patient care (University of Nigeria Teaching Hospital 2018).

Following reports about the critical health workforce shortage in developing countries, the World Health Organization (WHO) (2008) recommended "task-shifting," a public health approach to address the HIV epidemic, increase access to health services, and strengthen the overall health system of countries deficient in human resources for health. The goal was to enable existing healthcare workers such as nurse midwives to provide care according to an extended scope of practice at all levels of the national health system and to allow creation of new roles within the health workforce. In 2014, the Nigerian National Council of Health (Federal Ministry of Health 2018) approved the Task-Shifting Policy, and the implementation of task-shifting commenced especially in the rural and underserved areas (Federal Ministry of Health 2014). Task-shifting type II is the "extension of the scope of practice of nurses and midwives in order to enable them assume some tasks previously undertaken by medical doctors and non-physician clinicians *(professional health workers who are not trained as physicians but capable of many of the diagnostic and clinical functions of a medical doctors and have more clinical skills than generic nurses and are present both in high-income and low-income countries)*." (Federal Ministry of Health 2014) The task-shifting model from physicians to nurses has expanded the role of nurses as the primary medical care provider for mothers with HIV and AIDS. This model has been used successfully in treating HIV patients in Nigeria (Iwu and Holzemer 2014; Iwu et al. 2010), South Africa

(Sanne et al. 2010), and Rwanda (Shumbusho et al. 2009) and in reducing maternal and fetal mortality and morbidity in Ethiopia (Gessessew et al. 2011).

17.3   Pathways to the Role and Practice of CNS in Nigeria

The three existing pathways to specialized nursing education and training provide the platform on which the CNS role and practice would evolve in Nigeria. The pathways include (National Association of Clinical Nurse Specialists 2004) hospital-based pathway, (Hamric et al. 2009) university-based pathway, and (Gordon et al. 2012) task-shifting pathway. Each pathway is presented below.

17.3.1 Hospital-Based Pathway

The hospital-based generic or basic nursing diploma is a 3-year program and is the first step prior to obtaining specialized nursing education and training. After 1 or 2 years of clinical experience, a post-basic specialized training (PBST) that lasts between 12 and 24 months follows with the RN focusing on a specific area of nursing (majority choose midwifery). To obtain further specialized education, the RN may acquire multiple certifications in specialties of their choice (University of Nigeria Teaching Hospital 2018; Agbedia 2012). Upon completion of the PBST, graduates are certified, registered, and licensed by the N&MCN to practice in their areas of specialty that include intensive care, midwifery, burns and plastic, pediatric, accident and emergency care, ophthalmic, orthopedics, nephrology, mental and psychiatric health, perioperative, oncology, community health nursing, and anesthesiology. Research indicates that PBST nurses have impacted the Nigerian health system in the following ways: increased patient satisfaction, decreased medical complications, decreased frequency of emergency cases and deaths, improved pain management, and decreased length of hospital stay and costs to patients (Ojo and Onasoga 2009).

Although the majority of Nigeria nurses are trained in hospital-based programs, this form of education and training is devoid of liberal education, opportunities for creativity, accountability, independent clinical decision-making, and understanding and appropriate utilization of the nursing process, evidence-based practice, and advanced nursing practice skills (Agbedia 2012; Ojo and Onasoga 2009). Thus, the RN with PBST may enroll in a university-based 4-year program (also known as direct entry) to obtain a BNSc degree. Overall, a nurse that follows the hospital-based pathway spends a minimum of 8 years to obtain an RN license (3 years), a certification in one nursing specialty (1 year), and a BNSc in nursing (4 years). Hence, the saying goes "Nigerian nurses are over trained at the diplomate level due to unnecessary overlap in education between the diploma and baccalaureate programs." Consequently, many PBST nurses are slow in embracing university education (Agbedia 2012), so their specialized education and training are not obtained at the graduate level. However, with their minimum 8-year long training and many years of clinical experience, these nurses may provide nursing care that they were not formally trained for especially in rural and underserved areas of the country.

17.3.2 University-Based Pathway

To receive the university-based specialized education and training at the graduate level (master's and doctor of philosophy [PhD]), the potential candidate must as a first step complete a 5-year BNSc program. Upon completion of the BNSc, graduates are registered by the N&MCN as "generic" nurses (RN), registered midwives (RM), and registered public health nurses (RPHN). The next step would be to obtain a master's degree in one of the specialties, for example, maternal and child health, medical-surgical, mental health and psychiatric, administration and management, nursing education, and community health nursing. Upon completion of the master's or PhD program, graduates are equipped for careers in clinical settings, administration and management, and education and research at all levels of healthcare and educational institutions, as well as corporate organizations and other relevant agencies (University of Nigeria Teaching Hospital 2018). Although masters-prepared nurses should practice to the full extent their education and training, the majority of them are employed in academia because advanced clinical roles are non-existing and there is no national framework and guidelines to recognize and reward growth in clinical nursing practice in Nigeria (Chiegboka 2015).

17.3.3 Task-Shifting Pathway

Task shifting involves redistributing specific tasks, where appropriate, from highly qualified health workers to health workers with shorter training and fewer qualifications in order to make more efficient use of the available human resources for health (Federal Ministry of Health 2018). Nigerian nurses and nurse midwives have had their practice expanded in the treatment of HIV infection and reproductive, maternal, newborn, and child care (Federal Ministry of Health 2014). They:

- Provide early infant male circumcision.
- Repair cervical laceration and complex vaginal laceration.
- Assess client's readiness to commence antiretroviral therapy (ART).
- Manage severe pregnancy and labor complications (anemia, preeclampsia, eclampsia, malaria fetal malpresentations, prolonged and/or obstructed labor, hypertension, bleeding, and infection).
- Issue prescription for antiretroviral (ARV) regimen and refer to pharmacy.
- Diagnose severe HIV diseases and confirm HIV infection.

Further, research indicates that in Nigeria, task-shifting to nurses and nurse midwives decreased patients' wait times by 62%, decreased physician workload by 41% (Iwu et al. 2010; Udegboka and Moses 2009), improved job satisfactions for nurses, and retained more patients in HIV settings (Iwu and Holzemer 2014).

Although task-shifting is in the early stages of implementation in Nigeria, the medical and nursing regulatory bodies are yet to standardize recruitment, training, and evaluation criteria to assess its positive impact on the health system. Equally important are the development of (National Association of Clinical Nurse Specialists 2004) standard context-relevant curriculum (Iwasiw et al. 2008) for training and continual education (Hamric et al. 2009), regulatory framework to define CNS role and scope of practice for existing health workforce, and (Gordon et al. 2012) competencies for CNS and guidelines for (National Association of Clinical Nurse Specialists 2004) immediate opportunities for referral to medical doctors, (Hamric et al. 2009) regular supportive supervision and clinical mentoring from physicians and non-physician clinicians, and (Gordon et al. 2012) systematic collection of strategic information concerning the implementation of the task-shifting model. (Federal Ministry of Health 2018)

17.4   Moving Forward: Challenges and Opportunities

According to Ayandiran et al., there is a critical need to utilize nurses with higher education in Nigeria to promote critical thinking and increase use of evidence-based nursing practice (Ayandiran et al. 2013). The hallmarks of CNS practice are integrating evidence-based practice into healthcare, designing programs of care and innovative nursing interventions, and providing leadership and education to nurses (Gordon et al. 2012). Higher education is essential for moving forward with these core CNS responsibilities. According to Sun and Larson (2015), translation of evidence-based practice from research to frontline nursing is possible when there are well-trained scholars who usually receive their training from graduate programs. In 2008, the Fellows of West African College of Nursing (FWACN) (Madubuko n.d.) proposed the development of the advanced nurse practitioner role for the West African sub-region; however, not much has been achieved since the proposal was presented.

The challenges to developing advanced practice roles include professional rivalry between nurses and doctors and fear of losing earnings. In a study (Ugochukwu et al. n.d.) that explored the perception of 24 nurses about the factors that hinder the development of the advanced nurse practitioner role in five southeastern states of Nigeria, a chief nursing officer (participant) stated, "The doctors think that nurses will take over their jobs or replace them." Another challenge was from medical doctors who were concerned about unethical conduct, poor quality and management, and abuse of roles by nurses. Another hindrance was from medical organizations on the grounds that advanced nursing practice would negatively impact their role in Africa and that nurses had insufficient training for the expanded roles. Other challenges include limited resources and cost of training, mentoring, support, and supervision of expanded roles (Madubuko n.d.; Ugochukwu et al. n.d.; Oloo 2003; Mullan and Frehywot 2007; Dovlo 2004; The Nigerian Medical Association 2005).

Further, research with a clinical focus is among the most lacking in nursing and midwifery research in Africa (Sun and Larson 2015). In Nigeria, the majority of nurses who obtain graduate nursing degrees prefer to join academia; hence, nursing faculty conduct more research than nurses in clinical settings. There is, therefore, a dearth of research in the hospital setting related to the lack of masters- and doctorally prepared nurses in the clinical setting. It is vital to note that a handful of nurses who obtain their masters while providing direct patient care in the hospitals continue with direct patient care despite their advanced nursing degree and are neither recognized for professional growth nor rewarded by employers. Research indicates that barriers that hinder nurses from conducting research in health facilities include lack of understanding of research priorities; inadequate staff; lack of experienced nurse researchers, organizational support, and funding; absence of nursing research mentors; and lack of leadership in the dissemination of research findings (Ayandiran et al. 2013).

17.5 Conclusion

Regardless of the pathway, setting, or specialty, Nigeria is long overdue for the development, recognition, and legal inclusion of the CNS role and practice in the career structure of nurses at all levels of the health system. Nurses and nurse midwives in Nigeria may have achieved the CNS core competencies without formal master's education. Hence, the N&MCN should collaborate with professional nursing associations (National Association for Nigerian Nurses and Midwives (NANNM); National Association of Nigerian Nurses in North America (NANNNA); and other nursing specialty associations) and all stakeholders to push policy that would recognize advanced degree nurses in the clinical settings with appropriate salary scale, establish standards for CNS role and practice, and develop the CNS curriculum with master's level courses that include opportunities for content specific clinical experiences and preceptorship.

References

Agbedia C (2012) Re-envisioning nursing education and practice in Nigeria for the 21st century. Open J Nurs 2(3):226–230

Ayandiran EO, Irinoye OO, Faronbi JO, Mtshali NG (2013) Education reforms in Nigeria: how responsive is the nursing profession? Int J Nurs Educ Scholarsh 10(1):11–19

Chiegboka I (2015) Establishing a national framework and guidelines for professional development and recognition programme in Nigeria as a necessity for nursing clinical excellence. West Afr J Nurs [serial on the Internet] [cited May 18, 2018]; 26(1): 82–87

Dovlo D (2004) Using mid-level cadres as substitutes for internationally mobile health professionals in Africa. A desk review. Human Resources for Health [serial on the Internet] [cited May 18, 2018]; 27–12

Dunn L (1997) A literature review of advanced clinical nursing practice in the United States of America. J Adv Nurs [serial on the Internet]. [cited May 14, 2018]; 25(4): 814–819

Federal Ministry of Health (2014) Task-shifting and task-sharing policy for essential health care services in Nigeria. http://www.health.gov.ng/doc/TSTS.pdf

Federal Ministry of Health (2018) FG, partners to scale up family planning access. http://www.health.gov.ng/index.php/component/content/article/78-featured/465-fg-partners-to-scale-up-family-planning-access

Gessessew A, Barnabas G, Prata N, Weidert K (2011) Task shifting and sharing in Tigray, Ethiopia, to achieve comprehensive emergency obstetric care. Int J Gynecol Obstet [serial on the Internet] [cited May 18, 2018]; 113(1): 28–31

Gordon JM, Lorilla JD, Lehman CA (2012) The role of the clinical nurse specialist in the future of health care in the United States. Perioper Nurs Clin 7(3):343–353

Hamric AB, Spross JA, Hanson CM (2009) Advanced practice nursing: an integrative approach. Saunders Elsevier, St. Louis

Iwasiw C, Goldenberg D, Andrusyszyn MA (2008) Curriculum development in nursing education. Jones & Bartlett Publishers

Iwu EN, Holzemer WL (2014) Task shifting of HIV management from doctors to nurses in Africa: clinical outcomes and evidence on nurse self-efficacy and job satisfaction. AIDS Care 26(1):42–52

Iwu E, Ezebuihe I, Caroline O, Umaru E, Gomwalk A, Moen M, Riel R, Johnson J (2010) Task shifting-a strategic response to human resource for health crisis: qualitative evaluation of hospital-based HIV clinics in North Central Nigeria. International AIDS Conference, Vienna

Madubuko G (n.d.) Nurse practitioner/advanced nursing practice development in West Africa: a proposal. https://international.aanp.org/Content/docs/WestAfrica.pdf

Mullan F, Frehywot S (2007) Non-physician clinicians in 47 sub-Saharan African countries. Lancet [serial on the Internet] [cited May 18, 2018]; 370(9605): 2158–2163

National Association of Clinical Nurse Specialists (2004) Statement on clinical nurse specialist practice and education. NACNS

Ojo AA, Onasoga OA (2009) In: Current trends & issues in nursing in Nigeria pri RoyalBird ventures Ltd., Mushin, Lagos

Oloo A (2003) Upgrade skills in health care. The East African. http://www.nationaudio.com/News/DailyNation/09112003/Letters/Letters1.html

Sanne I, Orrell C, Fox M, Conradie F, Ive P, Orrell C, et al (2010) Nurse versus doctor management of HIV-infected patients receiving antiretroviral therapy (CIPRA-SA): a randomised non-inferiority trial. Lancet [serial on the Internet] [cited May 18, 2018]; 376 North American Edition (9734): 33–40

Shumbusho F, van Griensven J, Lowrance D, Turate I, Weaver M, Binagwaho A, et al (2009) Task shifting for scale-up of HIV care: evaluation of nurse-centered antiretroviral treatment at rural health centers in Rwanda. PLoS Med [serial on the Internet] [cited May 18, 2018]; 6(10): e1000163

Sun C, Larson E (2015) Clinical nursing and midwifery research in African countries: a scoping review. Int J Nurs Stud [serial on the Internet] [cited May 18, 2018]; 52(5): 1011–1016

The Nigerian Medical Association (2005) Communique issued at the end of the meeting of the National Executive Council of the Nigerian Medical Association held from 26–28 August, 2005 in Maiduguri, Borno State. http://www.nigeriannma.org

Udegboka N, Moses JH (2009) Reduction of client waiting time through task shifting in northern Nigeria. International AIDS conference on HIV pathogenesis, treatment and prevention, Cape Town

Ugochukwu CG, Nnabuenyi AI, Ndubuka C (n.d.) Advanced Practice Nursing challenges in developing countries: perception of nurses in selected health care facilities in SouthEast Nigeria. http://www.commonwealthnurses.org/conference2014/Documents/ChikaUgochukwu.pdf

University of Nigeria Teaching Hospital (2018) Specialized education and training. http://www.unthenugu.com.ng/education_training.html

World Health Organization (WHO) (2008) Task shifting: rational redistribution of tasks among health workforce teams: global recommendations and guidelines. WHO, Geneva. TTR-Task Shifting.pdf. Accessed 11 May 2014

Part VI

Oceania

The Role and Practice of CNS in Australia

18

Dale Pugh and Elizabeth Scruth

Abstract

The role of the clinical nurse specialist in the Australian context is only present in some states and territories. Although the role of the clinical nurse specialist (CNS) is filled by a registered nurse, the role itself is not regulated by the Nursing and Midwifery Board of Australia. This means that the title is not protected by the National Law, although the Nurse Practitioner title is. The role and scope of practice is articulated in employment awards and job descriptions developed by the employing organisation. Although the clinical nurse specialist role is not present in all states and territories, other advanced practice roles provide similar types and levels of 'specialist' nursing and midwifery care, including the clinical nurse consultant (CNC) role. The CNC position is also not regulated by the Nursing and Midwifery Board of Australia. In some states, the clinical nurse specialist has responsibility for direct patient care, whereas in other jurisdictions, the clinical nurse specialist has a specialist advisory and support role. A review of a number of CNS roles revealed the requirement for advanced, expert and specialised knowledge for the clinical speciality as detailed in the job descriptions. Not all jurisdictions require tertiary qualifications for preparation to practice as a CNS. The scope of practice for the reviewed positions presented in this chapter broadly includes the provision of advanced and specialised best practice clinical skills to assess, plan, organise, implement and evaluate care. Other key elements

This chapter has been written before the 2020 APN ICN guidelines were published and reflects the views of the authors.

D. Pugh (✉) · E. Scruth
Northern California Regional Quality/Accreditation/Regulation and Licencing Division,
Kaiser Permanente, Oakland, CA, USA
e-mail: Elizabeth.Scruth@kp.org

© Springer Nature Switzerland AG 2021
J. S. Fulton, V. W. Holly (eds.), *Clinical Nurse Specialist Role and Practice*,
Advanced Practice in Nursing, https://doi.org/10.1007/978-3-319-97103-2_18

include education to patients and family, other nurses and colleagues, participation in the development of evidence-based practice through research and policy evaluation and advocacy.

Keywords
Australia · Clinical nurse specialist · Clinical nurse consultant · Advanced practice · Nurse practitioner · Nursing · Midwifery

18.1   Brief History of the Role and Practice of CNS

18.1.1 Introduction

This chapter will present a discussion on the role and practice of the clinical nurse specialist (CNS) in Australia. The role of CNS was introduced in Australia in the late 1980s with the instigation of career structures driven with industrial reform of nursing with new position and clear career ladders (Health Department of WA). This chapter will introduce the broad nursing and healthcare system in Australia. The history of the CNS will be detailed. Definitions of the CNS role will be explored against the broader context of advanced practice nursing. A conceptualisation of the role will be presented along with key responsibilities, scope of duties, areas of practice, educational requirements and competencies. A number of example position are included to provide a fuller description of this view. A recent white paper on advanced practice nursing is presented to further highlight the CNS role against other advanced practice nurse roles (Australian College of Nursing n.d.).

Australia is comprised of 6 states and 2 territories, with a population of approximately 24 million people. The vastness of the land mass means that there are only two people per square kilometre with the majority of the population living in coastal areas (Australian Government n.d.). The Australian healthcare system is recognised as being complex as is the funding framework. The cost of healthcare is borne by all levels of government, non-government organisations, private health insurers and those individuals who pay for out-of-pocket expenses not fully subsidised or reimbursed (Australian Government Department of Health). The healthcare system in Australia is comprised of public and private providers, settings, participants and supporting processes (Australian Institute Health and Welfare 2016). Federal, state and territory and local governments have a shared responsibility for the development, delivery and governance of health. The Australian Government's funding contributions include a universal public health insurance scheme. Medicare was introduced in 1984 with the aim of providing free or subsidised access to public hospital services and to treatment by health professionals, including medical practitioners. The Medicare system extends to three areas, hospital care, medical and pharmaceuticals. Healthcare services receive funding under the National Healthcare Agreement but are primarily a state responsibility (Australian Institute Health and Welfare 2016). Healthcare providers and facilities are situated in metropolitan, regional areas and rural and remote areas. In parallel to each of these contexts, hospital sizes and capabilities will vary from large tertiary facilities providing a full range of services, including specialist paediatric and obstetric hospitals, decreasing in size and scope to regional hospitals and health services, which provide typically generalist services for a range of patient populations and presentations, to small rural hospitals with or without medical practitioners, to single nurse facilities. Private providers include private hospitals, allied health practices, medical practices and pharmacies (Australian Institute Health and Welfare 2016). Individuals who choose care in a private hospital can apply for private health insurance to fully or partially cover the cost of care (Private healthcare Australia n.d.). Individuals who obtain private health insurance may be eligible for a means tested rebate (Australian Government Department of Health). There is now a significant issue with individuals choosing not to have insurance or cancelling their policies, putting greater pressures on public health services (Lannin 2019).

A recent development to healthcare and funding is the implementation of the National Disability Insurance Scheme (NDIS n.d.) implemented in 2013. The NDIS is a major reform of and for disability support through an insurance scheme Buckmaster and Clark 2018). The NDIS is funded by the Commonwealth and State and Territory governments (Buckmaster n.d.). The NDIS allows for funding to be used for 'capacity building' nursing supports, including training by nurses to support independence, and actual nursing care to assist the individual to remain in their home (NDIS).

18.1.2 Nursing in Australia

Nursing in Australia has had a rich history with early nursing practice during colonial times being replicated from that seen in the British Empire (Grehan 2004). Over the following decades, a number of key milestones for nursing are noted. In 1868, a cohort of 'Nightingale' nurses arrived to work at the Sydney Hospital which provided the origins of nurse training (Grehan 2004). Nursing registration was first introduced to Tasmania in 1901 and by 1920 in the remaining states (Grehan 2004). Hospital-based training continued until it was decided to transfer nurse training to the tertiary sector. This was commenced in 1984 and completed in the early to mid-1990s (Australian Government Department of Health n.d.-a, n.d.-b). In 1992, a mutual recognition agreement was signed by Australia and New Zealand. This was extended to allow mutual recognition between the States and New Zealand (Council of Australian Governments n.d.), allowing nurses to move more freely to work in Australia or New Zealand without applying for individual country registration. In 2000, the first two nurse practitioners commenced practicing in Australia (Australian College Nurse Practitioners n.d.). Movement of nurses across state and territory borders was made easy with the 2010 national law and registration system (Australian Health Practitioners Regulatory Authority 2009).

Nursing and midwifery are practiced in all states and territories of Australia in a variety of clinical contexts. Nursing practice in Australia has been governed under a national registration system since 2010 (Duffield et al. 2011). Practice is legislated under the *Health Practitioners Regulation National Law Act 2009* (Australian Health Practitioners Regulatory Authority 2009). Nurses in Australia are registered to practice either as enrolled nurses, registered nurses, nurse practitioners and midwife, although registering as a midwife does not necessarily require registered nurse status with direct entry of midwifery course being available since 2000. Registrant data on September 30, 2019, revealed 301,069 registered nurses, 25,889 with dual registered nurse and midwife status, and 1904 nurse practitioners (Nursing and Midwifery Board of Australia n.d.). All nursing and midwifery positions are articulated in terms of a scope of practice and associated level through an industrial or employment award for all states and territories in government. Awards are defined as 'a comprehensive industrial agreement which defines the minimum employment states for a particular occupation, e.g. nursing or industry' (Roche et al. 2013).

18.1.3 History of the Role of CNS

The clinical nurse specialist (CNS) role first emerged in Australia in the late 1980s with the development of career structures (Duffield et al. 1995; Dunn et al. 2006) articulated in respective state employment awards, for example, the then NSW Nurses Award of 1986 (Duffield et al. 1995). In Western Australia (WA), the career structure provided four streams of nursing practice: management, clinical, education and research that a nurse could develop into and specialise in. Each stream contained different levels, denoting increasing knowledge, skill level and scope of practice. For example, in Western Australia (WA), level 1 denoted a registered nurse; level 2 a clinical nurse, staff development nurse or area manager; and level 3 the CNS or nurse manager (Health Department of WA 1990). The career structure differed for the states or territories where it was implemented, but all implemented a CNS role, although this position was titled clinical nurse consultant in the state of South Australia (Dunn et al. 2006). Over the years, there have been changes to roles and titles, but the structure continues to allow the opportunity to be promoted in a clinical stream rather than just management or education (Appel et al. 1996).

18.2   Definition of CNS

18.2.1 Advanced Practice Nursing

As early as 2002, it was acknowledged that there was no one definition or profile of the advanced practice nurse role. This position has changed with research and discourse provided by a number of authors and professional nursing organisations. The Nursing and Midwifery Board of Australia define advanced practice as a nursing practice that incorporates professional leadership, education, research and support of systems. Practice includes relevant expertise, critical thinking, complex decision-making and autonomous practice and is effective and safe. The advanced practice nurse can work within a generalist or specialist context, and they have responsibility and accountability for managing people who have complex healthcare needs (NMBA 2020).

In 2019, the Australian College of Nursing (ACN), the peak nursing body for Australia, published a white paper on advanced practice nursing (ACN n.d.). This paper was informed by three key nursing manuscripts (Gardner et al. 2016, 2017a, b). The ACN (n.d.: 6) defines advanced practice nursing as 'the experience, education and knowledge to practice at the full capacity of the registered nurse practice scope. It is neither a title nor a role: it is a level of clinical practice that involves cognitive and practical integration of knowledge and skills from the clinical, health systems, education and research domains of nursing. The nurse practising at this level is a leader in nursing and health care. Advanced practice nursing is enabled through education at master's level'. The ACN further define a 'nurse specialist' as 'a clinician with postgraduate education and practice in a speciality field' (ACN n.d.: 16).

In the Australian context, positions that are considered advanced practice positions for nursing and midwifery practice settings have been identified. These positions include nurse practitioner (NP), clinical nurse consultant (CNC), clinical nurse coordinator, nurse clinical practice consultant, clinical nurse and CNS (Gardner et al. 2016). The scope of practice for these roles, except the nurse practitioner position, being defined and protected by law, has similarities despite different titles. In some of the stated positions, there can be different grades of the position and associated different pay scales (Roche et al. 2013).

18.2.2 Clinical Nurse Specialist

Not all states and territories have a CNS position, but all have advanced practice positions (Gardner et al. 2016). CNS positions are defined in part by the state or territory employment award (Duffield et al. 2011) and elaborated on by the health service which employs the CNS and reflected in the respective job description. As such, a single definition of the CNS role in Australia does not exist. A number of identified descriptions provide illustration of the role.

In the state of New South Wales (NSW), the position of CNS or clinical midwife specialist (Grade 1) is defined as a registered nurse/midwife who applies a high level of clinical nursing knowledge, experience and skills in providing complex nursing/midwifery care directed towards a specific area of practice, a defined population or defined service area, with minimum direct supervision. The CNS, Grade 1, will possess as a minimum, a post-registration qualification and at least 12 months' experience in the respective clinical area since obtaining this qualification, or 4 years post-registration experience, with three in the nominated clinical speciality. The role of CNS, Grade 2, identifies the incumbent as a registered nurse/midwife who possesses relevant post-registration qualifications and at least 3 years' experience in the specified clinical area. The CNS in NSW is required to exercise extended autonomy of decision-making, professional knowledge and judgement in providing complex care requiring advanced clinical skills (NSW Government 2017). It is noted that the CNS position in NSW is not equivalent to the CNS position in the United States (Duffield et al. 2011).

In Victoria (VIC), the role description for the CNS in one tertiary hospital, as per the language in the Enterprise Bargaining Agreement[1] (EBA) for that state, provides the following definition. The CNS is a clinical expert in their area of specialisation and is responsible for professional responsibilities that support service delivery and the development of self and others (Royal Children's Hospital Melbourne 2016).

The Queensland registered nurse/midwife classification structure does not stipulate the CNS position; rather, this state employs clinical nurse consultants (CNC). The CNC has responsibility for coordinating clinical practice in a clinical specialty (Queensland Government Queensland Health n.d.). Clinical nurse consultants are also employed in NSW (Fry et al. 2012); WA, Victoria (Victorian Government 2016–2020); Tasmania (Tasmanian Government 2018); Northern Territory; and the ACT. The role of CNC is considered an advanced practice role (Cashin et al. 2014). It is suggested that the role of CNC has 'notable similarities' to that of the CNS role in the United States (USA) (Elsom et al. 2006) and by other authors as being 'equivalent' to the CNS role in the United Kingdom (UK) and the United States (Elsom et al. 2006; Roche et al. 2013). The similarity of the CNS and CNC is not relevant to WA, where the roles are different. The CNS provides a specialist service to a cohort of patients in the same location, e.g. intensive care or surgical ward, whereas the CNC provides consultancy for the area of speciality to a patient cohort, e.g. wound management or pain management.

A theme within the identified literature related to advanced practice in Australia is the ambiguity of the position and role titles (Duffield et al. 1995) and difficulty defining the roles (Dunn et al. 2006). It is evident from what has been presented and summarised in Table 18.1 that for those states and territories that have a CNS position, definitional variation exists.

18.3   Conceptualisations/Model(s) of CNS Practice

Minimal research has been conducted into the concept or model of CNS practice in Australia; however, a limited number of studies have profiled the CNS role and analysed role attributes and scope of practice (Duffield et al. 1995; Appel et al. 1996; Dunn et al. 2006; Gardner et al. 2016). The limitation of this research is that it is not recent, and the majority has been conducted in one state, NSW (Duffield et al. 1994, 1995; Appel et al. 1996; Luck et al. 2015). There is some difficulty conceptualising the CNS role for the Australian context because each state and territory has a different model of advanced practice nursing, which may not include the CNS role.

---

[1] An EBA is an employment award.

Table 18.1 Summary of defining domains of CNS positions for states and territories

	Western Australia	Northern Territory	Queensland	New South Wales	Australian Capital Territory	Victoria	Tasmania	South Australia
Definition of CNS as per employment award	Not specified in the award; but most CNSs are categorised as a Senior Registered Nurse Level 3 (some Level 4 if they provide a state-wide service which are detailed in the award	Not specified in the award; but as defined by the Department of Health—Nursing and Midwifery	Not specified in the award; details the CNC position	Grade 2: A RN/midwife who applies a high level of clinical nursing knowledge, experience and skills in providing complex nursing or midwifery care directed to a specific area of practice, a defined population or service with minimum direct supervision	Not specified in the award; but registered nurse/registered midwife—Level 3 means a RN/RM who may be referred to as:	A RN with a either specific post basic qualification and 12 months' experience in the clinical area of the post-basic qualification and is responsible for clinical nursing duties; or minimum of 4 years' post-registration experience including 3 years in the specialist field (Victorian Government 2016–2020)	Not specified in the award; but includes description for clinical nurse consultant who is:	Not specified in the award; but includes descriptions for Nurse/midwife consultant Level 3; and advanced nurse/midwife consultant Level 4 (South Australian Government 2016)

(continued)

Table 18.1 (continued)

Western Australia	Northern Territory	Queensland	New South Wales	Australian Capital Territory	Victoria	Tasmania	South Australia
Responsible for an expanded professional practice role, which may include, but is not limited to, the criteria outlined below	• Operates with substantial autonomy in providing direct client care and sound clinical advice and recommendations appropriate to the defined practice area which influence the decisions made by others. Is a resource for others	• A CNC is a RN/midwife who coordinates clinical practice in a clinical speciality (Queensland Health 2015)	Grade 2: Encompasses the clinical nurse specialist/clinical midwife specialist Grade 1 role criteria and is distinguished from a CNS Grade 1 by the following additional role characteristics:	• Clinical nurse or midwifery consultant		• A nurse who coordinates the delivery of care in a clinical unit and may provide direct care to selected patients/clients with complex care requirements and is accountable for standards of nursing care in a clinical unit (Tasmanian Government 2016)	

• A multidisciplinary role as team leader/ coordinator of health professionals	• Applies specialist knowledge, skills, attributes and abilities within a defined practice area in therapeutic and professional relationships with individuals, as well as with families, groups and communities. Is recognised by the team for this expertise, is a resource for others and engages in agreed independent practice under the supervision and management of the team (Northern Territory Government 2018)	• Exercises extended autonomy of decisior-making	• Nurse or midwifery educator, nurse manager

(continued)

Table 18.1 (continued)

Western Australia	Northern Territory	Queensland	New South Wales	Australian Capital Territory	Victoria	Tasmania	South Australia
• Clinical/professional responsibility for a multidisciplinary ward/unit, district or region providing complex or tertiary level services			• Exercises professional knowledge and judgement in providing complex care requiring advanced clinical skills and undertakes one of the following roles:	• Nurse coordinator			
• An expanded role of clinical practice and/or management/ leadership control			• Leadership in the development of nursing specialty clinical practice and service delivery in the ward/unit/ service	• Advanced practice nurse			

• Use of advanced problem solving strategies that influence, manage and coordinate patient care over and above the problem-solving skills required at SRN Level 3 (WA Health System-ANF 2018)	• Specialist clinical practice across a small or medium sized health facility/sector/service • Primary case management of a complete episode of care • Primary case management of a continuum of specialty care involving both inpatient and community-based services	• Clinical nurse Coordinator (Australian Capital Territory 2017)

(continued)

Table 18.1 (continued)

	Western Australia	Northern Territory	Queensland	New South Wales	Australian Capital Territory	Victoria	Tasmania	South Australia
				• An authorised extended role within the scope of registered nurse/midwifery practice (New South Wales Government 2017)				
Identification of CNS positions	Yes	Yes; nurse/midwife specialist (clinical) (Northern Territory Government 2018)	No	Yes	No	Yes	Yes	Yes

Key responsibilities or purpose as per example job description	Delivery of quality patient care, developing standards, implementing changes to clinical practice, initiating research and QI activities; provision of a consultation service within area of expertise and assigned area (Royal Perth Hospital 2018)	N/A	Accountable for providing sound professional advice and for assessment, planning, review, evaluation and coordination of comprehensive client care and/or case management for individuals, groups or communities within the speciality area across the healthcare episode (Northern Territory Government 2018)	Utilise specialised clinical knowledge, complex patient/client care management skills and leadership skills to ensure department is equipped with the resources needed for service provision associated with speciality clinical practice within a tertiary hospital environment, so as to maximise the health outcomes for the patient (New South Wales 2018)	N/A	CNS is a clinical expert in an area of nursing specialisation and accepts responsibility for professional activities that support service delivery and the professional development of self and others

(continued)

Table 18.1 (continued)

	Western Australia	Northern Territory	Queensland	New South Wales	Australian Capital Territory	Victoria	Tasmania	South Australia
Selection criteria to guide suitability for the position	• Eligible for registration in the category of registered nurse by the NMBA[b]	• Highly developed knowledge, skills and experience in the relevant area of clinical nursing/midwifery	N/A	• Registered nurse with current authority to practice with AHPRA	N/A	• Nursing registration with AHPRA		
	• Demonstrated significant knowledge, experience and leadership in area of speciality	• Well-developed nursing/midwifery leadership and management knowledge, skills and experience		• Post-registration qualifications and at least 3 years post-registration experience in speciality		• Evidence of ongoing professional development as reflected in professional practice portfolio		
	• Demonstrated knowledge and application of human resource principles in nursing	• Knowledge and application of adult learning principles. Experience teaching in small groups and application of competency-based assessment (Northern Territory Government 2018)		• Demonstrated application of professional and ethical boundaries when working with complex situations as part of a multidisciplinary team		• Demonstrate ability to meet key accountabilities		

• Demonstrated knowledge and application of quality improvement initiatives	• Demonstrated ability to analyse problems and apply a range of options to develop solutions to avoid future crises	• Demonstrate well-developed interpersonal skills
• Demonstrated knowledge of research principles to support evidence-based practice	• Demonstrated ability to proactively engaged with medical practitioners, peers and vendors to understand their needs enhance service delivery and act on situations when the norm is to wait for a situation to resolve itself	• Demonstrate effective working relationships

(continued)

Table 18.1 (continued)

Western Australia	Northern Territory	Queensland	New South Wales	Australian Capital Territory	Victoria	Tasmania	South Australia
• Demonstrated well-developed interpersonal and communication skills			• Demonstrated ability to identify and implement improvements in clinical service delivery		• Demonstrate flexibility and ability to prioritise workloads		
• Current knowledge of legislative obligations for equal opportunity, disability services and occupational safety and health (Royal Perth Hospital 2018)			• Demonstrated ability to apply and share professional expertise to immediate work and developments within field of expertise to enhance service delivery (New South Wales Government 2018)		• Demonstrate commitment to ensuring safe, quality care for all patients and their families (Royal Children's Hospital 2018)		

| Educational requirements; and length of time in speciality | Postgraduate qualifications are desirable but not mandated; 'significant' experience, actual length of time not specified | Graduate diploma or equivalent experience beyond entry to practice in speciality (Northern Territory Government 2018) | N/A | Grade 1: Relevant post-registration qualifications and at least 12 months' experience working in the relevant clinical area of their post-registration qualification; or 4 years' post-registration experience, including 3 years' experience in the relevant specialist field | N/A | Postgraduate qualification in specific nursing field, and 12 months' experience in clinical area |

(continued)

Table 18.1 (continued)

Western Australia	Northern Territory	Queensland	New South Wales	Australian Capital Territory	Victoria	Tasmania	South Australia
			Grade 2: RN/midwife appointed to a position classified as such with relevant post-registration qualifications and at least 3 years' experience working in the clinical area of their specified postgraduate qualification (NSW Government 2017)		A minimum of 4 years' post-basic registration experience including 3 years in the speciality (Royal Children's Hospital 2018)		

Direct patient care/load	No	N/A	N/A	Yes	N/A	Yes. Defined in the EBA[c] as responsibility for clinical nursing duties and thus provides direct care

[a]Current Tasmanian Agreement 2016, explains that a review of the CNS position is being conducted
[b]Nursing and Midwifery Board of Australia
[c]Enterprise bargaining agreement

18.3.1 Key Responsibilities and Scope of Duties

A review of three job descriptions, for WA, NSW and Victoria, provide detail around the key responsibilities of the CNS role. The job descriptions for CNS positions in the state WA tend to be generic but provide illustrative language of the scope of practice. In one tertiary hospital in WA (Royal Perth Hospital 2018), the CNS's key responsibilities include 'supervision of the delivery of quality patient care, developing standards of practice, implementing changes to clinical practice and initiating research and quality improvement activities; and the provision of a consultation service within their area of expertise/assigned area to all customers within the Hospital and Health Service'. The scope of duties of this CNS position is listed in Table 18.2.

This CNS position in Victoria (Royal Children's Hospital 2018) lists a number of domains of practice with 'key accountabilities', including direct and comprehensive care, support of systems, education, research and quality and professional leadership. With respect to actual care, the CNS is expected to 'conduct comprehensive patient assessments' and interpret the data from these assessments to develop and implement care. The scope of duties extends to conducting procedures specific to the speciality.

Table 18.2 CNS scope of duties: a tertiary hospital in WA[a]

1	Leads and manages the multidisciplinary ward/unit team
2	Provides clinical leadership and consultancy to medical, nursing and allied healthcare professionals and providers in the areas of speciality at a hospital and health service level
3	Provides advanced and complex patient care within the area of speciality at a hospital and health service level
4	Initiates and analyses the research to determine clinical management trends. Promotes excellence, and implements best practice that supports the delivery of appropriate clinical care and management in area of speciality
5	Maintains excellence in interpersonal skills and leadership to guide appropriate patient care in relation to area of speciality
6	Promotes and guides a multidisciplinary team approach to decision-making
7	Develops standards and policies for the areas of speciality using an evidenced-based approach, developing innovative methods and techniques for effective practice and change within the hospital and health service
8	Develops policies and monitors compliance with relevant industry acknowledged standards and legislative requirements
9	Coordinates and implements quality improvement activities recognising national safety and quality health service standards
10	Manages human and material resources to affect quality patient care
11	Implements and maintains performance management systems which support ongoing developments of staff
12	Develops, implements and evaluates educational and training programs related to the areas of speciality, hospital and community needs
13	Provides a public relations function for the area including where relevant investigation and management of questions from government ministers, enquiries and consumer complaints

[a]Royal Perth Hospital Job description form: Clinical nurse specialist. https://rph-healthpoint.hdwa.health.wa.gov.au/directory/CORPORATESERVICES/CorporateNursing/Nursing%20Job%20Description%20Forms%20JDFs/SRN%204%20Clinical%20Nurse%20Consultant%20-%20SAFE%20RP603057%20April%202017.pdf. Accessed 10 Jan 2018

The CNS is required to coordinate and collaborate with care requirements and ensure collaboration with other services to ensure the optimisation to meet the patient's needs. CNSs are expected to translate their expert knowledge to educational programs for their speciality.

A CNS position for the operating theatre in a health district (NSW Government Health 2018) is responsible for the utilisation of specialised clinical knowledge and skills for complex patient or client care. Leadership skills are required to ensure that the clinical area has the appropriate resources needed for service provision and to maximise the health outcomes for the patient cohort of this area. The job description for this position comprehensively lists key accountabilities. In relation to clinical care, the CNS uses advanced and specialised best practice clinical skills to assess, plan, organise, implement and evaluate care. The CNS is required to exercise professional knowledge and judgement to provide complex care which requires advanced clinical skills. The CNS also has responsibility for promoting an environment that encourages collaboration to effect positive patient outcomes and a positive workplace culture. Not unlike the previous two CNS positions, education development of others is also a requirement.

Components of the nurse specialist role were identified in one South Australian study (Dunn et al. 2006). These components were clinical, education, professional development, management and research. The subcomponents for clinical included procedures, consultation, outreach and community involvement, attendance at clinics and direct patient care, medication management and monitoring. The provision of education included patients and family and staff. The specialist nurse attended formal and informal development opportunities, including participation in professional organisations and committees. The subcomponents of management were much broader, including care and case coordination, human resource management, equipment management, and management of data and budgets.

18.3.2 Direct Versus Non-direct Care

The role of CNS articulated in the Victoria employment award provides further illustration of one CNS model, the 'Strong Model of Advanced Practice' detailed in the work by the following authors (Gardner et al. 2013). This model contains five domains which broadly depict the scope of practice for an advanced practice nurse. These are (1) direct comprehensive care, (2) support of systems, (3) education, (4) research and (5) publication and professional leadership. The first domain can be seen in the CNS role in Victoria which has responsibility for a patient caseload. This is similar in NSW where the CNS has responsibility for 'clinical bedside practice.' In WA, this position is fulfilled by the clinical nurse who has responsibility for direct patient care. In contrast, the CNS in WA does not generally have responsibility for the care of patients each shift; rather, the role provides expert and specialist advice to a specific patient cohort or clinical area, for example, intensive care patients.

18.3.3 Areas of Practice

Further illustration of the concept of the CNS role can be gleamed from the clinical practice areas which the CNS works. The CNS employed by a hospital is generally appointed to work in a clinical ward or area and can have a patient caseload or provide expert advice regarding the care of a particular patient without the caseload. In WA, CNSs are typically employed in all major clinical areas, including intensive care, coronary care, paediatrics, oncology, orthopaedics and operating theatres. In a South Australian study conducted in 2006, it was noted that CNSs were mostly employed in larger hospitals (Dunn et al. 2006). The CNS is also employed in community settings, including specialist areas within the community setting, for example, community mental health.

A number of other roles, while not necessarily titled CNS, fall into the broader domain of advanced practice due to the nature of the scope of practice and qualifications required for this determined practice. The first of these examples is the practice of the sexual health nurse. The Australasian Sexual Health and HIV Nurses Association (ASHHNA) is the peak Australasian sexual, reproductive health and human immunodeficiency virus (HIV) nurses' professional organisation and articulates a number of practice and professional competencies (Australasian Sexual Health and HIV Nurses Association n.d.). The association states that an advanced RN is a nurse who has acquired an expert knowledge base, complex decision-making skills and clinical competence to allow practice in an expanded and more autonomous scope. Further, the advanced RN in sexual and reproductive health and/or HIV can demonstrate (a) advanced level of theoretical knowledge and (b) educational preparation with postgraduate qualifications (Australasian Sexual Health and HIV Nurses Association). In some practice contexts for this speciality domain, medication competency is required. In QLD, as one example, Central Queensland University (Central Queensland University n.d.) offers a short course to allow sexual health nurses to obtain the necessary competency to safely supply and administer medications in accordance with the Drug Therapy Protocol—Sexual Health Program (including reproductive health), relevant approved Health Management Protocol and the Queensland Health (Drugs & Poisons) Regulation 1996.

The Queensland government instigated and manages the rural and isolated practice (scheduled medicine endorsement) registered nurse (RIPRN) course aimed at educating the nurse to practice using advanced decision-making and skills (Queensland Government Queensland Health) necessary for this practice context where there is significant professional and geographical isolation. Throughout Australia, 1181 registered nurse are endorsed by the Nursing and Midwifery Board to administer scheduled medications as per the RIPRN curriculum (Nursing and Midwifery Board 2019).

18.4 CNS Practice Competencies

The Nursing and Midwifery Board of Australia (2016) provides a set of competency standards for the registered nurse, which form the foundational competencies for registered nurses in all states and territories. Competency standards do not exist for the CNS role. Many competency standards have been developed for specialist nurse practice by the respective professional nursing organisation. In 2008, 20 Australian competency documents were identified (Chiarella et al. 2008). Two current examples are competency standards for specialist palliative care nursing practice (Canning et al. 2005) and for specialist breast cancer nursing practice (Yates et al. 2007).

18.5   Outcome Measures and Evaluation

Outcome measures and evaluation of nursing care are typically aligned to national standards relevant to inpatient care. The relevant standards are (1) clinical governance, (2) partnering with consumers, (3) preventing and controlling healthcare-associated infections, (4) medication safety, (5) comprehensive care, (6) communicating for safety, (7) blood management and (8) recognising and responding to acute deterioration (Australian Commission on Safety and Quality in Healthcare 2017). These standards detail key actions and criterion to ensure safe and high-quality care, including governance of healthcare practitioners through registration, credentialing and professional development requirements. Key performance indicators and associated reporting are aligned to relevant standards, for example, fall management, pressure injury management and medication safety. Clinical nurse specialists and other advanced practice nurses can have a key role ensuring that policy and practice standards, including necessary training, are enacted to minimise harm associated with each standard.

18.6   CNS Education

It has been proposed that the role of CNS requires formal specialist education (Daly and Carnwell 2003). The educational requirements for a CNS position fall into two categories, with some states stipulating a postgraduate qualification and others describing the obtainment of a qualification in the speciality as desirable, but not mandatory. In Australia, a postgraduate qualification can be a graduate certificate, graduate diploma and master's or doctoral-level qualifications. A study to identify advanced nursing practice conducted in 2016 with 5662 respondents provides insight to the extent of post-registration qualifications (Gardner et al. 2016). Although the findings do not discriminate the CNS position, 19% of respondents held a master's degree, with only 0.7% holding a doctoral degree. Approximately 10% had a hospital-based certificate.

18.7   Endorsement and Professional Recognition

The National Law in Australia allows for the registration and regulation of two levels of nurses: the registered nurse and the enrolled nurse (AHPRA 2009). The only advanced practice nursing role registered is the nurse practitioner role (Duffield et al. 2011). Although the clinical nurse specialist role is filled by a registered nurse, the role of the CNS itself is not regulated by the Nursing and Midwifery Board of

Australia. This means that the title is not protected by the National Law. Some nursing positions other than the NP position can require credentialing. The Queensland Health Service Directive requires, for example, that 'nurses and midwives intending to engage in a specific scope of practice are credentialed and have a current, documented scope of practice' (Queensland Health Service Directive 2020).

There is no professional nursing or midwifery organisation for the CNS in Australia or professional certification requirement for these positions. Governance of the role and the associated scope of practice primarily lies with employing health service. Nonetheless, credentialing has been explored and developed for some specialist practice in Australia. For example, the Australian College of Critical Care Nurses' (ACCCN) launched their inaugural credentialing model in 1998 (Chiarella et al. 2008). The latest edition was published in 2015 (Australian College of Critical Care Nurses 2015). Credentialing can be awarded to the critical care nurse who is deemed to practice at or above the level of the Competency Standards for Specialist Critical Care Nurses (Duffield et al. 2011). Credentialing is also available for mental health nurses through the Australian College of Mental Health Nurses. To be credentialed, the mental health nurse will be a specialist nurse who demonstrates registration, education, practice, professional development and professional integrity (The Australian College of Mental Health Nurses n.d.).

18.8   Moving Forward: Challenges and Opportunities

The CNS position is not found in all states and territories in Australia, although arguably there are equivalent roles, including the CNC position. The lack of national governance of the CNS role via the nursing regulatory authorities or single professional organisation and a dominance of industrial awards with respect to role definitions and titles means that a unified approach to the CNS role is not likely in the near future.

Much of what has been written about specialist and advanced roles demonstrates diversity in the positions and roles, including titles with resultant ambiguity and confusion (Duffield et al. 1995, 2011; Elsom et al. 2006). Furthermore, these positions and role responsibilities are determined industrially and not predominantly by the profession (Duffield et al. 2011). Although there is national regulation of registered nurse positions and nurse practitioners, other specialist and advanced practice positions are not. It is argued that an ad hoc approach to and a lack of coordination to the defining of clinical practice can result in a large number of 'highly specialised, small and potentially similar areas of practice' (Duffield et al. 2011). These authors argue that a more coordinated approach to these roles and positions may result in increased efficacy of resources. The authors of the 2006 study of specialist nurses in SA have also argued that 'formal description and evaluation of the role is an essential prerequisite to determining the role's impact on health care'. A more recent study argues that further research is required to (more clearly) articulate CNS role descriptors as the boundaries between the CNS and CNC descriptors are blurred (Luck et al. 2015).

Back in 2006, it was asserted in one study that while anecdotal evidence existed to support the nurse specialist role in Australia, empirical evidence is required to demonstrate clinical and educational outcomes and outputs (Dunn et al. 2006). The most recent and significant study of advanced practice nursing in the Australian context (Gardner et al. 2016) provides some guidance on the direction of practice and role development while noting that the CNS position is not specifically articulated. Nonetheless, the study demonstrates that advanced nursing practice can be measured as a 'level of nursing practice' as opposed to labelled roles or positions. The authors while further acknowledging the difficulty with robust definitions and profiles of the advanced practice nurse role argue that there is opportunity to address these needs by the development of a model for advanced nursing practice, including standardisation across Australian jurisdictions (Gardner et al. 2016, 2017a, b).

A further challenge is the lack of literature which addresses the impact on patient care and healthcare outcomes where a CNS is involved in the care (Dunn et al. 2006). Where the CNS role is explicitly stated, the focus of the literature has been in role definition, classification and profiles. With the new focus on the area of advance practice of nursing in Australia with the 2019 release of the ACN white paper, this deficit may be addressed. The ACN assert that this white paper provides a strategy for health service improvement for cohorts in the Australian population who receive less equitable and timely healthcare. An advanced practice nursing model is a viable solution to address this area of need. Further research will benefit measurement of new and expanded roles and areas of practice.

The literature provides a range of examples where patient and health needs have driven specialist nursing roles in the Australian context. The following two exemplars have emerged to address the complex health needs of patients with cancer. There is assertion that patients with complex needs have to be cared for by a multidisciplinary team including a specialist nurse. In one study, it was shown that the specialist gynaecological-oncology nurse was seen by the multidisciplinary team as 'being the glue in the team'. A key finding of this study revealed the view by participants that patients not cared for by a team with a specialist nurse were disadvantaged (Cook et al. 2019).

18.9   Exemplar of CNS Practice

18.9.1 Specialist Breast Nurse in Australia

In 2003, the National Breast Centre (NBCC) commenced a project aimed at defining a set of competencies for the specialist breast nurse (SBN) to improve the outcomes of women with breast cancer (Yates et al. 2007). The competencies complemented the existing nursing competency standards for breast cancer care. Over 60 stakeholders were involved in the development of the competency and education standards including registered nurses clinically involved in the specialty area and those holding management and academic positions. Medical and allied health personnel were also consulted along with a national consumer advocate. The SBN was defined as a registered nurse who applies advanced knowledge to manage women with breast cancer across the continuum of care. The scope of practice included diagnosis, treatment, rehabilitation, follow-up and palliative care. The domains of care were defined as supportive care, collaborative care, coordinated care, information provision and education and clinical leadership.

18.9.2 Prostate Cancer Specialist Nurse in Australia

In the early 2000s, it was recognised that prostate cancer rates in Australia were increasing (Sykes 2011). The treatment strategies for prostate cancer can have a significant impact on the quality of life. The role of this nurse to provide information and support is critical and acknowledged by the National Institute of Clinical Excellence in Improving Outcomes in Urological Cancer Document in 2002 (Sykes 2011). Cancer nurse coordinators are already established in Australia with a defined scope of practice including psychosocial assessment and supportive care. It was identified that there was not a designated role for the nurse providing exclusive support for prostate cancer patients. This leads to the development and roll out of national program of prostate cancer specialist nurses (Sykes 2011).The core capabilities of the prostate cancer specialist nurse included (1) professional practice at a systems level; (2) critical thinking and analysis, quality improvement and research; (3) provision and coordination of care including the assessment, planning, implementation and evaluation of care for people affected by cancer and disease and treatment-related care; and (4) collaborative and therapeutic practice. One university in Australia—La Trobe—conducts a specialised course of study that prepares registered nurses to care for men with prostate cancer (La Trobe University n.d.). It is a short course that is offered by the School of Nursing and Midwifery and includes a comprehensive overview of physiology, pathophysiology, treatment options and psychosocial care for the patient and family. It is offered as an online course of 52 contact hours. All registered nurses in Australia are qualified to undertake the course, and there is no minimum requirement of a bachelor's degree (La Trobe University n.d.).

The position of the prostate cancer specialist nurse is a new concept in Australia, and it is important to evaluate the role to measure the impact on both the patient and the healthcare system. A national program manager is now in place for the purpose of establishing the program nationwide in Australia and to evaluate outcomes.

18.10 Conclusion

This chapter has introduced and provided a discussion of the CNS role, as a subset of advanced practice nursing in the Australian context. This chapter highlights a number of nuances that provide a picture of the role, the nurse profiles and scope of practice. While all CNSs are registered nurses, the role itself is not a registrable position in the National Law. As such, the title and scope of practice is not regulated by the Nursing and Midwifery Board but rather is detailed in the respective Industrial Award with practice being governed by the employer. Where the specialist nurse chooses to be credentialed to enable expanded scope of practice, then the college of the speciality can have oversight if this has been established.

The CNS in Australia is not necessarily required to have postgraduate qualifications, although this can be viewed as supporting the assertion and requirement of possessing the required knowledge of the practice area. In keeping with the fact that the role is not regulated by the Nursing and Midwifery, there are not defined competencies for the CNS role, although specialist professional groups have defined their own. Minimal literature was identified that demonstrated exploration of the impact on patient or healthcare outcomes related to the practice or influence of the CNS role and should be addressed to ensure contemporaneous understanding of the role and effect and to ensure all advanced practice is assessed for efficacy, value and sustainability of this area of nursing. Some of the identified literature identified role titles which reflected specialist knowledge but omitted the word clinical, for example, as in the two provided examples, 'specialist breast nurse' and prostate cancer specialist nurse'. While there are differences in titles, there is a link to the overarching intent of these positions in that they provide an advanced level of skill and knowledge for the provision of expert and comprehensive care to

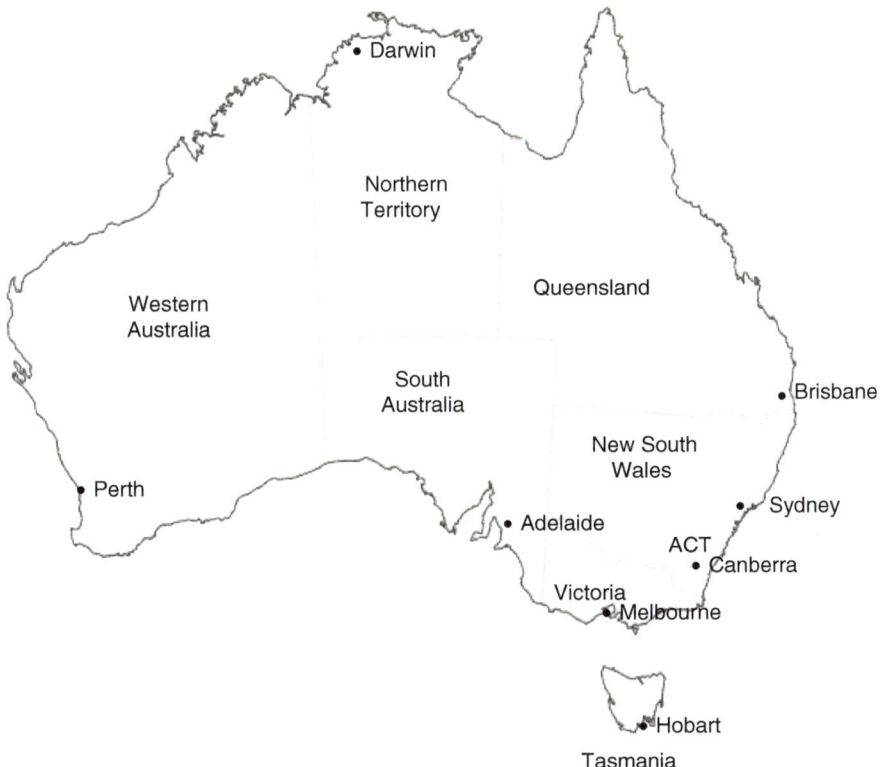

Fig. 18.1 Australian states/territory

patients. In the renewed focus on advanced practice nursing by the Australian peak nursing body, the ACN provides not only a challenge to nurses and practice but an invitation to governments and health organisations to see nursing practice as a viable option to address healthcare and service inequality in areas of Australia and for vulnerable populations (Fig. 18.1).

References

Appel A, Malcolm P, Nahas V (1996) Nursing specialisation in New South Wales. Australia Clinical Nurse Specialist 10(2):76–81

Australian College Nurse Practitioners (n.d.) History. https://www.acnp.org.au/history. Accessed 26 July 2020

Australian College of Nursing (n.d.) A new horizon for health services: optimizing advanced practice nursing. https://www.acn.edu.au/wp-content/uploads/white-paper-optimising-advanced-practice-nursing.pdf. Accessed 2 Feb 2020

Australian College of Critical Care Nurses. (2015) Practice standards for specialist critical care nurses. ACCCN. https://www.acccn.com.au/documents/item/934

Australian Commission on Safety and Quality in Healthcare (2017) National Safety and Quality Health Service Standards: guide for hospitals. ACSQH, Sydney

Australian Capital Territory (2017) ACT public sector nursing and midwifery enterprise agreement 2017–2019. https://www.cmtedd.act.gov.au/__data/assets/pdf_file/0003/1266186/Final-Draft-Nursing-Midwifery-Agreement-2017-2019.pdf

Australian Government (n.d.) About Australia. https://www.australia.gov.au/about-australia/facts-and-figures. Accessed 18 Mar 2018

Australian Government Department of Health (n.d.-a) The Australian health system. https://www.health.gov.au/about-us/the-australian-health-system#cost-of-health-care-in-australia. Accessed 2 Feb 2020

Australian Government Department of Health (n.d.-b) Appendix IV: history of the commonwealth involvement in the nursing and midwifery workforce. https://www1.health.gov.au/internet/publications/publishing.nsf/Content/work-review-australian-government-health-workforce-programs-toc~appendices~appendix-iv-history-commonwealth-involvement-nursing-midwifery-workforce. Accessed 2 Feb 2020

Australian Health Practitioners Regulatory Authority (2009) Health Practitioners Regulation National Law Act 2009. https://www.ahpra.gov.au/About-AHPRA/What-We-Do/Legislation.aspx. Accessed 18 Mar 2018

Australian Institute Health and Welfare (2016) How does Australia's health system work? https://www.aihw.gov.au/getmedia/f2ae1191-bbf2-47b6-a9d4-1b2ca65553a1/ah16-2-1-how-does-australias-health-system-work.pdf.aspx. Accessed 18 Mar 2018

Buckmaster L, Clark S (2018) The National Disability Insurance Scheme: A chronology. https://www.aph.gov.au/About_Parliament/Parliamentary_Departments/Parliamentary_Library/pubs/rp/rp1819/Chronologies/NDIS. Accessed 26 July 2020

Buckmaster L (n.d.) Paying for the National Disability Scheme. https://www.aph.gov.au/About_Parliament/Parliamentary_Departments/Parliamentary_Library/pubs/BriefingBook45p/NDIS. Accessed 26 July 2020

Canning D, Yates P, Rosenberg JP (2005) Competency standards for specialist palliative care nursing practice. Queensland University of Technology, Brisbane. https://www.health.qld.gov.au/__data/assets/pdf_file/0023/141188/compstand.pdf. Accessed 10 Mar 2018

Cashin A, Stasa H, Gullick J, Conway R, Cunich M (2014) Clarifying clinical nurse consultant work in Australia: a phenomenological study. Collegian 22:405–412

Central Queensland University (n.d.) Sexual and reproductive health—nurse authorisation course. https://www.cqu.edu.au/courses/sexual-and-reproductive-health-nurse-authorisation-course. Accessed 7 Feb 2020

Chiarella M, Thoms D, McInnes E (2008) An overview of the competency movement in nursing and midwifery. Collegian 15:49–53

Cook O, McIntyre M, Recoche M, Lee S (2019) Our nurse is the glue for our team—multidisciplinary team members' experiences and perceptions of the gynaecological oncology specialist nurse role. Eur J Oncol Nurs 41:7–15

Council of Australian Governments (n.d.) Trans-Tasman mutual recognition agreement. https://www.coag.gov.au/about-coag/agreements/trans-tasman-mutual-recognition-arrangement-arrangement-between-australian. Accessed 7 Feb 2020

Daly WM, Carnwell R (2003) Nursing roles and levels of practice: a framework for differentiating between elementary, specialist and advanced nursing practice. J Clin Nurs 12(2):158–167

Duffield C, Pelletier D, Donoghue J (1995) A profile of the clinical nurse specialists in one Australian state. Clin Nurse Spec 9(3):149–154

Duffield CM, Gardner G, Chang AM, Fry M, Stasa H (2011) National regulation in australia: a time for standardisation in roles and titles. Collegian. 18;45–49

Duffield CM, Pelletier D, Donoghue J (1994). Role overlap between clinical nurse specialists and nursing unit managers. JONA 24(11), 34–63

Dunn S, Pretty L, Martin M, Gassner L (2006) A framework for description and evaluation of the nurse specialist role in South Australia. Collegian 13(1):23–30

Elsom S, Happell B, Manias E (2006) The clinical nurse specialist and nurse practitioner roles: room for both or take your pick? Aust J Adv Nurs 24(2):56–59

Fry M, Duffield C, Baldwin R, Roche M, Stasa H, Solman A (2012) Development of a tool to describe the role of the clinical nurse consultant in Australia. J Clin Nurs 22:1531–1538

Gardner C, Chang A, Duffield C, Doubrovsky A (2013) Delineating the practice profile of advanced practice nursing: a cross sectional survey using the modified strong model of advanced practice. J Adv Nurs 69(9):1931–1942. https://eprints.qut.edu.au/56458/. Accessed 2 Feb 2020

Gardner G, Duffield C, Doubrovsky A, Adams M (2016) Identifying advanced practice: a national survey of a nursing workforce. Int J Nurs Stud 55:60–70

Gardner G, Duffield C, Doubrovsky A, et al. (2017a) The structure of nursing: a national examination of titles and practice profiles. INR Jun 64(2):233–241

Gardner G, Duffield C, Gardner A, Batch M (2017b) The Australian advanced practice nursing self-appraisal tool. https://doi.org/10.6084/m9.figshare.4669432

Grehan M (2004) From the sphere of Sarah Gampism: the professionalism of nursing and midwifery in the colony of Victoria. Nurs Inq 11(3):192–201

Health Department of WA. WA Nurses' Career Structure Evaluation Committee (1990) Report of the Nurses' Career Structure Evaluation Committee

Jamieson L, Mosel Williams L (2002) Confusion prevails in defining advanced practice nursing. Collegian 9(4):29–33

La Trobe University (n.d.). https://www.latrobe.edu.au/short-courses/nursing. Accessed 25 Apr 2018

Lannin C (2019) Private health insurance at a 'tipping point', with Australians dropping cover in droves. Australian Broadcasting Commission. https://www.abc.net.au/news/2019-08-01/private-health-insurance-heading-for-the-emergency-ward/11371286. Accessed 2 Feb 2020

Luck L, Wilkes L, O'Baugh J (2015) Treading the clinical pathway: a qualitative study of advanced practice nurses in a local health district in Australia. BMC Nurs 14:52

NDIS (n.d.) Supports funded by the NDIS. https://www.ndis.gov.au/understanding/supports-funded-ndis. Accessed 26 July 2020

Northern Territory Government (2018) Public sector nurses and midwives' 2018–2022 enterprise agreement. https://www.fwc.gov.au/document/agreement/AE501953

NSW Government (2017) Public Health system nurses' and midwives (state) award. http://www.nswnma.asn.au/wp-content/uploads/2013/07/Public-Health-System-Nurses-and-Midwives-State-Award-2017-1-July-2017.pdf. Accessed 10 Mar 2018

NSW Government Health (2018) Clinical nurse specialist job description. https://nswhealth.erecruit.com.au/ViewPosition.aspx?id=385670. Accessed 25 Feb 2018

Nursing and Midwifery Board of Australia. (2016) Registered Nurse Standards for Practice. file:///C:/Users/Dale%20Pugh/Downloads/Nursing-and-Midwifery-Board---Standard---Registered-nurse-standards-for-practice---1-June-2016.PDF

Nursing and Midwifery Board of Australia (2020) Advanced nursing practice and specialty areas within nursing: Fact sheet. file:///C:/Users/Dale%20Pugh/Downloads/Nursing-and-Midwifery-Board---Fact-sheet---Advanced-nursing-practice-and-specialty-areas-within-nursing---May-2020.PDF. Accessed 26 July 2020

Nursing and Midwifery Board of Australia (n.d.) Registrant data: reporting period: 01 July 2019 to 30 September 2019. https://www.nursingmidwiferyboard.gov.au/About/Statistics.aspx. Accessed 6 Feb 2020

Private healthcare Australia (n.d.) Benefits for you 2015. https://www.privatehealthcareaustralia.org.au. Accessed 18 Mar 2018

Queensland Health (2015) Nursing and Midwifery Structure. https://www.qnmu.org.au/DocumentsFolder/QNMU%20DOCUMENTS/General/About%20Us/Nursing%20classification%20FINAL%20CORRECT.pdf

Queensland Government Queensland Health (n.d.) Remote and isolated practice (scheduled medications) registered nurse course. https://www.health.qld.gov.au/cunninghamcentre/html/courses/022. Accessed 8 Feb 2020

Queensland Government (2020) Credentialling and defining the scope of clinical practice. Queensland Health Service Directorate. https://www.health.qld.gov.au/__data/assets/pdf_file/0038/670979/qh-hsd-034.pdf

Roche M, Duffield C, Wise S, Fry M, Solman A (2013) Domains of practice and advanced practice nursing in Australia. Nurs Health Sci 15:497–503

Royal Children's Hospital Melbourne (2016) Clinical nurse specialist: application guide. https://www.rch.org.au/uploadedFiles/Main/Content/nursing/CNS%20Application%20Guide%20V1%20June%202016%20(002).pdf. Accessed 26 Feb 2018

Royal Children's Hospital (2018) Position Description: Clinical Nurse Specialist. https://www.rch.org.au/uploadedFiles/Main/Content/nursing/CNS%20Position%20Description%20V2.pdf

Royal Perth Hospital (2018) Job description: clinical nurse specialist. Rph nursing division

South Australian Government (2016) Nursing and Midwifery (South Australian Public Sector) Enterprise Agreement. Appendix 7—career structure. http://www.sahealth.sa.gov.au/wps/wcm/connect/public+content/sa+health+internet/about+us/about+sa+health/our+workforce/enterprise+bargaining/nursing+and+midwifery+ea+negotiations+2016. Accessed 10 Mar 2018

Sykes J (2011) Future directions for the prostate cancer specialist nurse in Australia. Int J Urol Nurs 5(3):139–145

Tasmanian Government (2018) https://www.tic.tas.gov.au/award_history/nurses_tasmanian_public_sector_award_2005

Tasmanian Government (2016) Nurses and midwives (Tasmanian state service) agreement. http://www.tic.tas.gov.au/__data/assets/pdf_file/0019/371251/T14480_of_2017_Nurses_and_Midwives_TSS_Agreement_2016.pdf. Accessed 10 Mar 2018

The Australasian Sexual Health and HIV Nurses Association (n.d.) Competency Standards for sexual and reproductive health and HIV nurses. http://ashhna.org.au/wp-content/uploads/2014/12/ASHHNA_Competency-Standards-for-sexual-and-reproductive-health-and-HIV-nurses.pdf. Accessed 7 Feb 2020

The Australian College of Mental Health Nurses (n.d.) What is credentialing. http://www.acmhn.org/credentialing/what-is-credentialing. Accessed 4 Feb 2020

Victorian Government (2016–2020) Nurse and midwives (Victoria public Health sector Enter-
    prise agreement). http://www.anmfvic.asn.au/~/media/files/ANMF/EBA%202016/Nurses-and-
    Midwives-Vic-PS-SIE-EA-2016-2020-amended. Accessed 25 Feb 2018
Western Australian Government (2016) WA Health System—Australian Nursing Federation—
    Registered Nurses, Midwives, Enrolled (Mental Health) and Enrolled (Mothercraft) Nurses—
    Industrial Agreement. http://forms.wairc.wa.gov.au/Pages/AwardsAgreements/Agreements.
    aspx?agreements=w. Accessed 10 Mar 2018
WA Health System – Australian Nursing Federation (2018) Registered Nurses, Midwives, Enrolled
    (Mental Health) and Enrolled (Mothercraft) Nurses Industrial Agreement. https://ww2.health.
    wa.gov.au/-/media/Files/Corporate/general-documents/Awards-and-agreements/Nurses-Reg-
    istered-and-Enrolled-Mental-Health/Australian-Nursing-Federation-Registered-Nurses-Mid-
    wives-Enrolled-and-Enrolled-Nurses-Industrial-Agreement-2018.pdf
Yates P, Evans A, Moore A, Heartfield M, Gibson T, Luxford K (2007) Competency standards and
    educational requirements for specialist breast nurses. Collegian 14(1):11–15

Clinical Nurse Specialist Role and Practice in New Zealand

19

Glynis Cumming, Rachael Haldane, and Jan Ipenburg

Abstract

A number of factors have influenced the embedding of the clinical nurse specialist (CNS) role in New Zealand (NZ) since its first inception in the 1970s. The last 20 years has seen a proliferation of CNS roles, and it is now the most common of the two advanced nursing practice roles in NZ. The CNS role is not title-protected and is regulated within the registered nurse scope of practice. Individual CNS roles are determined by employers, which has resulted in confusion about the function and nature of the role. What is lacking is a clear national definition, competency assessment and educational pathway that is agreed on by CNS's, employers, nursing organisations and Nursing Council of New Zealand. The development of a CNS model, which reflects the diverse nature of the role, is crucial for the full potential of the CNS role to be realised.

Keywords

Clinical nurse specialist · CNS · Advanced nursing practice · ANP · Nurse Specialist · Scope of practice · New Zealand

This chapter has been written before the 2020 APN ICN guidelines were published and reflects the views of the authors.

G. Cumming · R. Haldane (✉) · J. Ipenburg
Clinical Nurse Specialist Society New Zealand Inc., Canterbury, New Zealand

© Springer Nature Switzerland AG 2021
J. S. Fulton, V. W. Holly (eds.), *Clinical Nurse Specialist Role and Practice*,
Advanced Practice in Nursing, https://doi.org/10.1007/978-3-319-97103-2_19

Abbreviations

ANP   Advanced Nursing Practice
CCP   Clinical Career Pathway
CNS   Clinical Nurse Specialist
DHB   District Health Board
MECA   Multi Employment Collective Agreement
MOH   Ministry of Health
NCNZ   Nursing Council of New Zealand
NENZ   Nurse Executives of New Zealand
NP   Nurse Practitioner
NS   Nurse Specialist
NZ   New Zealand
NZNA   New Zealand Nursing Association
NZNO   New Zealand Nursing Organisation
PDRP   Professional Development Recognition Pathway
RN   Registered Nurse
SCN   Specialty Clinical Nurse

19.1   Clinical Nurse Specialist: New Zealand

The role of the clinical nurse specialist in New Zealand (NZ) needs to be considered in the unique context of biculturalism and the principals of the *Te Tiriti o Waitangi* (Treaty of Waitangi). This founding document between the government and Maori (indigenous people) is enshrined in legislation (Ministry of Justice 2016). Nursing and, therefore, the clinical nurse specialist role (CNS) incorporates the principles of partnership, protection and participation, which provides a framework for cultural safety, with the aim of reducing health inequities (New Zealand Nursing Organisation [NZNO] 2011).

Government funding is provided to 20 District Health Boards (DHB's) based on population data. Each DHB is responsible for implementing government strategies and meeting national targets determined by the government. NZ has a dual healthcare system of publicly and privately funded healthcare (New Zealand Parliment 2009). The majority of CNS positions sit within the DHBs. A key focus for employers and nursing is to ensure that all nurses are working to their full scope of practice in order to contribute to meeting health targets and improving the health and well-being of the NZ population.

Whilst there are many key stakeholder organisations within NZ that influence the nursing to a varying degree, there is a lack of coherent professional nursing and political strategies that foster the development of advanced nursing roles other than the NP. Some of these key organisations include the Nursing Council of NZ (NCNZ, est. 1903), National Nursing Organisation (NNO), Nurse Executives New Zealand (NENZ), New Zealand Nurses Organisation (NZNO), College of Nurses and Ministry of Health (MOH).

19.1.1 Clinical Nurse Specialist Role: New Zealand History

New Zealand's first documented clinical nurse specialist (CNS) role was an 18-month pilot undertaken in the early 1970s (Jollands 1975). The aim of this pilot was to develop a role that provided advanced nursing care to increasingly complex patients. The outcomes of the research were aimed at developing a career structure that recognised the importance of clinical experts at the bedside. The evaluation of this pilot demonstrated the benefits of the CNS role, with recommendations for increased CNS positions (Jollands 1975).

Over the next 20 years, healthcare underwent restructuring and reform, creating a turbulent environment. During this time, advanced nursing practice (ANP) roles, including that of the CNS, were developed in an ad hoc way, which resulted in limited embedding (Christensen 1999; Isles 2005). Whilst the concept of clinical career pathways (CCP) was discussed in 1976, it wasn't until 1989 that New Zealand Nursing Association (New Zealand Nurse Association 1976) introduced an advanced certification which specifically excluded specialist credentialing. This was a voluntary process that provided professional recognition, but did not reflect changes to the nurse's employment conditions (Isles 2005; Bloomer 2010). In 1991, the political reform with the introduction of the Employment Contract Act resulted in further fragmentation of the nursing profession due to the disestablishment of collective bargaining.

By the late 1990s, the CNS role started to proliferate in New Zealand. In 1998, the Ministerial Taskforce report highlighted the importance of the CNS role and its contribution to improved patient outcomes. Furthermore, they recommended these roles be "recognised and endorsed by Nursing Council" (Ministry of Health [MOH] 1998: 28). This key report goes on to advocate that NCNZ "develop competencies linked to nationally consistent nursing titles, so that all nurses using a particular title can be recognised as having particular competencies" (Ministry of Health [MOH] 1998: 38). NENZ reinforced this viewpoint with their position statement in 1998, which proposed two ANP roles: the CNS and nurse practitioner (NP) (as cited by Jacobs, 1998). This position remains unchanged (Nursing Executives of New Zealand [NENZ] 2014).

In juxtaposition to NENZ and MOH, a workshop of nurse leaders (1999) recommended that only one regulated ANP title be endorsed, that of the NP (Christensen 1999). In response, NCNZ (Nursing Council of New Zealand [NCNZ] 2001) developed a framework for post-registration education, which specified standards for specialty and ANP, but specifically did not align these to titles. The NP role was subsequently regulated in 2001 (Nursing Council of New Zealand [NCNZ] 2017). The literature shows that the focus of nursing organisations and NCNZ has been on the development of the NP role (Roberts 2009).

Despite this focus on the NP role, their numbers have been slow to grow with only 242 practicing NPs in 2017 (Nursing Council of New Zealand [NCNZ] 2015). In contrast, the CNS position has continued to proliferate with approximately 1500 CNSs' employed in the DHB sector alone in 2015. This is nearly 6% of the registered nursing workforce, twice that identified in 2007 (Coleman, 2015). It is interesting that Coleman (Minister of Health) collated this data, as Nursing Council collects yearly statistics on the number of registered nurses (RN) and NPs but not CNSs.

19.1.2 NZ Definition of a Clinical Nurse Specialist Role

Internationally and in NZ, there is confusion and lack of clarity surrounding the CNS role (Carryer 2014; Holloway 2011). Whilst it is acknowledged as an ANP role in NZ by nursing academics, MOH, nursing organisations and employers (Ministry of Health [MOH] 1998; Nursing Executives of New Zealand [NENZ] 2014; NZNO 2015; South Island Alliance 2018), a consensus on a national definition has not been reached (Isles 2005; Roberts 2009; Carryer 2014; Holloway 2011; Cumming 2008). Confusion exists around defining a specialist level of practice and the distinct role of the CNS. This leads to variable interpretation of titles such as specialty clinical nurse, nurse specialist and CNS. Concepts for the CNS role were identified from the grey literature as outlined in Table 19.1. These concepts include advanced nursing practice, specialist care and knowledge, research, evidence-based practice and leadership.

19.1.3 Conceptualized Models of Clinical Nurse Specialist Practice

Currently within NZ, there is no national model that conceptualises CNS practice and the three spheres of influence: organisational, nursing practice and patients/whanau (National Clinical Nurse Specialist Competency Task Force 2010). Several DHBs have undertaken reviews of nursing roles and have developed their own model of practice, which may include a nurse specialist or CNS. Frameworks developed by Holloway (Holloway 2011), South Canterbury DHB (South Canterbury District Health Board 2017) and NNO (National Nursing Organisation [NNO] 2004) present nursing roles in a hierarchical framework, based on specialisation and postgraduate attainment. The NZNO model of care document suggest CNSs should work at the full scope of their practice, which is currently the RN scope of practice (New Zealand Nursing Organisation [NZNO] 2011).

The New Zealand Nursing Specialist Framework (NZNSF) developed by Holloway (Holloway 2011) is the foundation for a national process to endorse specialty standards. Prior to this, individual specialty groups were developing their own frameworks, and there was little consistency (Cassie 2011). The NZNSF has been developed on the basis of capability rather than competency, with three components, namely, role adequacy (level of practice), role legitimacy (legitimate specialty) and role support (specialty nursing group to set and authorise standards). Holloway (Holloway 2011) suggests a nurse specialist may demonstrate the required capabilities, but not hold a designated CNS title (p 145, Table 19.1). This creates further confusion surrounding specialist practice and the CNS role.

Table 19.1 Overview of the definitions provided by the independent professional bodies

Professional body	Date	Definition of CNS role
NZNO	2011	Defined advanced nursing practice (ANP) and included roles of NP and CNS. "The scope of ANP is distinguished by autonomy to practice at the edges of the expanding boundaries of nursing. It is firmly grounded in the unique body of knowledge that is nursing. In ANP the nurse makes use of the scientific theories, drawn from nursing and other disciplines, as well as current research which enable articulation of sound rationale for the selection of nursing actions" (p1. Para5.)
NZNO MECA	2015	"Focus on care delivery, Providing specialist nursing/midwifery care and expertise, both in direct care delivery and in support to other staff in the management of a defined patient group/area of specialty practice Researching, evaluating, developing and implementing standards of nursing/midwifery practice in the specific area of practice. Leads the development of pathways, protocols and guidelines in the specific area of practice" (p75.)
National Professional Development Working Party (PDRP)	2005	Provides specialist nursing care, teaching, specialist care coordination, research evidence-based-practice implementation. Describes ANP of which the CNS is recognised within this role
National Nursing Organisations	2014	Expert nurses working in specific areas of practice with advanced knowledge and skills, providing mentorship. Often has additional educational qualifications and designated prescriber status
Nurse Executives NZ (NENZ)	2014	"The CNS is a registered nurse who uses advanced specialised clinical knowledge to practice within a defined specialty or specialties" (p3. para1.) CNS works within ≥ 1 of 3 spheres of nursing influence—patient/client nursing practice, nursing standards, nursing personnel and organisation/systems. Advanced specialist and nursing knowledge. Key role components include clinical expertise, collaboration, consultation, education, research and leadership
South Island Alliance	Accessed 2018	"Defines specialist area of practice with specific skills or interventions related to management of disease or health issues." (p1.) ANP, specialist care – may include designated medical responsibilities, diagnostics and implementation of treatment protocols. Extended/Expanded roles dependent on patient need. Education. Maybe involved in leadership and policy

19.1.4 Clinical Nurse Specialist Practice Competencies

Although the Ministerial Taskforce (1998) urged the NCNZ to develop CNS competencies, this never occurred (Roberts 2009; Cumming 2008; Jacobs 2000). In 2007, the multi-employer collective agreement (MECA) developed role descriptors for designated senior nurses including the CNS. Results of a survey of participants, at the inaugural national CNS forum in 2009, showed that CNS role components matched with MECA descriptions (Cumming 2012). However, although being used

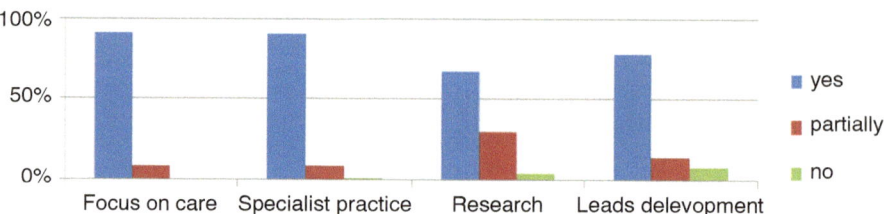

Fig. 19.1 Role components: how CNS practice matched with MECA definitions (2009). ****Table** *provided with permission from Cumming (2012: 22)*

by many employers, the MECA descriptors fail to show the depth and breadth of the role (Fig. 19.1).

In research undertaken by Roberts (2009: 2), thematic analysis showed four areas of CNS practice: leader, clinical expert, coordinator and educator. She clearly identifies that the CNS role goes beyond the Nursing Council RN scope and urged NCNZ to develop a separate scope of practice for the CNS. This is supported by current research illustrating domains of practice for ANP roles including direct care, support of systems, research, education and professional leadership (Carryer et al. (2018). An important finding was the similar profile between the NP and the CNS with both sitting within the advanced practice scope. Carryer (Carryer et al. 2018) also suggests that the employer's choice of creating either of these two ANP roles should be based on service needs.

19.1.5 Clinical Nurse Specialist Education and Credentialing

Nursing Council is responsible for setting standards for nursing scopes of practice, as well as monitoring and accrediting nursing education programmes. The only formal credentialing requirement for a CNS is to hold a current RN practicing certificate (Nursing Council of New Zealand [NCNZ] 2016), which includes an approved nursing qualification and current assessment of NCNZ RN competencies. The Professional Development and Recognition Programme (PDRP) includes competent, proficient and expert RN, as well as a senior nursing level. There is no mandatory requirement to complete PDRP at any level; however, some employers mandate that CNSs participate at the senior nurse level (New Zealand Nursing Organisation [NZNO], College of Nursing Aoteroa NZ 2012; PDRP Document Review Project Team 2017).

The NZ MOH Strategy (Minister of Health 2016) strongly advocates for educational development of the nursing workforce. Specific funding is allocated for postgraduate study to meet increasingly complex healthcare needs and health inequities. Health Workforce NZ was established in 2007 to reduce the barriers to nurses accessing funding for postgraduate education. This is supported by literature in which Barnhill et al. (2012), recognised that a key aspect of ANP is postgraduate education. This fosters critical components of ANP such as critical thinking, increased confidence and development of a broader understanding of nursing practice.

There is no nationally agreed educational qualification for the CNS position. Individual employers determine prerequisites for these roles, which has led to inconsistencies. Roberts (2009) reviewed 15 job descriptions, which showed varied postgraduate requirements. She identified that only 60% of employers required the RN to either be working towards or hold some form of postgraduate qualification. However, postgraduate nursing education has gained momentum, with Carryer et al. (2014) research reporting 43% ($n = 420$) of CNS respondents hold a master's degree. Key stakeholder documents are now reflecting the need for a CNS to hold a minimum of a postgraduate qualification (Nursing Executives of New Zealand [NENZ] 2014; South Island Alliance 2018; South Canterbury District Health Board 2017).

Postgraduate programmes have been developed in accordance with requirements of the Health Practitioners Competence Assurance Act (2003) and NCNZ Competencies for the RN Scope of Practice (Health Workforce New Zealand [HWNZ] 2017). There is only one NCNZ accredited master's degree programme for registration as an NP (Nursing Council of New Zealand [NCNZ] 2017). Although here is no formalised postgraduate educational programme for the CNS, many have undertaken the same master's education as the NP.

19.1.5.1 Nurse Prescribing

Jacobs and Boddy (2008) claim the first discussion occurred in 1992 in relation to RN prescribing. In 1998, the intention to enable limited prescribing was met with concerns by both nursing and medicine. The NP role gained authorised prescribing status in 2005 (Walton 2006), and in 2014, NCNZ mandated that all new NPs had to prescribe (Nursing Council of New Zealand [NCNZ] 2014). Discussion has ensued looking at other RN prescribing, and in 2015, there was agreement that limited prescribing rights would be offered to suitably qualified and experienced RNs, working in primary care and specialty practice (Ministry of Health [MOH] 2016). These prescribing rights were not allocated to any specific title, rather to those working within a collaborative team (New Zealand Nursing Organisation [NZNO] 2013). Diabetes nurse specialists (DNS) undertook the first RN prescribing pilot in 2011 (Philips and Wilkinson 2015). This trial was demonstrated to be safe and clinically effective with no adverse events reported (Budge and Snell 2013).

A limitation of NZNO's current 2018–2023 nursing strategy is its lack of recognition around the CNS role. It does, however, identify prescribing as an essential area for advanced practice and the need to apply sufficient support and funding for this to occur (New Zealand Nursing Organisation [NZNO] 2018). Given NZNO's lack of acknowledgement of the CNS role, it is surprising that the NZNO Chief Executive, Musa, was quoted as stating that prescribing will enable CNS's to work at their full scope (Unknown 2018).

19.1.6 Outcome Measures and Evaluation

There is increasing pressure on healthcare services to deliver timely, accessible and equitable care within an increasingly complex healthcare system (Ryall 2007). It is essential that CNS's demonstrate their value and place within the healthcare environment. Currently, key performance indicators are determined by employers within job descriptions. However, improved service delivery and patient outcomes from CNS interventions are starting to emerge in NZ literature, as evidenced by the following examples. The findings of a CNS-led glaucoma clinic audit showed a marked reduction in waiting list numbers and wait times for a first specialist appointment (Slight et al. 2009). Similarly, increased cost effectiveness and accessibility to retinal medical treatments in an ophthalmology service were achieved by CNS's undertaking intravitreal injections of anti-vascular endothelial growth factor, for macular degeneration, with minimal complications (Samalia et al. 2016). A gerontology nurse specialist (GNS) utilised a geriatric assessment tool to identify at-risk older people in primary health. Whilst this research showed no statistically significant results in terms of the expected outcomes, i.e. hospital admissions, it did enable the GNS to initiate significantly more multidisciplinary referrals and care coordination for those at risk (King et al. 2018). These examples illustrate some of the contributions CNS's make to improve health outcomes and to highlight the importance of CNS's demonstrating their practice and publishing research.

19.1.7 Moving Forward: Challenges and Opportunities

The confusion that surrounds the CNS role is not confined to NZ (Isles 2005; Cumming 2008). One aim of the NZNO MECA (New Zealand Nursing Organisation [NZNO] 2007) was to reduce the number of nursing titles. However, we would argue that this has added to the confusion due to the similarity between the specialty clinical nurse (SCN) and CNS titles (Roberts et al. 2011). NCNZ's development of guidelines for expanded practice for the RN adds further to this confusion for employers and nurses. These guidelines include educational requirements, competencies and a framework for employers. Given the work NCNZ has put into developing these expanded practice guidelines, it is surprising NCNZ has not been able to provide the same level of clarity for the CNS.

The opportunity therefore lies in reaching consensus with key stakeholders, nursing organisations, employers and CNS's in defining the CNS role. It is essential that we utilise international models of CNS practice (European Specialist Nurses Organisation 2015; Tazim Virani and Associates 2012), alongside local literature to open discussions. The challenge, however, will be in getting agreement from all parties (Roberts 2009) on a definition, approved postgraduate educational qualification pathway and competency assessment for the CNS, similar to that provided for the NP. This would strengthen the role and provide role clarity for employers, tertiary providers, CNS's and the consumer (Roberts 2009; Cumming 2008).

19.1.7.1   Development of a National CNS Group

In 2009, the first CNS national forum was held. A survey undertaken of participants identified that CNS's wanted a national group and a defined scope of practice (Cumming 2012). At the CNS conference in 2013, participants signed a charter for the development of a national CNS group. From this, a working committee was formed to lead an independent national group, later to become the Clinical Nurse Specialist Society New Zealand (CNSSNZ, 2015). With the development of CNSSNZ came opportunities for supporting CNS's across NZ as a professional body. This in turn has its own unique opportunities and challenges in terms of engagement both with CNS's and key stakeholders. The overall aim of the society is to increase visibility and to give CNS's a voice in addressing the challenges previously described. Similar to that undertaken internationally, an evidence-based approach will be taken to address these issues.

19.1.8   Exemplar of Clinical Nurse Specialist Practice

19.1.8.1   Quality Initiative: CNS Exemplar

Across child health, children experience a number of anxiety provoking and painful procedures including the placement of intravenous (IV) needles. Procedural preparation includes using age appropriate words to reflect the necessity of the procedure, engaging the child through utilisation of play and distraction (Bray et al. 2015) and appropriate analgesia. Commonly, topical anaesthetic creams are used to numb the site of injection. This intervention has its own complications, is expensive and can take an hour for optimal effect.

RW is a paediatric oncology CNS who observes the pain and distress children experience due to IV insertions, injections and accessing implantable ports. RW identified an alternative to the current practice of using topical anaesthetics to numb injection sites in an article published in a Children's Healthcare Australasia newsletter. The article reported on the use of a handheld device that acts almost immediately (10 seconds) to cool and numb an injection site, resulting in patients experiencing reduced pain with IV insertions.

Realising this could greatly improve the experience for her patients, RW contacted the Australian Hospital medical imaging team that had successfully used the device for over 5000 cannulations. She also contacted the Australasian distributor who offered to loan a device for a trial period and provide staff education on its use. With the information gathered, RW discussed the device with relevant key stakeholders including the quality coordinator. A decision was made to undertake a pilot study of the device in one paediatric ward. RW worked closely with the nurse educator to develop the education plan prior to implementing the pilot.

Prior to use, the device was assessed by the medical physics and bioengineering department and the infection prevention and control team. Instructions for safe use and cleaning of the device were written. A qualitative evaluation survey was designed to capture the parents/child's experiences of the device. The cooling device was applied to sites prior to intravenous cannulation venepuncture, accessing implantable ports and injections. The overall results from the survey demonstrated that the device provided an improved patient and family experience by reducing pain associated with treatment and reducing waiting times.

RW undertook an economic analysis of the device and estimated that this change in practice has potential savings of $8750 per 1000 + applications. The successful pilot study findings and predicted cost savings have led to the device being introduced throughout the paediatric department and the wider hospital.

This quality initiative is closely aligned to the organisation's vision to deliver better outcomes for the patient. This supports the overarching commitment of the regional alliance partners and central government policies, for improved quality, safety and experience of care whilst ensuring best value from public health system resources (South Island Alliance 2018; Minister of Health 2016). RW has presented this quality initiative at a number of national conferences; as a result, the device is at various stages of being introduced across other DHBs and in the private healthcare sector in NZ.

This exemplar illustrates how RW meets several of the advanced practice capabilities within the New Zealand Child Health Nursing Knowledge and Skills Framework (College of Child and Youth Nurses NZNO, Royal New Zealand Plunket Society 2014). Examples of this include advocacy for service development where needs are identified and provision of an environment that promotes safety, security and optimal health for children and families, including therapeutic relationships.

19.1.9 Conclusion

A number of factors have influenced the embedding of the CNS role in New Zealand since it was first introduced in the 1970's. The last 20 years have seen a steady increase in CNS numbers; it is now the most common of the two ANP roles in NZ. A key challenge for CNS's across NZ is in addressing the invisibility of the CNS role (Cumming 2008; Roberts et al. 2011). Litchfield (2002) forecasts the negative effect of creating a "professional elite", which has occurred through the development of a hierarchical nursing paradigm, following the creation of a single regulated NP role (Nursing Council of New Zealand [NCNZ] 2017; New Zealand Nursing Organisation [NZNO] 2018). It is now critical that CNS's challenge the perception by some, that the NP role is the pinnacle of nursing practice (Holloway 2011; Carryer et al. 2018; Roberts et al. 2011; Ministry of Health [MOH] 2002) and that the CNS is a stepping stone to NP.

With the growth and development of the CNS role, the MOH recommendations (1998) to develop competencies for the CNS role deserves serious consideration by NCNZ. Research supports the recognition of the CNS as an ANP role in NZ (Roberts 2009; Carryer et al. 2018); however, a clear national definition, competency assessment and educational pathway that are endorsed by key stakeholders are lacking. It is acknowledged that with approximately 1500 CNS's in NZ, the task of credentialing these nurses will require significant resources and commitment by

NCNZ. Finally, the challenge is to create a model that reflects the depth and diversity of the CNS role; without this, the full potential of the role will not be realised.

References

Barnhill D, McKillop A, Aspinall C (2012) The impact of postgraduate education on registered nurses working in acute care. Nursing Praxis in New Zealand. 28(2): 27–36

Bloomer H (2010) The canterbury and west coast district health boards' professional development and recognition programme for nurses: a comparative study of participants and non-participants [Dissertation]. University of Otago, Christchurch

Bray L, Snodin J, Carter B (2015) Holding and restraining children for clinical procedures within an acute care setting: an ethical consideration of the evidence. Nurs Inq 22(2):157–167

Budge C, Snell H (2013) Registered nurse prescribing in diabetes care: 2012 managed national roll out. Health Workforce New Zealand, New Zealand Society for the Study of Diabetes, Palmerston North

Carryer J (2014) Clarifying nursing titles—editorial letter. Kai Tiaki Nursing New Zealand 20(8):3

Carryer J, Wilkinson J, Towers A, Gardner G (2018) Delineating advanced practice nursing in New Zealand: a national survey. Int Nurs 65:24–32

Cassie F (2011) So you are a nurse specialist—What does that mean again? Health Central NZ

Christensen J (1999) Integrating the terminology and titles or nursing practice roles: quality, particularity and levelling. Nurse Praxis in New Zealand. 14(1):4–12

College of Child and Youth Nurses NZNO, Royal New Zealand Plunket Society (2014) New Zealand child health nursing knowledge and skills framework. New Zealand Nursing Organisation, Wellington

Cumming G (2008) From a generic to a gynaecological oncology clinical nurse specialist: an evolving role [Dissertation]. Otago Polytechnic, Dunedin

Cumming G (2012) Clinical nurse specialist survey: understanding the issues facing clinical nurse specialists New Zealand. Kai Tiaki: Nursing New Zealand: 26

European Specialist Nurses Organisation (2015) Competences of the clinical nurse specialist (CNS): common plinth of competences for the common training framework of each specialty. European Specialist Nursing Organisation, Brussels

Health Workforce New Zealand [HWNZ] (2017) HWNZ postgraduate nursing training specification. Ministry of Health, Wellington

Holloway KT (2011) Development of a specialist nursing framework for New Zealand [PhD]. Sydney University of Technology, Sydney

Isles V (2005) The development and role of the clinical nurse specialist in New Zealand [Dissertation]. Otago Polytechnic, Dunedin

Jacobs S (2000) Credentialing: setting standards for advanced nursing practice. Nursing Praxis in New Zealand. 16(2):38–46

Jacobs S, Boddy JM (2008) The genesis of advanced nursing practice in New Zealand: policy, politics and education. Nursing Praxis in New Zealand. 24(1):11–23

Jollands E (1975) Clinical specialist trial. New Zealand Nursing Journal. (Oct):23–4

King A, Boyd M, Raphael D, Jull A (2018) The effect of a geontology nurse specialist for high needs older perolpe in the community on healtcare utilisation: a controlled before-after study. Biomed Central Geriatr. 18–22

Litchfield M (2002) Nurse practitioner role limits the profession. Kai Tiaki Nursing New Zealand. (Nov):20–3

Minister of Health (2016) New Zealand health strategy future direction 2016. Ministry of Health, Wellington. p42

Ministry of Health [MOH] (1998) Report of the ministerial taskforce on nursing: releasing the potential of nursing. Ministry of Health, Wellington

Ministry of Health [MOH] (2002) Nurse practitioners in New Zealand. Ministry of Health, Wellington

Ministry of Health [MOH] (2016) Registered nurse prescribing. Ministry of Health, Wellington

Treaty of Waitangi [Internet]. Ministry of Justice. 2016 [cited 26/05/2018]. https://www.justice.govt. nz/about/learn-about-the-justice-system/how-the-justice-system-works/the-basis-for-all-law/ treaty-of-waitangi/

Coleman J (2015) More opportunities for specialist nurses [press release]. Ministry of Health, Wellington

National Clinical Nurse Specialist Competency Task Force (2010) Clinical nurse specialist core competencies: executive summary 2006–2008. National Association of Clinical Nurse Specialists, Harrisburg

National Nursing Organisation [NNO] (2004) National framework for nursing professional development & recognition programmes & designated role titles. New Zealand Nursing Organisation

New Zealand Nurse Association (1976) Policy statement on nursing in New Zealand. New Zealand Nurses Association, Wellington

New Zealand Nursing Organisation [NZNO] (2007) District Health Boards/NZNO nursing and midwifery multi-employer collective agreement. New Zealand Nursing Organisation, Wellington

New Zealand Nursing Organisation [NZNO] (2011) Beyond 2020: a vision for nursing. New Zealand Nursing Organisation, Wellington

New Zealand Nursing Organisation [NZNO] (2013) Nursing council wants community and specialist nurses to prescribe. Kai Tiaki Nursing New Zealand 19(2):5

New Zealand Nursing Organisation [NZNO] (2018) NZNO strategy for nursing 2018–2023. Advancing the health of the nation. Hei oranga motuhake mō ngā whānau, hapū, iwi. New Zealand Nursing Organisation, Wellington.

New Zealand Nursing Organisation [NZNO], College of Nursing Aoteroa NZ (2012) Articulating the difference between PDRP level 4 RN roles and those advanced practice roles requiring not only nursing expertise but also positional authority. New Zealand Nursing Organisation, Wellington

New Zealand Parliment (2009) New Zealand health systems reforms. Wellington: Parliament Library

Nursing Council of New Zealand [NCNZ] (2001) Framework for post-registration nursing practice education. New Zealand Nursing Council, Wellington

Nursing Council of New Zealand [NCNZ] (2014) Nurse practitioner: changes coming into effect on 1 July 2014. New Zealand Nursing Council, Wellington

Nursing Council of New Zealand [NCNZ] (2015) The New Zealand nursing workforce: a profile of nurse practitioners, registered nurses and enrolled nurses 2014–2015. Wellington

Nursing Council of New Zealand [NCNZ] (2016) Competencies for registered nurses. New Zealand Nursing Council, Wellington

Nursing Council of New Zealand [NCNZ] (2017) Competencies for the nurse practitioner scope of practice. New Zealand Nursing Council, Wellington

Nursing Executives of New Zealand [NENZ] (2014) Position statement: advanced clinical practice roles. Nursing Executives New Zealand

District Health Boards/NZNO nursing and midwifery multi-employer collective agreement 2015–2017, NZNO (2015)

PDRP Document Review Project Team (2017) National framework and evidential requirements: New Zealand nursing professional development & recognition programmes for registered and enrolled nurses. Nurse Executives New Zealand

Philips H, Wilkinson J (2015) Non-prescribing diabetes nurse specialist views of nurse prescribing in diabetes health. Nursing Praxis in New Zealand. 31(1):5–17

Roberts J (2009) The characteristics of the clinical nurse specialist role in new zealand [Dissertation]. Eastern Institute of Technology, Taradale

Roberts J, Floyd S Thompson S (2011) The clinical nurse specialist in New Zealand: how is the role defined. Nursing Praxis in New Zealand. 27(2):24–34

Ryall HT (2007) Better, sooner, more convenient: health discussion paper. Ministry of Health, Wellington

Samalia P, Garland D, Squirrell D (2016) Nurse specialists for the administration of anti-vascular endothelial growth factor intravitreal injections. NZ Med J 129(1438):32–38

Slight C, Marsden J, Raynel S (2009) The impact of a glaucoma nurse specialist role on glaucoma waiting lists. Nursing Praxis in New Zealand. 25(1):38–47

South Canterbury District Health Board (2017) South Canterbury district health board: a framework for the clinical nursing workforce. South Canterbury District Health Board, Southland

South Island Alliance (2018) Advanced nursing roles—differentiation and development. Work Force Development Hub.

Tazim Virani & Associates (2012) Strengthening the role of the clinical nurse specialist: background paper. Canadian Nurses Association, Ottawa

Unknown (2018) New Zealand: new laws empower nurses to utilise full scope—Editorial. Australian Nurs Midwifery J 25(8):44

Walton L (2006) Nurse practitioner prescribing. Health Policy Monitor

Challenges and Opportunities for CNS Practice Globally

20

Janet S. Fulton and Vincent W. Holly

Abstract

Clinical nurse specialists (CNS) are an advanced practice nursing role. CNSs have expert knowledge, complex decision-making abilities, and enhanced skills for expanded practice in a specialty area. This book describes the CNS role and practice as it exists in 15 selected countries and identifies how CNS practice is shaped by the context in which practice takes place. The CNS role is well-established in some countries and is in varying stages of development in other countries. Regardless of the level of establishment, evidence demonstrates that CNSs are making an impact on the health and well-being of people. The chapters explore the common characteristics of CNS practice, education, and regulation. Areas of commonality include role definition, practice competencies, and expectations for improved clinical and fiscal outcomes. Greater variations reflect the educational and regulatory structure of a country. Our contributing authors, writing from the perspective of their country, have identified opportunities and challenges for the continuing growth and success of the CNS role. This closing chapter summarizes and reflects on the information from the chapter contributors representing geographic areas from North America, Europe, Middle East, Asia, and Oceania.

J. S. Fulton (✉)
Indiana University School of Nursing, Indianapolis, IN, USA
e-mail: jasfulto@iu.edu

V. W. Holly
Critical Care Services, Indiana University Health Bloomington Hospital, Bloomington, IN, USA
e-mail: vholly@iuhealth.org

© Springer Nature Switzerland AG 2021
J. S. Fulton, V. W. Holly (eds.), *Clinical Nurse Specialist Role and Practice*,
Advanced Practice in Nursing, https://doi.org/10.1007/978-3-319-97103-2_20

Keywords

Clinical nurse specialist · Advanced practice nurse · Advanced nursing practice · Advanced practice registered nurse · Global · International

20.1   Introduction

Globally, nursing developed as a profession following different paths. Local, regional, and national policies, politics, norms, and traditions all played a part in shaping how nursing is practiced in any country. Nonetheless, nursing has continued to develop in response to a common denominator, the health and well-being of the public we serve. Nursing practice assures care and comfort for our fellow humans by preventing or reducing risk of disease and harm, relieving distressing symptoms, promoting physical and cognitive functioning, and maximizing quality of life. Nursing interventions are universal in scientific grounding and unique in application. All nurses, regardless of educational preparation, regulatory title, or professional credentials, are dedicated to the same mission.

In response to the public's need for expanded, advanced, and complex care interventions, the nursing profession is creating clinicians who practice at advanced levels. Advanced practice nurse roles are established in some countries, evolving in additional countries and still emerging in other countries. Advanced practice nurses have expert knowledge, complex decision-making abilities, and enhanced skills for an expanded scope of practice that is shaped by the country and context in which a nurse is credentialed for practice (International Council of Nurses 2020). Advanced practice nurses are graduates of a nursing program holding legal or other required credentials for practice as a generalist registered nurse. Building upon generalist scope of practice, an advanced practice nurse earns a graduate degree in nursing from a program that prepared graduates for an advanced nursing role. Where graduate nursing degrees are not available, transition programs can fill in the gap between generalist education and advanced practice educational standards. Preparation and recognition of advanced practice nursing roles vary globally.

The most recognized advanced nursing practice roles are clinical nurse specialist, nurse practitioner, and nurse anesthetist. In some countries, nurse midwives are recognized as advanced practice nurses, depending on educational preparation and scope of practice. Several countries, including Australia, the United Kingdom, and Hong Kong, use the title clinical nurse consultant (CNC) to designate a practice role consistent with CNS practice (International Council of Nurses 2020; Bryant-Lukosius and Wong 2019).

A "nurse specialist" is defined by the International Council of Nurses as a nurse prepared beyond the level of a generalist and authorized to practice in a specialty area with advanced expertise (International Council of Nurses 2009). These specialist nurses have extensive experience, complete specialized courses, modules, and/or on-the-job training. The scope of practice may include clinical, teaching,

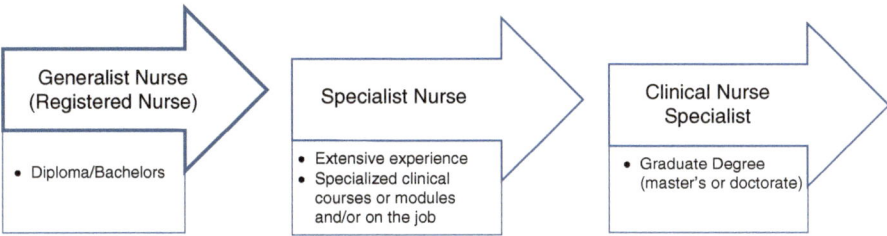

Fig. 20.1 Progression from generalist nurse to clinical nurse specialist (ICN 2020)

administration, research, and consultant competencies. However, while not an advanced practice role, the nurse specialist role is considered a step in the progression toward achieving the CNS role (International Council of Nurses 2020). See Fig. 20.1.

The emergence of advanced practice nursing roles is an important and essential initiative for the nursing profession in fulfilling the social mandate to meet the public's need for nursing services. In moving forward with developing advanced roles, we should acknowledge the important contributions all nurses make to the health of the populations we serve, support our colleagues at all levels and in different roles, and seek pathways for more nurses to advance their education.

20.2   Role Definition, Practice Competencies, Outcomes

Clinical nurse specialist is an advanced practice role. Role is defined as a set of expected functions of a person and is characterized by a pattern of behavior in a given social context (Fulton 2020). Nursing has many different functional roles such as those for advanced practice nurses and still others for educators, administrators, and informaticists to name just a few examples. Practice is the act of applying role-specific knowledge and skill to achieve desired outcomes. Practice competencies are statements of actions a person in the role uses to achieve desired outcomes. The CNS role, like other advanced roles, is guided by CNS-specific practice competencies that delineate expected practice behaviors. Role competencies are developed by professional organizations and other stakeholders with deep knowledge about the functions of and expected outcomes for the role. Role competencies for advanced practice nurses are learned through formal academic preparation at the graduate level that includes knowledge acquisition, skill development, and competency attainment through supervised clinical experiences (Fulton 2020).

CNS practice competencies are organized by practice domains. In 1998, the National Association of Clinical Nurse Specialists in the United States, using a rigorous and iterative process, proposed and has since recognized CNS practice in three domains: direct patient care, advanced nursing practice, and system-level changes for improved outcomes (Baldwin et al. 2009; National Association of Clinical Nurse Specialists 2019). A three-domain model has been supported by findings from an extensive literature review that identified three substantive areas of CNS practice: managing care of complex and vulnerable populations, educating and supporting nursing and interdisciplinary staff, and facilitating change and innovation within healthcare systems (Lewandowski and Adamle 2009). In Finland, CNS practice is organized into four domains – advanced clinical practice; practice development, consultation, and staff education; organizational leadership, and; scholarship (see Chap. 9). The Canadian Nurses Association organized CNS practice competencies into four domains: clinical care, systems leadership, advancement of nursing practice, and evaluation and research (Canadian Nurses Association 2014). The United Kingdom's Position Statement on Advanced Level Nursing identifies four domains for all advanced practice roles—direct clinical care, leadership and collaborative practice, improving quality in developing practice, and developing self and others (UK Department of Health 2010). Except for the National Association of Clinical Nurse Specialists in the United States, no other professional organization has developed CNS practice outcome statements corresponding to the practice domains (National Association of Clinical Nurse Specialists 2019). Outcome statements establish expectations and provide CNSs, other providers, employers, and the public with a foundation for evaluating CNS contributions to health outcomes and establishing the value of the CNS role in healthcare.

Three countries have professional CNS organizations: the National Association of Clinical Nurse Specialists in the United States, the Clinical Nurse Specialist Organization of New Zealand, and the Japanese Association of Certified Nurse Specialists. In many other countries, CNSs comprise discrete units, such as a council, within larger nursing organizations, or may be included in units dedicated to the interests of advanced practice nursing roles. The nurse practitioner/advanced practice nursing network of the International Council of Nurses (ICN) is an example of a unit dedicated to advanced practice roles, including CNSs, within a larger organization, ICN.

Table 20.1 is a summary of the description, competencies, education, and credentialing of CNSs across the countries discussed in this book.

20.3 Educational Standards

Each advanced practice role, including CNS, should have a unique curriculum designed to provide graduates with the academic content to achieve role competencies. Through formal, higher education, CNSs learn to analyze, synthesize, and apply nursing knowledge, theory, and research evidence to improve patient outcomes through direct care delivery and indirectly through system-wide changes and the advancement of specialty nursing care and the nursing profession. Ideally, the graduate program includes supervised clinical experiences designed to support knowledge application and skill development necessary to achieve beginner-level CNS competencies.

Globally, CNS education is influenced by the structure of nursing education in a country. In Taiwan, a CNS receives a master's degree after progressing through four

Table 20.1 Summary of the description, competencies, education, and credentialing of CNSs across representaive countries

Countries with recognized CNS roles

Country	Definition	Competencies	Education	Credentialing	Comments
Australia	The CNS role is not present in all states and territories; however, other advanced roles provide similar types and levels of "specialist" nursing care including the clinical nurse consultant (CNC).	No nationally defined competencies. CNS scope and practice generally includes direct clinical care in the specialty, patient and family education, development of evidence-based practice through research and policy evaluation, and advocacy	Varies by state and territory.	Neither the CNS nor CNC role is regulated by the Nursing and Midwifery Board of Australia. Government nursing position levels and scope are defined in respective industrial Awards and Agreements. Each state or territory aligns job scope and essential criteria with requirements for a position. CNS jobs descriptions demonstrate common scope and practice responsibilities.	In Australia, a post-graduate qualification can be a graduate certificate (hospital-based) or a graduate diploma, master's or doctoral degree.
Canada	A CNS is a registered nurse who holds a graduate degree in nursing and has a higher level of expertise in a clinical specialty (Canadian Nurses Association).	Pan-Canadian competencies for the CNS (64 total competencies) are organized into four categories related to clinical care, systems leadership, advancement of nursing practice, and evaluation and research.	Master's degree in nursing; no graduate programs specific to CNS role and competencies.	Regulation of nurses occurs at the provincial/ territorial level and is governed by a nursing college or association. Title protection is not consistent.	Lack of CNS specific programs contributes to shortage of CNSs in areas of need. Limited specialty certification options, particularly at the advanced level.

(continued)

Table 20.1 (continued)

Countries with recognized CNS roles

Country	Definition	Competencies	Education	Credentialing	Comments
Finland	CNS is defined as an experienced master's or doctoral prepared registered nurse whose central focus of practice is advanced clinical nursing.	Competencies cover the spheres of patient, nursing, organization, and scholarship. Development of CNS practice competency descriptions is ongoing.	Master's or doctoral degree in nursing. Master's level education prepares nurses for advanced clinical nursing roles and practice. No national curriculum for advanced practice. Doctoral education is not clinically focused but prepares CNSs to better achieve the scholarship aspects of the CNS role.	No legislative or regulatory mechanisms or protected titles are in place for advanced nurse providers.	Research in CNS role development and implementation is expanding rapidly.
France	Clinical nurse specialist (in French the term was translated as "infirmière spécialiste clinique" in France which means "nurse specialist in clinical nursing") the transformative power of this function is emphasized within nursing teams in order to change the organization of care and the practice of nurses.	1. Assess the health status of patients as a relay for medical consultations for identified pathologies. 2. Define and implement the patient's care plan based on the overall assessment of the patient's state of health. 3. Design and implement prevention and therapeutic education actions. 4. Organizing patient care and health pathways in collaboration with all stakeholders. 5. Implement and conduct actions to evaluate and improve professional practices by exercising clinical leadership. 6. Research, analyze and produce professional and scientific data	The modular curriculum, spread over several years, is followed by the nurses on the job, which favors the integration of the contents.	Final certification is organized before a jury of peers, which was initially international in nature.	An advanced practice nurse is certified in one of the four areas of intervention: - Stabilized chronic disease, prevention, and common pathologies in primary care - Oncology and hematology-oncology - Chronic kidney disease, dialysis, kidney transplantation - Psychiatry-mental health

Ireland	A CNS is defined as a nurse specialist in clinical practice who has undertaken formal recognized post-registration education relevant to his/her area of specialist practice at level 8 or above on the National Qualification Authority of Ireland (NQAI) framework.	The core competencies of the CNS are shared by all who practice at specialist level based on the core concepts of the role. The core concepts are: Client focus, Patient/client advocate, Education and training, Audit and research, and Consultancy. Specific competencies are those identified as specific to the practice role and setting.	The framework for education since 2010 includes academic qualifications and professional experience. The CNS must have 5 years post-registration experience, 2 years practice in specialty area, and a post registration diploma minimum level 8 of NQAI related to specialty area.	To become a CNS there is a requirement to fulfill the requirements determined by the NCPDNM framework for the establishment of CNS posts. The responsibility for CNS approval lies with the Health Service Executive (HSE) Office of the Nursing and Midwifery Services Director (ONMSD)	The CNS has an expanded scope of practice that incorporates the interpretation and application of advanced nursing theory and research, higher-level decision-making and autonomy in practice, which are consistent with their education level and clinical experience.
Japan	CNS provides efficient, high-level nursing care to individuals, families, and groups that have complex nursing problems (Japanese Nursing Association)	Competencies are attained through an educational program and supervised clinical experiences; however, there are no standard core CNS competencies applying to CNSs in all specialties.	CNSs are master's degree prepared; Japanese Association of Nursing Programs in Universities accredit education programs preparing CNS students.	There is no separate license or regulatory recognition for CNSs. Japanese Nursing Association certifies individual CNSs.	The USA CNS was the model for developing the Japanese CNS. Japanese Association of Certified Nurse Specialists http://jpncns.org/

(continued)

Table 20.1 (continued)

Countries with recognized CNS roles

Country	Definition	Competencies	Education	Credentialing	Comments
New Zealand	Advanced nursing practice (ANP) includes the role of CNS and nurse practitioner. The scope of ANP is distinguished by autonomy to practice at the edges of the expanding boundaries of nursing. It is firmly grounded in the unique body of knowledge that is nursing. In ANP the nurse makes use of the scientific theories, draws form nursing and other disciplines, as well as current research, which enable articulation of sound rational for the selection of nursing actions. (New Zealand Nursing Organization).	CNSs provide specialist nursing care and expertise both in direct care delivery and in support to other staff in the management of defined patient group/area of special practice. CNSs research, evaluate, develop, and implement standards of nursing practice in specialty areas of practice. CNSs lead the development of pathways, protocols, and guidelines in specific area of practice. (New Zealand Nursing Organization, Multi-Employer Collective Agreement).	Post-graduate education recommended. Employers may mandate a specific level of education/credential.	No formal credentialing mechanism for CNS; regulated within the registered nurse scope of practice.	In 1998 the Ministry of Health recognized the CNS as a crucial member of the healthcare team and recommended the role be recognized and endorsed by Nursing Council. CNSs consistently follow the 2006 Multi-Employer Collective Agreement. Clinical Nurse Specialist Organization of New Zealand https://www.cnssnz.org/

Taiwan	A clinical APN, including CNSs, use professional knowledge to manage complex situations, make decisions, and expand professional competencies. APNs function as expert clinicians and leader in advancing nursing practice by caring, teaching consulting, coordinating, leading, and researching.	Core competencies developed by Taiwan Nurses Association, including: Direct care, coaching, consultation, systems leadership, research and innovation.	The CNS is recognized as an APN, which is the top level of nursing recognition in a clinical ladder system. APNs are prepared with master's and doctoral degrees in nursing.	A state issued APN credential and license are not officially required by the Taiwanese government, but the Taiwan Nurses Association accredits APN certification.	The Taiwan Nursing Accreditation Council has been established to evaluate nursing education programs.
Turkey	Use the title Specialist Nurse. An expert (specialist) nurse specializes in post-graduate education related to their profession and whose diploma is registered with the Ministries. Nurses completing post-graduate education are titled Nurse Specialist.	Nurse Specialist competencies include: Direct clinical care, consult with nurses on clinical care, support nursing professional development, patient education, consultant to individuals, institutions and organizations related to specialty expertise and ethical issues.	Specialist nursing education is provided through post-bachelor's master's or doctorate in nursing.	Nurse specialist is officially recognized title in Turkey.	Specialist education is provided by graduate programs in universities; certificate programs are available but are not academic and duration, content and adequacy varies.

(continued)

Table 20.1 (continued)

Countries with recognized CNS roles

Country	Definition	Competencies	Education	Credentialing	Comments
United Kingdom	No specific definition of CNS role across UK. Scotland is the only UK country to have formalized the CNS role, defined as a "registered nursing professional who has acquired additional knowledge, skills and experience together with a professionally and/or academically accredited post-registration qualification (if available) in a clinical specialty. They practice at an advanced level and may have sole responsibility for care episode or defined client/group) (Information Services Division, Scottish Government).	No nationally agreed upon competencies for CNS role. Many specialties have developed specialty-focused competencies. Existing competencies based on job roles such as case manager, consulting specialist, procedure-focused specialist, clinical education, physician extender (working under supervision), clinical care coordinator.	Master's degree is recommended.	No regulatory or legal credentialing. CNS title is not protected.	The lack of a regulatory framework presents a risk to patient safety; however, there is little to impede the development of CNS practice and innovative approaches to meeting patient needs for advanced nursing care.

United States of America	A CNS as an advanced practice nurse who diagnoses, treatments, and provides ongoing management of patients; provides [specialty] expertise and support to nurses caring for patients; helps drive practice changes throughout the organization; and ensures use of best practices and evidence-based care to achieve the best possible patient outcomes (American Nurses Association).	Core competencies for CNSs regardless of specialty defined by the National Association of Clinical Nurse Specialists.	Graduate education (master's or doctorate) required. The curriculum must incorporate the CNS core competencies and prepare graduates to practice as CNSs.	CNSs are regulated at the state level. Professional certification as a CNS available from several nursing organizations.	CNSs are recognized as one of the four advanced practice registered nurse (APRN) roles, the other roles being nurse practitioner, nurse midwife, and nurse anesthetist. National Association of Clinical Nurse Specialists www.nacns.org
Countries with emerging CNS roles					
China	Although CNS title has been introduced as an advanced practice role in China, Specialty Nurse is more common.	No consistent core competencies for CNSs. Specialty nurse competencies include specialty practice skills, clinical teaching skills, clinical research abilities, and ability to organize, manage and collaborate.	Specialist nurses receive on-the-job training. Master's degrees for CNSs were introduced in 2010.	No national entry criteria for specialty nurses. Specialty certificates may be issued by national or provincial government or nursing organizations.	University-based academic nursing programs have been slow to emerge. Less than 20% nurses earn an academic degree in nursing.
Germany	APN roles are not well established or delineated. Most APN roles are comparable to clinical nurse specialists practicing in 3 spheres – direct patient care, nursing and nursing staff, and organization.	Competencies identified in job descriptions include guidance and coaching, consultation, evidence-based practice, leadership, collaboration, ethical decision making.	Education beyond basic training is recommended; however, few programs are available. APN curricula are not standardized.	Title protection is not available; APN is used to distinguish advanced roles from other, non-academically qualified nurses; however, there is no distinction between APN roles.	University-based academic nursing programs have been slow to emerge. Academic courses were first established in the 1990s.

(continued)

Table 20.1 (continued)

Countries with recognized CNS roles

Country	Definition	Competencies	Education	Credentialing	Comments
Nigeria	Select groups of nurses have expanded practice in specialty areas essential to addressing health problems dominant among the population.	Educated with graduate degrees to work in clinical settings, most graduate prepared nurses are employed in academia due to lack of formal advanced clinical roles.	Three pathways to nursing specialty practice – hospital diploma, "task-shifting" specialty training, and university degree (master's with specialty focus)	Graduates of all nursing programs are professionally registered and licensed by the Nursing & Midwifery Council of Nigeria.	Expanded and advanced practice is occurring to address population health problems; formal standards with alignment of education and credentialing is needed.
Saudi Arabia	No formal definition: commonly understood definition is a master's prepared nurse working at a higher level than an RN with greater responsibility and accountability.	No nationally agreed upon competencies – currently use UK's four domains for nurse consultants: Expert clinical practice, leadership, research, and education.	Limited educational opportunities in the country. Saudi nurses are supported to travel outside the country for advanced education. CNSs and other APNs currently practicing in Saudi Arabia were educated in USA, UK and Australia.	The Saudi Commission for Health Specialties registers nurses to practice in Saudi Arabia; does not regulate nursing practice or protect nursing titles. No official credentialing for CNSs or other APNs.	The CNS title is in job descriptions for clinical nurses working in specialty populations with higher level of accountability than staff nurses.

levels of education (see Chap. 14). The ladder steps are basic nursing (1 year), clinical care nursing (2 years), coaching and holistic care training (3 years), and research and specialized training (4 years). Graduates are prepared to practice as system leaders by providing high levels of direct care to complex patients, consulting with and coordinating interprofessional teams, and conducting research and evidence-based innovation projects.

Like Taiwan, Turkey has a structured educational pathway. The title "nurse specialist" is used in Turkey to designate a practice role consistent with CNS practice. Specialist nurses in Turkey must complete a master's degree consisting of specified courses, a research study in a specialty subject, and clinical practice hours. Graduates are prepared to provide direct care, assist other nurses in professional development, and consult with other providers, institutions, and organizations related to their specialty expertise (see Chap. 15).

In Canada, Finland, and the United States, a graduate degree, either master's or doctorate, is expected. Graduates practice in the domains of patient care, nursing practice, and systems/leadership. In Australia, New Zealand, and the United Kingdom, opportunities for graduate education are limited, and various configurations of post-generalist education are used to prepare CNSs. In Australia, for example, a postgraduate qualification can be a graduate certificate (hospital based) or a graduate degree (master's or doctorate). In Canada, where both graduate education and the CNS role have existed for many years, there are still no specific CNS educational programs (see Chap. 6).

The CNS role is emerging in Nigeria where the majority of nurses obtain their education through hospital-based nursing programs. To progress to a graduate degree, diploma-prepared nurses must first complete the 5-year baccalaureate program. Since there are limited opportunities for advanced clinical practice, most nurses prepared with graduate degrees are employed in academia. Specialty practice is provided by generalists under an initiative known as task-shifting. Task-shifting involves providing specialty courses and/or training to experienced nurses who are then provided with increased access to specialized care and help improve health outcomes in selected populations. Task-shifting for the AIDS/HIV populations is one example of specialty nurses filling a high care need in Nigeria. Task-shifting to specialty nurses is an example of the process of nursing progression from generalist to advanced practice nurse (see Chap. 17).

Some countries are struggling to implement academic programs for nursing. Germany, for example, did not offer a baccalaureate nursing degree until 2004. While most advanced practice nurses in Germany practice in a role comparable to the CNS, graduate curricula for advanced practice is not standardized with courses varying in content and depth. Expanding advanced practice education is further hindered by the lack of faculty with advanced clinical practice work experience (see Chap. 11).

Given the diversity of educational systems for nurses, standards for CNS education will need to be broad and flexible; however, common elements have emerged. First, CNS education should be post-generalist and acquired at an academic degree-granting university or school. A graduate degree is preferred at the master's or doctoral level (International Council of Nurses 2020). Second, the educational program should prepare graduates for advanced practice and include theoretical and scientific nursing content, scientific knowledge from related disciplines, supervised clinical practice for application of knowledge, and achievement of CNS practice competencies. Third, CNS education must include a specialty focus. In Japan, for example, the Japanese Association of Nursing Programs in Universities (JANPU) accredits CNS educational programs at the master's level and recognizes 13 specialties—oncology, psychiatric-mental health, community health, gerontology, child health, women's health, chronic care, critical care, infection control, family health, home care, genetics, and disaster nursing (see Chap. 12). CNS specialty options should reflect the needs for the community, leaving the university to develop specialty curricula that will fulfill a community's need for advanced nursing services. For example, where a region or jurisdiction is experiencing increasing maternal-infant mortality, greater emphasis should be directed toward preparing clinical nurse specialists in maternal-infant care to work within these vulnerable communities. Fourth, graduates should be prepared to practice in domains related to direct clinical care, advancement of nursing practice, and systems leadership (National Association of Clinical Nurse Specialists 2019; Canadian Nurses Association 2014). Fifth, every curriculum should include knowledge and application of evaluation and research methods. Graduates should demonstrate ability to monitor their practice outcomes and analyze, synthesize, and present data to demonstrate their value to clinical care of patients and the healthcare system (Fulton et al. 2015; Bryant-Lukosius and Kiekoetter 2020).

20.4 Credentialing and Scope of Practice

Credentials are a form of evidence used to support a person's authority, status, and/or privileges. Nursing credentials can include academic degrees, professional certifications, specialty skills training (e.g., cardiopulmonary resuscitation), some types of continuing education, and others. Government agencies and private organizations may require nurses to hold specified credentials to obtain a license or otherwise be endorsed by a governmental or private agency. Because advanced practice nurses, including CNSs, practice in a scope expanded beyond generalist nursing practice, additional credentials are required to demonstrate authority to practice in an expanded scope. A graduate degree from a program that prepared CNSs in a specialty area is the foundational credential.

Professional specialty certification is offered by nursing organizations as evidence of having achieved competency within a specialty area of practice. Professional nursing organizations represent the body of expertise in a delineated area and are therefore an authoritative agent for validating competency. For example, the Oncology Nursing Society, through their certification agency, and the Oncology Nursing Certification Corporation, offers several different certifications for nurses in the specialty area of cancer care. Each exam has education and experience eligibility requirements (Oncology Nursing Certification Corporation n.d.). CNS certification is available from the American Nurses Association and American Nurses Credentialing Center immediately upon graduation from an approved CNS program (American Nurses Credentialing Center: Certifications n.d.). The Japanese Nursing Association certifies CNSs; candidates are not eligible to take the examination until 6 months after earning a graduate degree (see Chap. 12).

The credential(s) required for endorsement to practice, the agency that issues the credential, and the process for obtaining the credential vary by country and jurisdiction. In the United States, professional certification is required in many jurisdictions to achieve legal recognition to practice at an advanced level (see Chap. 5). While required for legal recognition to practice, professional certification by a nursing organization, which involves examination by a professional certification board, is not the same as legal license.

Certification examinations are costly and not available for all specialties. CNSs should achieve professional certification when possible, but requiring professional certification for legal recognition or endorsement to practice as a CNS is not practical or possible as a global standard at this time because of the lack of universal access to certification and the limited specialty options.

Governmental mechanisms for advanced practice recognition are not well developed globally and processes for legally recognize nurses at both generalist and advanced levels vary widely. For example, Saudi Arabia does not regulate nursing practice or protect nursing titles (see Chap. 16). In Australia, the only advanced practice role regulated is the nurse practitioner; CNS and midwifery roles are not regulated (see Chap. 18). In the United Kingdom, there are no specific certification requirements and no regulatory framework for clinical nurse specialists. The scope of practice and educational levels vary, and the role as practiced is not always advanced nursing (see Chap. 7). In Turkey, specialist nurses are registered by the Ministry of Health, which recognizes nurses with post-generalist education in an approved area of specialty (see Chap. 15). In Japan, the Japanese Nurses Association certifies individual CNSs in approved specialty areas, whereas the Japanese Association of Nursing Programs in Universities accredits education programs preparing CNSs in recognized areas of specialty. Japanese law does not require certification as a specialist and there is no separate license for CNSs (Chap. 12). In the United States, generalist nurses are licensed by a state government. Currently, efforts are underway to similarly license advanced practice nurses, including CNSs. While national standards for licensing advanced practice nurses have been proposed, they have yet to be implemented in all 50 states, and some states have modified the proposed standards (see Chap. 5).

A license is a legal recognition to autonomously practice in a designed scope. A license to practice as a generalist includes an autonomous scope of practice. Licensing advanced practice nurses, including CNSs, grants authority for an expanded scope of practice. Granting advanced practice recognition is not a priority in many countries. However, as individual countries move forward with educational opportunities and build capacity for advanced practice, mechanisms for legal recognition of advanced practice nurses, including CNSs, should be included.

In the absence of a nationally recognized legal scope of practice, employers determine CNS performance expectations. Professional competencies should be used to structure employer-based job descriptions. Given the lack of legal recognition for CNS practice globally, and the difficulties in achieving legal recognition, the urgent need is for professional nursing organizations to develop CNS competencies for guiding CNS practice and establishing expectations for CNS job performance.

20.5   Research and Evaluation

Research studies are urgently needed regarding the CNS role and practice. The CNS competencies developed by the National Association of Clinical Nurse Specialists (NACNS) have been validated, as have the corresponding practice outcome statements (National Association of Clinical Nurse Specialists 2019; Fulton et al. 2015). International initiatives are needed to develop and validate CNS practice competencies and outcome statements. Clearly defined competencies and outcomes will inform curricula preparing CNSs for practice and will provide a framework for measuring, monitoring, evaluating, and disseminating CNS outcomes.

Theoretical models and frameworks are needed to support research by clearly identifying the domains of practice and demonstrating the linkages between and among practice competencies and clinical outcomes. Much of the existing research involving CNS practice and outcomes lacks theoretical grounding, and well-done studies have rarely been developed beyond an initial, limited participation study.

CNSs, as expert clinicians, use work processes that are often invisible because expert work, done well, is largely invisible. CNS work has been identified as articulation work (Fulton et al. 2019). Articulation work involves the artful management of the intersections among the social worlds of people, technology, and organizations. Articulation work is invisible and therefore goes unrecognized or undervalued. It is incumbent upon CNSs to conduct research that helps with identifying and understanding the nuanced, expert work of the CNS and the contributions to individuals, nursing practice, and the healthcare system.

In addition to research, evaluation measures and methods are needed. The chapters in this book include examples of CNS practice. These rich descriptions demonstrate the contributions of CNSs to clinical and fiscal outcomes. However, there are no descriptions of measuring, monitoring, evaluating, or disseminating the outcomes of CNS work. Simple measures such as numeric counts and categorical descriptions are required to demonstrate CNS practice and related outcomes. Aligning data with competencies and outcome statements validates the scope of CNS's expertise and the significant outcomes for patients, employers, and the public.

One challenge for CNSs in researching and evaluating CNS practice is the lack of a clear articulation of generalist nursing practice. CNSs practice nursing in an expanded but mostly traditional nursing frame, making it ever so much more challenging to explain nursing practiced at an advanced level when that practice does not include diagnostics and procedures usually performed by physicians, even more reason for CNSs to measure, evaluate, and disseminate practice outcomes.

The International Council of Nurses supports the work of the International Classification for Nursing Practice (ICNP) initiative in providing terms that can be used to record the observations and interventions of nurses across the world (International Council of Nurses adds new content and updates the International Classification for Nursing Practice (ICNP) 2020). ICNP also provides a framework for sharing data about nursing and for comparing nursing practice across settings. CNSs need to reach out to ICNP for assistance in developing terms and structures for describing CNS practice.

20.6   Organizational Support and Advocacy

National and international networking of advanced practice nurses, including CNSs, will help facilitate wider, global implementation of the CNS role. National and international standards for definitions, competencies, outcome statements, education/curricula, and credentialing would help create a supportive framework for advancing the CNS role and practice. The International Council of Nurses and its NP/APN network are an essential resource for advancing CNS practice globally. The network's goal is to become an international resource for nurses practicing in nurse practitioner (NP) or advanced practice nursing (APN) roles and interested others (e.g., policy-makers, educators, regulators, health planners) by:

1. Making relevant and timely information about practice, education, role development, research, policy and regulatory developments, and appropriate events widely available
2. Providing a forum for sharing and exchange of knowledge expertise and experience
3. Supporting nurses and countries in the process of introducing or developing NP or ANP roles and practice
4. Accessing international resources that are pertinent to this field (ICN n.d.)

In addition to the international network, national organizations representing the advanced practice roles provide leadership and advocacy. Countries with a small number of advanced practice nurses and those developing the role can work with others to advance options for CNSs and other advanced roles in the context of their social and political contexts. A coalition of advanced practice nurses provides larger membership, shared resources, and common identity as advanced practice regardless of role.

Each advanced practice nursing role is a unique functional role in nursing. Any efforts to create competition among roles diminish the contributions of each. The CNS role must be preserved while working in collaboration with the larger advanced practice nursing network. Multiple global health challenges demand multiple advanced roles.

National organizations supporting CNSs exist in several countries including Canada, Japan, New Zealand, and the United States. These organizations establish standards, guidelines, and strategies to advance the CNS role. In addition, these organizations serve to represent CNS practice interests and influence national policy decisions. CNSs in countries without a professional CNS organization but having a substantial cohort of CNSs should form a professional nursing organization and develop goals and strategies for promoting advancement of the CNS role and recognizing the unique contribution of CNS practice.

CNSs must continue a trajectory of strong leadership and advocacy within the nursing profession and public policy arenas by being politically savvy, visible, and influential at decision-making forums within healthcare organizations, professional nursing associations, and government. Additional work is needed to keep CNSs involved in advocacy related to legislation affecting CNS practice. CNS leadership is needed on public and private boards of directors for agencies and organizations that influence health and healthcare delivery systems. CNSs can strengthen their voice through collaboration with nursing organizations in forming a unified response.

20.7   Final Thoughts

The future holds promise for advanced practice nursing and for the CNS role. More than 50 years ago, the impetus for the nursing profession to create the CNS role was to fill a need for clinical nurse experts at the point of nursing care. CNSs provide expert clinical care of complex and vulnerable patients and leadership for specialty care. CNSs advance nursing care and the profession through teaching, mentoring and coaching nurses, designing and evaluating care protocols, and supporting the professional development of nurses and nursing staff. In addition, CNSs work within systems to change care delivery methods and develop programs of care that improve quality and remove barriers to best practices. The exemplars in this book demonstrate the important contributions of CNSs to the health and well-being of the public. Wherever nursing is practice, regardless of country or community, there will always be a need to advance the profession of nursing for the improvement of health outcomes. As advanced practice nurses, CNSs are responsible for leading nurses and advancing nursing practice wherever and however it is practiced. The CNS is truly a role for global health.

References

American Nurses Credentialing Center: Certifications (n.d.). https://www.nursingworld.org/our-certifications/. Accessed 13 Aug 2020

Baldwin KL, Clark AP, Fulton JS, Mayo A (2009) National validation of the NACNS clinical nurse specialist core competencies. J Nurs Scholarsh 41:193–201. https://doi.org/10.1111/j.1547-5069.2009.01271.x

Bryant-Lukosius D, Kiekoetter S (2020) Nurse-sensitive outcomes. In: Fulton JS, Goudreau KA, Swartzell KL (eds) Foundations of clinical nurse specialist practice. Springer Publishing Company, New York, pp 45–69

Bryant-Lukosius D, Wong FKY (2019) International development of advanced practice nursing. In: Tracy MF, O'Grady ET (eds) Advanced practice nursing: an integrative approach. Elsevier, St. Louis, MO, pp 129–141

Pan-Canadian core competencies for the clinical nurse specialist. Canadian Nurses Association. 2014. https://cna-aiic.ca/~/media/cna/files/en/clinical_nurse_specialists_convention_handout_e.pdf. Accessed 13 Aug 2020

Fulton JS (2020) Evolution of the clinical nurse specialist role and practice in the United States. In: Fulton JS, Goudreau KA, Swartzell KL (eds) Foundations of clinical nurse specialist practice. Springer Publishing Company, New York, pp 1–19

Fulton JS, Mayo A, Walker J, Urden L (2015) Core practice outcomes for clinical nurse specialists: a revalidation study. J Prof Nurs 32:271–282. https://doi.org/10.1016/j.profnurs.2015.11.004

Fulton JS, Mayo A, Walker J, Urden LD (2019) Description of work processes used by clinical nurse specialists to improve patient outcomes. Nurs Outlook 67(5):511–522

ICN nurse practitioner/advanced practice nurse network. Aims and objectives. (n.d.). http://icn-apnetwork.org/. Accessed 13 Aug 2020

International Council of Nurses (2009) Framework of competencies for the nurse specialist. https://siga-fsia.ch/files/user_upload/08_ICN_Framework_for_the_nurse_specialist.pdf. Accessed 13 Aug 2020

International Council of Nurses (2020) Guidelines on advanced practice nursing. https://www.icn.ch/system/files/documents/2020-04/ICN_APN%20Report_EN_WEB.pdf. Accessed 6 Aug 2020

International Council of Nurses adds new content and updates the International Classification for Nursing Practice (ICNP) (2020). https://www.icn.ch/news/international-council-nurses-adds-new-content-and-updates-international-classification-nursing. Accessed 13 Aug 2020

Lewandowski W, Adamle K (2009) Substantive areas of clinical nurse specialist practice: a comprehensive review of the literature. Clin Nurse Spec 23:73–90

National Association of Clinical Nurse Specialists (2019) Statement on clinical nurse specialist practice and education, 3rd edn. Reston, VA: National Association of Clinical Nurse Specialists: Author 41(2), 193–201

Oncology Nursing Certification Corporation (n.d.). https://www.oncc.org/. Accessed 13 Aug 2020

Advanced level nursing: a position statement. UK Department of Health. 2010. https://assets.publishing.service.gov.uk/government/uploads/system/uploads/attachment_data/file/215935/dh_121738.pdf. Accessed 13 Aug 2020